6ᵀᴴ EDITION

Winningham's
CRITICAL THINKING CASES IN NURSING
Medical-Surgical, Pediatric, Maternity, and Psychiatric

Mariann M. Harding, PhD, RN, CNE
Associate Professor
Department of Nursing
Kent State University at Tuscarawas
New Philadelphia, Ohio

Julie S. Snyder, MSN, RN-BC
Quality Initiative Coordinator
Chesapeake Regional Medical Center
Chesapeake, Virginia;
Adjunct Faculty
School of Nursing
Old Dominion University
Norfolk, Virginia

Barbara A. Preusser[†]**,** PhD, FNPC
Family Nurse Practitioner
Veterans Administration Medical Center
Salt Lake City, Utah

[†]*Deceased*

3251 Riverport Lane
St. Louis, Missouri 63043

WINNINGHAM'S CRITICAL THINKING CASES IN NURSING: MEDICAL-SURGICAL,
PEDIATRIC, MATERNITY, AND PSYCHIATRIC, SIXTH EDITION   ISBN: 978-0-323-28961-0

Notices

Knowledge and best practice in this field are constantly changing. As new research and experience broaden our understanding, changes in research methods, professional practices, or medical treatment may become necessary.

Practitioners and researchers must always rely on their own experience and knowledge in evaluating and using any information, methods, compounds, or experiments described herein. In using such information or methods they should be mindful of their own safety and the safety of others, including parties for whom they have a professional responsibility.

With respect to any drug or pharmaceutical products identified, readers are advised to check the most current information provided (i) on procedures featured or (ii) by the manufacturer of each product to be administered, to verify the recommended dose or formula, the method and duration of administration, and contraindications. It is the responsibility of practitioners, relying on their own experience and knowledge of their patients, to make diagnoses, to determine dosages and the best treatment for each individual patient, and to take all appropriate safety precautions.

To the fullest extent of the law, neither the Publisher nor the authors, contributors, or editors, assume any liability for any injury and/or damage to persons or property as a matter of products liability, negligence or otherwise, or from any use or operation of any methods, products, instructions, or ideas contained in the material herein.

International Standard Book Number: 978-0-323-28961-0

Executive Content Strategist: Lee Henderson
Traditional Content Development manager: Billie Sharp
Associate Content Development Specialist: Samantha Taylor
Publishing Services Manager: Deborah L. Vogel
Project Manager: Pat Costigan
Book Designer: Margaret Reid

Printed in the United States of America
Last digit is the print number: 9   8   7   6   5   4   3

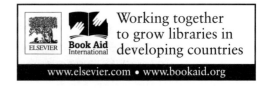

To Drs. Maryl L. Winningham and Barbara A. Preusser

Drs. Winningham and Preusser, authors of this text for the first four editions, dedicated their lives to the care of others and the pursuit of excellence in nursing practice. They have bequeathed a nursing heritage of integrity, excellence, courage, and service to their students, colleagues, and readers.

Contributors

Ann Campbell, RN, MSN, PNP
Senior Director of Education
Operation Smile
Virginia Beach, Virginia

Sherry D. Ferki, RN, MSN
Adjunct Faculty
School of Nursing
Old Dominion University
Norfolk, Virginia

Sara B. Forbus, MSN, RN, WHNP-BC
Lecturer
School of Nursing
Old Dominion University
Norfolk, Virginia

Contributors to Previous Editions

Elizabeth Jane Bell, MSN, ANPc
Lesley A. Black, BSN, MS, ANPc, CWOCN
Kent Blad, MS, FNPc, ACNP-C, FCCM
Jamie Clinton-Lont, BSN, FNPc
Susan L. Croft, BSN, MS
Joyce Foster, PhD, CNM, FACNM, FAAN
Shellagh Gutke, BSN, CWOCN
Nancy Hayden, MSN, FNPc
Sondra Heaston, MS, FNPc, CEN
Janice Hulbert, RN, MS
Lisa Jensen, BSN, MS, APRN, CS
Stephanie C. Kettendorf, MS, RN, CNS, NCBF
Julie Killebrew, BSN, MS
Karen Kone, BSN, ACRN
Kathleen Kuntz, MSN, APRN, SANE

Janet G. Madsen, PhD
Debra Ann Mills, RN, MS
Jeanie O'Donnell, MSN
Deb Plasman-Coles, PAc
Laura Lee Scott, MSN, FNPc
Mary Seegmiller, MSN
Sandra Smeeding, MS, FNPc
Deborah D. Smith, BSN
Ann Speirs, BSN
Ronald Ulberg, BSN, MSN
Kristy Vankatwyk, MSN, FNPc
Annette S. Wendel, BSN
Wendy Whitney, MSN, FNPc, CANP
Mary Youtsey, BSN, CDE

Reviewers

Diane K. Daddario, MSN, ACNS-BC, RN-BC, CMSRN
Adjunct Faculty
Pennsylvania State University
University Park, Pennsylvania

Sara B. Forbus, MSN, RN, WHNP-BC
Lecturer
Old Dominion University
Norfolk, Virginia

Mimi Haskins, MS, RN, CNS, CMSRN
Clinical Assistant Professor
School of Nursing
SUNY at Buffalo
Buffalo, New York

LaWanda Herron, PhD, MSA, MSN, FNP-BC
Director, Associate Degree Nursing
Holmes Community College
Goodman, Mississippi

Jamie L. Jones, MSN, RN, CNE
Assistant Professor, Nursing
University of Arkansas at Little Rock
Little Rock, Arkansas

Tamara M. Kear, PhD, RN, CNS, CNN
Assistant Professor of Nursing
Villanova University, College of Nursing
Villanova, Pennsylvania

Cheryl A. Lehman, PhD, RN, CNS-BC, RN-BC, CRRN
Clinical Professor, BSN Program
Director–Retired
The University of Texas Health Science Center
at San Antonio
San Antonio, Texas

Cynthia W. Ward, DNP, RN-BC, CMSRN, ACNS-BC
Surgical Clinical Nurse Specialist
Carilion Roanoke Memorial Hospital
Roanoke, Virginia

Introduction

There is an urgent need for nurses with well-practiced critical thinking skills. As new graduates, you will make decisions and take actions of an increasingly sophisticated nature. You will encounter problems you have never seen or heard about during your classroom and clinical experiences. You are going to have to make complex decisions with little or no guidance and limited resources.

We want you to be exposed to as much as possible during your student days, but more importantly, we want you to learn to *think*. You cannot memorize your way out of any situation, but you can *think* your way out of any situation. We know that students often learn more and faster when they have the freedom to make mistakes. This book is designed to allow you to experiment with finding answers without the pressure of someone's life hanging in the balance. We want you to do well. We want you to be the best. It is our wish for you to grow into confident, competent professionals. After all, someday we will be one of those people you care for, and when that day comes, we want you to be very, very good at what you do!

What Is Critical Thinking?

Critical thinking is *not* memorizing lists of facts or the steps of procedures. Instead, critical thinking is an analytical process that can help you think through a problem in an organized and efficient manner. Five steps are involved in critical thinking. Thinking about these steps may help you when you work through the questions in your cases. Here are the five steps with an explanation of what they mean.

1. Recognize and define the problem by asking the right questions: Exactly what is it you need to know? What is the question asking?
2. Select the information or data necessary to solve the problem or answer the question: First you have to ask whether all the necessary information is there. If not, how and where can you get the additional information? What other resources are available? This is one of the most difficult steps. In real clinical experiences, you rarely have all of the information, so you have to learn where you can get necessary data. For instance, patient and family interviews, nursing charting, the patient medical chart, laboratory data on your computer, your observations, and your own physical assessment can help you identify important clues. Of course, information can rapidly become outdated. To make sure you are accessing the most current and accurate information, you will occasionally need to use the Internet to answer a question.
3. Recognize stated and unstated assumptions; that is, what do you think is or is not true? Sometimes answers or solutions seem obvious; just because something seems obvious doesn't mean it is correct. You may need to consider several possible answers or solutions. Consider all clues carefully and *do not dismiss a possibility too quickly*. Remember, "*You never find an answer you don't think of.*"
4. Formulate and select relevant and/or potential decisions. Try to think of as many possibilities as you can. Consider the pros and cons of the consequences of making each decision. What is the best answer/solution? What could go wrong? This requires considering many different angles. In today's health care settings, decision-making often requires balancing the well-being needs of the patient, the preferences and concerns of the patient and caregiver, and financial limitations imposed by the reimbursement system. In making decisions, you need to take into account all relevant factors. Remember, you may need to explain why you rejected other options.

5. Draw a valid, informed conclusion: Consider all data; then determine what is relevant and what makes the most sense. Only then should you draw your conclusion.

It may look as if this kind of thinking comes naturally to instructors and experienced nurses. You can be certain that even experienced professionals were once where you are now. The rapid and sound decision-making that is essential to good nursing requires years of practice. The practice of good clinical thinking leads to good thinking in clinical practice. This book will help you practice the important steps in making sound clinical judgments until the process starts to come naturally.

The practice of good clinical thinking leads to good thinking in clinical practice.

The "How to" of Case Studies

When you begin each case, read through the whole story once, from start to finish, getting a general idea of what it is about. Write down things you have to look up. This will help you move through the case smoothly and get more out of it. How much you have to look up will depend on where you are in your program, what you know, and how much experience you already have. Note that questions related to the Quality and Safety Education for Nurses (QSEN) competency of Safety are highlighted a "bull's-eye" icon 🎯. Preparing cases will become easier as you advance in your program.

Acknowledgments

We would like to express our appreciation to the editorial Elsevier staff for their professional support and contributions in guiding this text to publication. Thank you to Samantha Taylor for picking up the work in mid-production and guiding us to the finish. We extend a special thanks to our reviewers who gave us helpful suggestions and insights as we developed this edition.

Mariann's gratitude goes to the most important people in her life—her husband, Jeff, and her daughters, Kate and Sarah—for their love and understanding during the months of writing. She gives a special thanks to her students, colleagues, and patients; each has taught her much and fueled her passion for nursing and education. Lastly, Mariann praises God, who has given her an incredible gift in this opportunity to serve others.

Julie thanks her husband, Jonathan, for his love, support, and patience during this project. She is grateful for the encouragement from daughter Emily, son-in-law Randy, and parents Willis and Jean Simmons. Julie appreciates the hard work of colleagues Ann Campbell, Sara Forbus, and Sherry Ferki as contributors to this edition. She is especially thankful to the students, whose eagerness to learn is an inspiration. Most importantly, Julie gives thanks to God, our source of hope and strength.

Contents

CONTENTS

PART ONE *Medical-Surgical Cases*
Cardiovascular Disorders

Case Study 1

Name _____ Class/Group _____ Date _____

Group Members _____

▶ **Scenario**

M.G., a "frequent flier," is admitted to the emergency department (ED) with a diagnosis of heart failure (HF). She was discharged from the hospital 10 days ago and comes in today stating, "I just had to come to the hospital today because I can't catch my breath and my legs are as big as tree trunks." After further questioning, you learn that she is strictly following the fluid and salt restriction ordered during her last hospital admission. She reports gaining 1 to 2 pounds every day since her discharge.

1. What error in teaching most likely occurred when M.G. was discharged 10 days ago?

CASE STUDY PROGRESS

During the admission interview, the nurse makes a list of the medications M.G. took at home.

Chart View

Nursing Assessment: Medications Taken at Home	
Enalapril (Vasotec)	5 mg PO bid
Pioglitazone (Actos)	45 mg PO every morning
Furosemide (Lasix)	40 mg/day PO
Potassium chloride	20 mEq/day PO

2. Which of these medications may have contributed to M.G.'s HF? Explain.

3. How do angiotensin-converting enzyme (ACE) inhibitors, such as enalapril (Vasotec), work to reduce HF? Select all that apply. ACE inhibitors:
   a. prevent the conversion of angiotensin I to angiotensin II.
   b. cause systemic vasodilation.
   c. promote the excretion of sodium and water in the renal tubules.
   d. reduce preload and afterload.
   e. increase cardiac contractility.
   f. block sympathetic nervous system stimulation to the heart.

CASE STUDY PROGRESS

After reviewing M.G.'s medications, the physician writes the following medication orders.

Chart View

Medication Orders

Enalapril (Vasotec)	5 mg PO bid
Carvedilol (Coreg)	3.125 mg PO twice daily
Glipizide (Glucotrol)	10 mg PO every morning
Furosemide (Lasix)	80 mg intravenous push (IVP) now, then 40 mg/day IVP
Potassium chloride (K-Dur)	20 mEq/day PO

4. What is the rationale for changing the route of the furosemide (Lasix)?

5. You administer furosemide (Lasix) 80 mg IVP. Identify three parameters you would use to monitor the effectiveness of this medication.

6. What laboratory tests should be ordered for M.G. related to the order for furosemide (Lasix)? Select all that apply.
   a. Magnesium level
   b. Sodium level
   c. Complete blood count (CBC)

    d. Serum glucose level
    e. Potassium level
    f. Coagulation studies

7. What is the purpose of the beta blocker carvedilol? It is given to:
    a. increase the contractility of the heart.
    b. cause peripheral vasodilation.
    c. increase urine output.
    d. reduce cardiac stimulation from catecholamines.

 8. You assess M.G. for conditions that may be a contraindication to carvedilol. Which condition, if present, may cause serious problems if the patient takes this medication?
    a. Angina
    b. Asthma
    c. Glaucoma
    d. Hypertension

CASE STUDY PROGRESS

One day later, M.G. has shown only slight improvement, and digoxin (Lanoxin) 125 mcg PO daily is added to her orders.

9. What is the action of the digoxin? Digoxin:
    a. causes systemic vasodilation.
    b. promotes the excretion of sodium and water in the renal tubules.
    c. increases cardiac contractility and cardiac output.
    d. blocks sympathetic nervous system stimulation to the heart.

10. Which findings from M.G.'s assessment would indicate an increased possibility of digoxin toxicity? Explain your answer.
    a. Serum potassium level of 2.2 mEq/L
    b. Serum sodium level of 139 mEq/L

    c. Apical heart rate of 64 beats/minute
    d. Digoxin level 1.6 ng/mL

11. When preparing to give the digoxin, you notice that it is available in milligrams (mg) not micrograms (mcg). Convert 125 mcg to mg.

12. M.G.'s symptoms improve with intravenous diuretics and the digoxin. She is placed back on oral furosemide (Lasix) once her weight loss is deemed adequate for achievement of a euvolemic state. What will determine whether the oral dose will be adequate for discharge to be considered?

13. M.G. is ready for discharge. According to the mnemonic *MAWDS*, what key management concepts should be taught to prevent relapse and another admission?

14. After the teaching session, which statement by M.G. indicates a need for further education?
    a. "I will weigh myself daily and tell the doctor at my next visit if I am gaining weight."
    b. "I will not add salt when I am cooking."
    c. "I will try to take a short walk around the block with my husband three times a week."
    d. "I will use a pill calendar box to remind me to take my medicine."

CASE STUDY OUTCOME

After 3 days, the STOP Heart Failure Nurse calls M.G. to ask about her progress. M.G. reports that her weight has not changed since she has been home.

Case Study 2

Name _____   Class/Group _____   Date _____

Group Members _____

▶ **Scenario**

M.P. is a 65-year-old African American woman who comes to your clinic for a follow-up visit. She was diagnosed with hypertension (HTN) 2 months ago and was given a prescription for a thiazide diuretic but stopped taking it 2 weeks ago because "it made me dizzy and I kept getting up during the night to empty my bladder." During today's clinic visit, she expresses fear because her mother died of a cerebrovascular accident (CVA, stroke) at M.P.'s age, and M.P. is afraid she will suffer the same fate. She states, "I've never smoked and I don't drink, but I am so afraid of this high blood pressure." You review the data from her past clinic visits.

Chart View

Family History

Mother, died at age 65 years of CVA
Father, died at age 67 years of myocardial infarction (MI)
Sister, alive and well, age 62 years
Brother, alive, age 70 years, has coronary artery disease (CAD), HTN, type II diabetes mellitus (DM)

Patient Past History

Married for 45 years, two children, alive and well, six grandchildren
Cholecystectomy, age 42 years
Hysterectomy, age 48 years

Blood Pressure Assessments

January 2: 150/92
January 31: 156/94 (Given prescription for hydrochlorothiazide [HCTZ] 25 mg PO every morning)
February 28: 140/90

1. According to the most recent guidelines from the Joint National Committee on Prevention, Detection, Evaluation, and Treatment of High Blood Pressure, M.P.'s blood pressure (BP) falls under which classification?

2. What could M.P. be doing that is causing her nocturia?

CASE STUDY PROGRESS

During today's visit, M.P.'s vital signs are as follows: BP: 162/102; P: 78; R: 16; T: 98.2° F (36.8° C). Her most recent basic metabolic panel (BMP) and fasting lipids are within normal limits. Her height is 5 ft, 4 in, and she weighs 110 lb. She tells you that she tries to go on walks but does not like to walk alone and so has done so only occasionally.

3. What risk factors does M.P. have that increase her risk for cardiovascular disease?

CASE STUDY PROGRESS

Because M.P.'s BP continues to be high, the internist decides to put her on another drug and recommends that she try again with the HCTZ.

4. According to the JNC 8 national guidelines, what drug category or categories are recommended for M.P. at this time?

5. M.P. goes on to ask whether there is anything else she should do to help with her HTN. She asks, "Do I need to lose weight?" Look up her height and weight for her age on a body mass index (BMI) chart. Is she considered overweight?

6. What nonpharmacologic lifestyle alteration measures might help M.P. control her BP? List two examples and explain.

CASE STUDY PROGRESS

The internist decreases M.P.'s HCTZ dose to 12.5 mg PO daily and adds a prescription for benazepril (Lotensin) 5 mg daily. M.P. is instructed to return to the clinic in 1 week to have her blood work checked. She is instructed to monitor her BP at least twice a week and return for a medication management appointment in 1 month with her list of BP readings.

7. Why did the internist decrease the dose of the HCTZ?

8. You provide M.P. with education about the common side effects of benazepril, which can include which of these? Select all that apply.
   a. Headache
   b. Cough
   c. Shortness of breath
   d. Constipation
   e. Dizziness

9. It is sometimes difficult to remember whether one has taken one's medication. What techniques might you teach M.P. to help her remember to take her medications each day? Name at least two.

10. After the teaching session, which statement by M.P. indicates a need for further instructions?
    a. "I need to rise up slowly when I get out of bed or out of a chair."
    b. "I will leave the salt shaker off the table and not salt my food when I cook."
    c. "It's okay to skip a few doses if I am feeling bad as long as it's just for a few days."
    d. "I will call if I feel very dizzy, weak, or short of breath while on this medicine."

CASE STUDY PROGRESS

M.P. returns in 1 month for her medication management appointment. She tells you she is feeling fine and does not have any side effects from her new medication. Her BP, checked twice a week at the senior center, ranges from 132 to 136/78 to 82 mm Hg.

11. When someone is taking HCTZ and an angiotensin-converting enzyme (ACE) inhibitor, such as benazepril, what laboratory test results would you expect to be monitored?

Chart View

Laboratory Test Results (Fasting)

Potassium	3.6 mEq/L
Sodium	138 mEq/L
Chloride	100 mEq/L
CO_2	28 mEq/L
Glucose	112 mEq/L
Creatinine	0.7 mg/dL
Blood urea nitrogen (BUN)	18 mg/dL
Magnesium	1.9 mEq/L

12. What laboratory test results, if any, are of concern at this time?

13. You take M.P.'s BP and get 134/82 mm Hg. She asks whether these BP readings are okay. On what do you base your response?

14. List at least three important ways you might help M.P. maintain her success.

CASE STUDY PROGRESS

M.P. tells you she was recently at a luncheon with her garden club and that most of those women take different BP pills than she does. She asks why their pills are different shapes and colors.

15. How can you explain the difference to M.P.?

16. During the visit, you ask M.P., "When was your last eye examination?" She answers, "I'm not sure, probably about 2 years ago. What does that have to do with my blood pressure?" What is your response?

CASE STUDY OUTCOME

M.P. comes in for a routine follow-up visit 3 months later. She continues to do well on her daily BP drug regimen, with average BP readings of 130/78 mm Hg. She participates in a senior citizens' group walking program at the local mall. She admits she has not done as well with decreasing her salt intake but says she is trying.

Case Study **3**

Name _____ Class/Group _____ Date _____

Group Members _____

▶ Scenario

You are a nurse at a freestanding cardiac prevention and rehabilitation center. Your new patient in risk-factor modification is B.T., a 41-year-old traveling salesman, who is married and has three children. He tells you that his work does not let him slow down. During a recent evaluation for chest pain, he underwent a cardiac catheterization procedure that showed moderate single-vessel disease with a 50% stenosis in the mid right coronary artery (RCA). He was given a prescription for sublingual (SL) nitroglycerin (NTG), told how to use it, and referred to your cardiac rehabilitation program for sessions 3 days a week. B.T.'s wife comes along to help him with healthy lifestyle changes. You take a nursing history, as indicated in the following.

Chart View

Family History

Father died suddenly at age 42 of a myocardial infarction (MI)
Mother (still living) had a quadruple coronary artery bypass graft (CABG × 4) at age 52

Past History and Current Medications

Metoprolol (Lopressor)	25 mg PO every 12 hours
Aspirin (ASA)	325 mg per day PO
Simvastatin (Zocor)	20 mg PO every evening

Lifestyle Habits

Has smoked an average of $1^1/2$ packs of cigarettes per day (PPD) for the past 20 years
Drinks an "occasional" beer and "a six-pack every weekend when watching football"
Dietary history: High in fried and fast foods because of his traveling
Exercise: "I don't have time to take walks."

General Assessment

White Male	
Weight	235 lb
Height	5 ft, 8 in
Waist circumference	48 in
Blood Pressure	148/88 mm Hg
Pulse	82 beats/min
Respiratory rate	18 breaths/min
Temperature	98.4° F (36.9° C)

1 Cardiovascular Disorders

1. Calculate B.T.'s smoking history in terms of pack-years.

2. There are several risk factors for coronary artery disease (CAD). For each risk factor listed, mark whether it is nonmodifiable or modifiable.
   a. Age
   b. Smoking
   c. Family history of CAD
   d. Obesity
   e. Physical inactivity
   f. Gender
   g. Hypertension
   h. Diabetes mellitus
   i. Hyperlipidemia
   j. Ethnic background
   k. Stress
   l. Excessive alcohol use

3. Circle the nonmodifiable and modifiable risk factors that apply to B.T.

CASE STUDY PROGRESS

You review B.T.'s most recent laboratory results.

Chart View

Laboratory Testing (Fasting)

Total cholesterol	240 mg/dL
HDL	35 mg/dL
LDL	112 mg/dL
Triglycerides	178 mg/dL

4. Which laboratory values are of concern at this time? Explain your answers.

5. B.T. asks you, "So, how is my 'good cholesterol' doing today?" Which is considered the "good cholesterol," and why? What do his HDL and LDL levels indicate to you?

CASE STUDY PROGRESS

B.T. laughingly tells you he believes in the five all-American food groups: salt, sugar, fat, chocolate, and caffeine.

6. Identify health-related problems in this case description; the problem that is potentially life-threatening should be listed first.

7. Of all of B.T.'s behaviors, which one is the most significant in promoting cardiac disease?

8. What interventions would you recommend to assist B.T. in addressing this behavior?

9. Because B.T. has several other problems, how will you determine what the priorities are that you need to address with B.T.?

10. Name a second problem you would work with B.T. to change. Identify an appropriate strategy to resolve the problem.

1 Cardiovascular Disorders

11. B.T.'s wife takes you aside and tells you, "I'm so worried for B. I grew up in a really dysfunctional family where there was a lot of violence. B. has been so good to the kids and me. I'm so worried I'll lose him that I have nightmares about his heart stopping. I find myself suddenly waking up at night just to see if he's breathing." How are you going to respond?

CASE STUDY PROGRESS

Six weeks after you start working with B.T., he admits that he has been under a lot of stress. He is walking on the treadmill and rubs his chest and says, "It feels really heavy on my chest right now." You feel his pulse and note that his skin is slightly diaphoretic and that he is agitated and appears to be anxious.

12. What is the first action you are going to do? What other information will you obtain? Explain.

13. B.T. is still uncomfortable, and he has an unopened bottle of sublingual nitroglycerin (SL NTG) tablets. His blood pressure is 158/98, and his pulse is 122. You decide to give him one tablet. After 5 minutes, which is the appropriate action to take?
    a. If the chest discomfort is relieved, call 911.
    b. If the chest discomfort is not relieved, give another SL NTG tablet, and wait 5 minutes more.
    c. If the chest discomfort is not relieved, have someone else call 911 while you give B.T. another SL NTG tablet.
    d. If the chest discomfort is not relieved, obtain a 12-lead electrocardiogram (ECG) to look for ischemic changes, and call 911.

14. What other actions will you take at this time?

15. Five minutes after the first NTG tablet, B.T. states that the discomfort is still there and only slightly relieved. Explain what you can expect to be doing while waiting for emergency medical system (EMS) personnel to arrive.

16. After taking the second NTG SL tablet, B.T. complains of a "terrible headache" and worries that he is getting worse. What is happening, and what should you tell him?

CASE STUDY OUTCOME

B.T. is transported to the emergency department of a local hospital and undergoes another cardiac catheterization with coronary stent placement.

Case Study **4**

Name _____ Class/Group _____ Date _____

Group Members _____

▶ Scenario

You are working in the internal medicine clinic of a large teaching hospital. Today your first patient is 70-year-old J.M., a man who has been coming to the clinic for several years for management of coronary artery disease (CAD) and hypertension (HTN). A cardiac catheterization done a year ago showed 50% stenosis of the circumflex coronary artery. He has had episodes of dizziness for the past 6 months and orthostatic hypotension, shoulder discomfort, and decreased exercise tolerance for the past 2 months. On his last clinic visit 3 weeks ago, a chest x-ray (CXR) examination revealed cardiomegaly, and a 12-lead electrocardiogram (ECG) showed sinus tachycardia with left bundle branch block (LBBB). You review J.M.'s morning blood work and initial assessment.

Chart View

Laboratory Results

Chemistry

Sodium	142 mEq/L
Chloride	95 mEq/L
Potassium	3.9 mEq/L
Creatinine	0.8 mg/dL
Glucose	82 mg/dL
BUN	19 mg/dL

Complete Blood Count

WBC	5400/mm^3
Hgb	11.5 g/dL
Hct	37%
Platelets	229,000/mm^3

Initial Assessment

Complains of increased fatigue and shortness of breath, especially with activity, and "waking up gasping for breath" at night, for the past 2 days.

Vital Signs

Temperature	97.9°F (36.6°C)
Blood pressure (BP)	142/83 mm Hg
Heart rate	105 beats//min
Respiratory rate	18 breaths/min

1. As you review these results, which ones are of possible concern, and why?

2. Knowing his history and seeing his condition this morning, what further questions are you going to ask J.M. and his daughter?

CASE STUDY PROGRESS

J.M. tells you he becomes exhausted and has shortness of breath climbing the stairs to his bedroom and has to lie down and rest ("put my feet up") at least an hour twice a day. He has been sleeping on two pillows for the past 2 weeks. He has not salted his food since the physician told him not to because of his high blood pressure, but he admits having had ham and a small bag of salted peanuts 3 days ago. He states that he stopped smoking 10 years ago. He denies having palpitations but has had a constant, irritating, nonproductive cough lately.

3. You think it's likely that J.M. has heart failure (HF). From his history, what do you identify as probable causes for his HF?

4. You are now ready to do your physical assessment. For each potential assessment finding for HF, indicate whether the finding indicates left-sided HF (L) or right-sided HF (R).

_____ 1. Fatigue, weakness, especially with activity
_____ 2. Jugular (neck) vein distention
_____ 3. Dependent edema (legs and sacrum)
_____ 4. Hacking cough, worse at night
_____ 5. Enlarged liver and spleen
_____ 6. Exertional dyspnea
_____ 7. Distended abdomen
_____ 8. Weight gain
_____ 9. S_3/S_4 gallop
_____ 10. Crackles and wheezes in lungs

Chart View

Medication Orders

Enalapril (Vasotec) 10 mg PO twice a day
Furosemide (Lasix) 20 mg PO every morning
Carvedilol (Coreg) 6.25 mg PO twice a day
Digoxin (Lanoxin) 0.5 mg PO now, then 0.125 mg PO daily
Potassium chloride (K-Dur) 10 mEq tablet PO once a day

CASE STUDY PROGRESS

The physician confirms your suspicions and indicates that J.M. is experiencing symptoms of early left-sided heart failure. A two-dimensional (2D) echocardiogram is ordered. Medication orders are written.

5. For each medication listed, identify its class and describe its purpose for the treatment of HF.

6. When you go to remove the medications from the automated dispensing machine, you see that carvedilol (Coreg CR) is stocked. Will you give it to J.M.? Explain.

1 Cardiovascular Disorders

7. As you remove the digoxin tablet from the automated medication dispensing machine, you note that the dose on the tablet label is 250 mcg. How many tablets would you give?

8. Based on the new medication orders, which blood test or tests should be monitored carefully? Explain your answer.

9. When you give J.M. his medications, he looks at the potassium tablet, wrinkles his nose, and tells you he "hates those horse pills." He tells you a friend of his said he could eat bananas instead. He says he would rather eat a banana every day than take one of those pills. How will you respond?

10. The 2D echocardiogram shows that J.M.'s left ventricular ejection fraction (EF) is 49%. Explain what this test results mean with regard to J.M.'s heart function.

CASE STUDY PROGRESS

This is J.M.'s first episode of significant HF. Before he leaves the clinic, you want to teach him about lifestyle modifications he can make and monitoring techniques he can use to prevent or minimize future problems.

11. List five suggestions you might make and the rationale for each.

12. You tell J.M. that the combination of high-sodium foods he had during the past several days might have contributed to his present episode of HF. He looks surprised. J.M. says, "But I didn't add any salt to them!" To what health care professional could J.M. be referred to help him understand how to prevent future crises? State your rationale.

13. You also include teaching about digoxin toxicity. When teaching J.M. about the signs and symptoms of digoxin toxicity, which should be included? Select all that apply.
    a. Dizziness when standing up
    b. Visual changes
    c. Loss of appetite or nausea
    d. Increased urine output
    e. Diarrhea

CASE STUDY OUTCOME

J.M.'s condition improves after 5 days of treatment, and he is discharged to home. He has a follow-up appointment with a cardiologist in 2 weeks. He is enrolled in the clinic's STOP Heart Failure program, and a heart failure nurse will contact him in a few days to check his progress.

Case Study **5**

Name _____ Class/Group _____ Date _____

Group Members _____

▶ **Scenario**

It is midmorning on the cardiac unit where you work, and you are getting a new patient. G.P. is a 60-year-old retired businessman who is married and has three grown children. As you take his health history, he tells you that he began feeling changes in his chest about 10 days ago. He has hypertension (HTN) and a 5-year history of angina pectoris. During the past week, he has had frequent episodes of mid-chest discomfort. The chest pain responds to nitroglycerin (NTG), which he has taken sublingually about 8 to 10 times over the past week. During the week, he has also experienced increased fatigue. He states, "I just feel crappy all the time." A cardiac catheterization done several years ago revealed 50% stenosis of the right coronary artery (RCA) and 50% stenosis of the left anterior descending (LAD) coronary artery. He tells you that both his mother and his father had coronary artery disease (CAD). He is currently taking amlodipine (Norvasc), metoprolol (Lopressor), atorvastatin (Lipitor), and aspirin 81 mg/day.

1. What other information are you going to obtain about his episodes of chest pain?

2. What are common sites for radiation of ischemic cardiac pain?

3. You know that G.P. has atherosclerosis of the coronary arteries. You need to know his risk factors for CAD to plan teaching for lifestyle modifications. What will you ask him about?

4. Although he has been taking sublingual nitroglycerin (SL NTG) for a long time, you want to be certain he is using it correctly. Which actions are correct when taking SL NTG for chest pain? (Select all that apply.)
   a. Stop the activity and lie or sit down.
   b. Call 911 immediately.
   c. Call 911 if the pain is not relieved after taking one SL tablet.
   d. Call 911 if the pain is not relieved after taking three SL tablets, 5 minutes apart.
   e. Chew the tablet slowly then swallow.
   f. Place the NTG tablet under the tongue.

5. You review the use and storage of SL NTG with G.P. Which statement by G.P. indicates a need for further education? Explain your answer.
   a. "I will discard any open bottle of nitroglycerin after a year."
   b. "I will not store other pills in the nitroglycerin bottle."
   c. "I carry the tablets with me at all times."
   d. "I will keep the pills in their original brown bottle."

CASE STUDY PROGRESS

When you first admit G.P., you place him on telemetry and observe his cardiac rhythm.

6. Identify the rhythm:

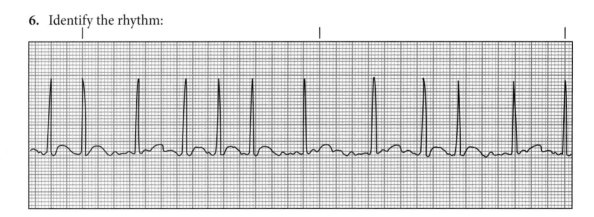

7. Explain the primary complication that could occur if this heart rhythm were not treated.

8. Review G.P.'s history. What conditions may have contributed to the development of this dysrhythmia?

9. You review G.P.'s laboratory test results and note that all of them are within normal range, including troponin and creatinine phosphokinase (CPK) levels. His potassium level is 4.7 mEq/L. Given this and his current dysrhythmia, what is the likely cause of the symptoms he has been experiencing this past week?

CASE STUDY PROGRESS

Within the hour, G.P. converts with intravenous diltiazem (Cardizem) to sick sinus syndrome with long sinus pauses that cause lightheadedness and hypotension.

10. What risks does the new rhythm pose for G.P.? Explain the reasons for your answers.

CASE STUDY PROGRESS

Because G.P.'s dysrhythmia is causing unacceptable symptoms, he is taken to surgery and a permanent DDDR pacemaker is placed and set at a rate of 70 beats/min.

11. What does the code *DDDR* mean?

 12. The pacemaker insertion surgery places G.P. at risk for several serious complications. List three potential problems that you will monitor for as you care for him.

13. G.P. will need some education regarding his new pacemaker. What information will you give him before he leaves the hospital?

14. G.P.'s wife approaches you and anxiously inquires, "My neighbor saw this science fiction movie about this guy who got a pacemaker and then he couldn't die. Is that for real?" How are you going to respond to her?

 15. G.P. and his wife tell you they have heard that people with pacemakers can have their hearts stop because of microwave ovens and cell phones. Where can you help them find more information?

CASE STUDY PROGRESS

After discharge, G.P. is referred to a cardiac rehabilitation center to start an exercise program. He will be exercise tested, and an individualized exercise prescription will be developed for him, based on the results of the exercise test.

16. What information will be obtained from a graded exercise (stress) test, and what is included in an exercise prescription?

Case Study 6

Name _____ Class/Group _____ Date _____

Group Members _____

▶ Scenario

S.P. is a 68-year-old retired painter who is experiencing right leg calf pain. The pain began approximately 2 years ago but has become significantly worse in the past 4 months. The pain is precipitated by exercise and is relieved with rest. Two years ago, S.P. could walk two city blocks before having to stop because of leg pain. Today, he can barely walk across the yard. S.P. has smoked two to three packs of cigarettes per day (PPD) for the past 45 years. He has a history of coronary artery disease (CAD), hypertension (HTN), peripheral artery disease (PAD), and osteoarthritis. Surgical history includes quadruple coronary artery bypass graft (CABG × 4) 3 years ago. He has had no further symptoms of cardiopulmonary disease since that time, even though he has not been compliant with the exercise regimen his cardiologist prescribed, continues to eat anything he wants, and continues to smoke two to three PPD. Other surgical history includes open reduction internal fixation of a right femoral fracture 20 years ago.

S.P. is in the clinic today for a routine semiannual follow-up appointment with his primary care provider. As you take his vital signs, he tells you that in addition to the calf pain, he is experiencing right hip pain that gets worse with exercise, the pain doesn't go away promptly with rest, some days are worse than others, and his condition is not affected by a resting position.

Chart View

General Assessment

Weight	261 lb
Height	5 ft, 10 in
Blood pressure (BP)	163/91 mm Hg
Pulse	82 beats/min
Respiratory rate	16 beats/min
Temperature	98.4° F (36.9° C)

Laboratory Testing (Fasting)

Cholesterol	239 mg/dL
Triglycerides	150 mg/dL
HDL	28 mg/dL
LDL	181 mg/dL

Current Medications

Ramipril (Altace)	10 mg/day
Metoprolol (Lopressor)	25 mg twice a day
Aspirin	81 mg/day
Simvastatin (Zocor)	20 mg/day

1. What are the likely sources of his calf pain and his hip pain?

2. S.P. has several risk factors for PAD. From his history, list two risk factors, and explain the reason they are risk factors.

3. You decide to look at S.P.'s lower extremities. What signs do you expect to find with PAD? Select all that apply.
   a. Cool or cold extremity
   b. Thin, shiny, and taut skin
   c. Brown discoloration of the skin
   d. Decreased or absent pedal pulses
   e. Ankle edema
   f. Thick, brittle nails

4. You ask further questions about the clinical manifestations of PAD. Which of these would you expect S.P. to have, given the diagnosis of PAD? Select all that apply.
   a. Dependent rubor
   b. Paresthesia
   c. Constant, dull ache in his calf or thigh
   d. Rest pain at night
   e. Pruritus of the lower legs
   f. Elevation pallor

5. What is the purpose of the daily aspirin listed in S.P.'s current medication?

CASE STUDY PROGRESS

S.P.'s primary care provider has seen him and wants you to schedule him for an ankle-brachial index (ABI) test to determine the presence of arterial blood flow obstruction. You confirm the time and date of the procedure and then call S.P. at home.

6. What will you tell S.P. to do to prepare for the tests?

CASE STUDY PROGRESS

S.P.'s ABI results showed 0.43 right (R) leg and 0.59 left (L) leg. His primary care provider discusses these results with him and decides to wait 2 months to see whether his symptoms improve with medication changes and risk factor modification before deciding about surgical intervention. S.P. receives a prescription for clopidogrel (Plavix) 75 mg daily and is told to discontinue the daily aspirin. In addition, S.P. receives a consultation for physical therapy.

7. What do these ABI results indicate?

8. You counsel S.P. on risk factor modification. What would you address, and why?

9. How will the physical therapy help?

10. In addition to risk factor modification, what other measures to improve tissue perfusion or to prevent skin damage should you recommend to S.P.?

11. S.P. tells you his neighbor told him to keep his legs elevated higher than his heart and asks for compression stockings to keep swelling down in his legs. How should you respond?

12. S.P. has been on aspirin therapy but now will be taking clopidogrel instead. What is the most important aspect of patient teaching that you will emphasize with this drug?

CASE STUDY OUTCOME

S.P. asks for nicotine patches to assist with smoking cessation and makes an appointment for a physical therapy evaluation and a nutritional assessment. He assures you he does not want to lose his leg and will be more careful in the future.

Case Study **7**

Name _____ Class/Group _____ Date _____

Group Members _____

▶ **Scenario**

You are the nurse working in an anticoagulation clinic. One of your patients is K.N., who has a long-standing history of an irregular heartbeat, known as *atrial fibrillation* or *A-fib,* for which he takes the oral anticoagulant warfarin (Coumadin). Recently K.N. had his mitral heart valve replaced with a mechanical valve.

1. How does atrial fibrillation differ from a normal heart rhythm?

2. What is the purpose of the warfarin (Coumadin) in K.N.'s case?

CASE STUDY PROGRESS

K.N. calls your anticoagulation clinic to report a nosebleed that is hard to stop. You ask him to come into the office to check his coagulation levels. The laboratory technician draws a PT/INR test.

3. What is a PT/INR test, and what are the expected levels for K.N.? What is the purpose of the INR?

4. When you get the results, his international normalized ratio (INR) is critical at 7.2. What is the danger of this INR level?

CASE STUDY PROGRESS

The health care provider does a brief focused history and physical examination, orders additional laboratory tests, and determines that there are no signs of bleeding other than the nosebleed, which has stopped. The provider discovers that K.N. recently started to take daily doses of an over-the-counter proton pump inhibitor (PPI), omeprazole (Prilosec OTC), for heartburn.

5. What happened when K.N. began taking the PPI?

6. What should K.N. have done to prevent this problem?

7. The provider gives K.N. a low dose of vitamin K orally, asks him to hold his warfarin dose that evening, and asks him to come back tomorrow for another prothrombin time (PT) and INR blood draw. Why is K.N. instructed to take the vitamin K?

8. You want to make certain K.N. knows what "hold the next dose" means. What should you tell him?

9. K.N. asks you why his PT/INR has to be checked so soon. How will you respond?

CASE STUDY PROGRESS

K.N.'s INR the next day is 3.7, and the health care provider makes no further medication changes. K.N. is instructed to return again in 7 days to have another PT/INR drawn.

10. Why should the INR be checked again so soon instead of the usual monthly follow-up?

11. K.N. grumbles about all of the laboratory tests but agrees to follow through. You provide patient education to K.N. and start with reviewing the signs and symptoms (S/S) of bleeding. What are potential S/S of bleeding that should be taught to K.N.? (Select all that apply.)
    a. Black, tarry stool
    b. Stool that is pale in color
    c. New onset of dizziness
    d. Insomnia
    e. New joint pain or swelling
    f. Unexplained abdominal pain

12. Identify two other patient education needs that you need to stress at this time.

13. Four months later, K.N. informs you that he is going to have a knee replacement next month. What will you do with this information?

CASE STUDY PROGRESS

You know that sometimes the only needed action is to stop the warfarin (Coumadin) several days before the surgery. Other times, the provider initiates "bridging therapy," or stops the warfarin and provides anticoagulation protection by initiating low-molecular-weight heparin. After reviewing all of his anticoagulation information, the provider decides that K.N. will need to stop the warfarin (Coumadin) 1 week before the surgery and in its place be started on enoxaparin (Lovenox) therapy.

14. Compare the duration of action of warfarin (Coumadin) and enoxaparin (Lovenox) and explain the reason the provider switched to enoxaparin at this time.

CASE STUDY PROGRESS

K.N. is in the office and ready for his first enoxaparin (Lovenox) injection.

15. Which nursing interventions are appropriate when administering enoxaparin? Select all that apply.
    a. Monitor activated partial thromboplastin time (aPTT) levels.
    b. Administer via intramuscular (IM) injection into the deltoid muscle.
    c. The preferred site of injection is the lateral abdominal fatty tissue.
    d. Massage the area after the injection has been given.
    e. Hold extra pressure over the site after the injection.

CASE STUDY PROGRESS

K.N. undergoes knee surgery without complications. Just before his discharge, his physician reviews the instructions and gives him a new prescription for warfarin (Coumadin). K.N. tells his doctor, "I saw this commercial for a new blood thinner called Xarelto. I'd like to take that instead because I wouldn't need to have all this blood work done."

16. How do you expect the physician to respond?

CASE STUDY OUTCOME

K.N. is discharged to a rehabilitation facility where he makes a quick recovery from the knee replacement surgery. He does not experience any thrombotic events or bleeding episodes during his recovery.

Case Study 8

Name _____ Class/Group _____ Date _____

Group Members _____

▶ Scenario

You are assigned to care for L.J., a 70-year-old retired bus driver who has just been admitted to your medical floor with right leg deep vein thrombosis (DVT). L.J. has a 48–pack-year smoking history, although he states he quit 2 years ago. He has had pneumonia several times and frequent episodes of atrial flutter or fibrillation. He has had two previous episodes of DVT and was diagnosed with rheumatoid arthritis 3 years ago. Two months ago he began experiencing shortness of breath on exertion and noticed swelling of his right lower leg that became progressively worse until it extended up to his groin. His wife brought him to the hospital when he complained of increasingly severe pain in his leg. When a Doppler study indicated a probable thrombus of the external iliac vein extending distally to the lower leg, he was admitted for bed rest and to initiate heparin therapy. His basic metabolic panel was normal; other laboratory results were as follows.

Chart View

Laboratory Testing

PT	12.4 sec
INR	1.11
aPTT	25 sec
Hgb	13.3 g/dL
Hct	38.9%
Cholesterol	206 mg/dL

1. List six risk factors for DVT.

2. Identify at least five problems from L.J.'s history that represent his personal risk factors.

3. Something is missing from the scenario. Based on his history, L.J. should have been taking an important medication. What is it, and why should he be taking it?

4. Keeping in mind L.J.'s health history and admitting diagnosis, what are the most important assessments you will make during your physical examination and assessment?

5. What is the most serious complication of DVT?

6. List at least eight assessment findings you should monitor closely for in the development of the complication identified in Question 5.

7. You review the literature for DVT and see the abbreviation *VTE*. What does VTE mean?

CASE STUDY PROGRESS

Your assessment of L.J. reveals bibasilar crackles with moist cough; normal heart sounds; blood pressure (BP) 138/88 mm Hg; pulse 104 beats/min; 3+ pitting edema of right lower extremity; mild erythema of right foot and calf; and severe right calf pain. He is awake, alert, and oriented but a little restless. His Spo_2 is 92% on room air. He denies chest pain but does have shortness of breath with exertion. He states he is anxious about missing his grandson's wedding. He denies any voiding problems.

8. Your institution uses electronic charting. Based on the assessment noted previously which of the following systems would you mark as "abnormal" as you document your findings? For abnormal findings provide a brief narrative note.
   X Abnormal
   ☐ Neurologic:
   ☐ Respiratory:
   ☐ Cardiovascular:
   ☐ Genitourinary:
   ☐ Skin:
   ☐ Psychosocial:
   ☐ Pain:

CASE STUDY PROGRESS

L.J. is placed on 72-hour bed rest with bathroom privileges and given acetaminophen (Tylenol) for pain. The physician writes orders for enoxaparin (Lovenox) injections.

9. L.J. asks, "Why do I have to get these shots? Why can't I just get a Coumadin pill to thin my blood?" What would be your response?"
   a. "Good idea! I will call to ask the physician to switch medications."
   b. "It would take the Coumadin pills several days to be effective."
   c. "Your physician prefers the injections over the pills."
   d. "The enoxaparin will work to dissolve the blood clot in your leg."

10. The order for the enoxaparin reads: Enoxaparin 70 mg every 12 hours subcut. L.J. is 5 ft, 6 in tall and weighs 156 lb. Is this dose appropriate?

11. What special techniques do you use when giving the subcutaneous injection of enoxaparin? Select all that apply.
    a. Rotate injection sites.
    b. Give the injection near the umbilicus.
    c. Expel the bubble from the prefilled syringe before giving the injection.
    d. After inserting the needle, do not aspirate before giving the injection.
    e. Massage the injection site gently after the injection is given.

12. True or False: Enoxaparin dosage is directed by monitoring aPTT levels. Explain your answer.

13. What instructions will you give L.J. about his activity?

14. What pertinent laboratory values and measurements would you expect the physician to order and the results of which you will monitor? Explain the reason for each test.

15. You identify pain as a key issue in the care of L.J. List four interventions you will choose for L.J. to address his pain.

16. You evaluate L.J.'s electrocardiogram (ECG) strip. Name this rhythm, and explain what consequences it could have for L.J.

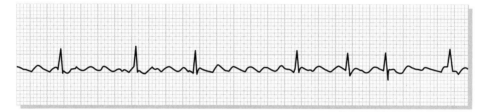

CASE STUDY PROGRESS

A week has passed. L.J. responded to heparin therapy and was bridged to oral warfarin therapy. His heart dysrhythmia converted to sinus rhythm after he started taking cardiac medications, and he is being discharged to home with home care follow-up. "Good," he says, "just in time to fly out west for my grandson's wedding. His wife, who has come to pick him up, rolls her eyes and looks at the ceiling.

17. Although you are surprised at his comment, you realize he is serious about going to the wedding. What are you going to tell him?

CASE STUDY OUTCOME

L.J. listens to you, and his wife is quite relieved. L.J.'s son arranges to record the wedding ceremony, and guests at the reception record special greetings for him. It's been 2 weeks, and he seems quite pleased. He watches the recording daily and points out his favorite parts to the home care nurse every time she visits.

Case Study **9**

Name _____   Class/Group _____   Date _____

Group Members _____

▶ Scenario

A.H. is a 70-year-old retired construction worker who has experienced lumbosacral pain, nausea, and upset stomach for the past 6 months. He has a history of heart failure, high cholesterol, hypertension (HTN), sleep apnea, and depression. His chronic medical problems have been managed over the years with oral medications: benazepril (Lotensin) 5 mg/day, fluoxetine (Prozac) 40 mg/day, furosemide (Lasix) 20 mg/day, Potassium chloride (KCl) 20 mEq bid, and lovastatin (Mevacor) 40 mg with the evening meal.

A.H. has just been admitted to the hospital for surgical repair of a 6.2-cm abdominal aortic aneurysm (AAA) that is now causing him constant pain. On arrival on your floor, his vital signs (VS) are 109/81, 61, 16, and 98.3°F (36.8°C). When you perform your assessment, you find that his apical heart rhythm is regular and his peripheral pulses are strong. His lungs are clear, and he is awake, alert, and oriented. There are no abnormal physical findings; however, he hasn't had a bowel movement for 3 days. His electrolytes, blood chemistries, and clotting studies are within normal range, except his hematocrit is 30.1%, and hemoglobin is 9 g/dL.

1. A.H. has several common risk factors for AAA that are evident from his health history. Identify and explain three factors.

2. Angiography reveals an aneurysm with a shape as in the accompanying illustration. What type of aneurysm is this?

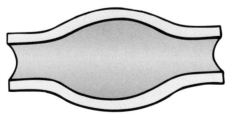

   a. Saccular aortic aneurysm
   b. Fusiform aortic aneurysm
   c. Aortic dissection
   d. False aortic aneurysm

CASE STUDY PROGRESS

While A.H. awaits his surgery, it is important that you monitor him carefully for decreased tissue perfusion.

3. Identify five things you would assess for, and state your rationale for each.

4. What is the most serious, life-threatening complication of AAA and why?

5. What single problem mentioned at the beginning of this case study presents a risk for AAA rupture? Why?

6. During your assessment you notice a pulsation in A.H.'s upper abdomen, slightly left of the midline, between the umbilicus and the xiphoid process. True or False: You will need to palpate this mass as part of your physical assessment. Explain your answer.

CASE STUDY PROGRESS

The resection of A.H.'s aneurysm is successful, but for the first 3 postoperative days he is delirious and requires one-to-one nursing care before he becomes coherent and oriented again. He is transferred back to your floor.

7. What assessments should be made that are specific to his postoperative care?

8. List five problems that are high priorities in A.H.'s postoperative care.

9. During the postoperative period after an aneurysmectomy, the nurse will implement which actions? Select all that apply.
   a. Keep the head of the bed (HOB) elevated at 60 degrees.
   b. Keep firm pressure on the abdominal incision during coughing exercises.
   c. Change dressings as ordered with aseptic technique.
   d. Monitor peripheral pulses of both lower extremities.
   e. Use the bed's knee gatch to allow for knee flexion during bed rest.

CASE STUDY PROGRESS

When A.H. is being prepared for discharge, you talk to him about health promotion and lifestyle change issues that are pertinent to his health problems.

10. Identify four health-related issues you might appropriately address with him and what you would teach in each area.

11. A.H. will be receiving follow-up visits from the home health care nurse to change his dressing and evaluate his incision. What can you discuss with A.H. before discharge that will help him understand what the nurse will be doing?

12. Which statement by A.H. indicates a need for further education?
    a. "I will report any fever greater than 100° F."
    b. "I will avoid heavy lifting for 3 more weeks."
    c. "I will call my doctor right away if I notice redness or swelling at the incision."
    d. "I will look for color changes in my feet and lower legs."

Case Study **10**

Name _____ Class/Group _____ Date _____

Group Members _____

▶ Scenario

You are working at the local cardiac rehabilitation center and R.M. is walking around the track. He summons you and asks if you could help him understand his recent laboratory report. He admits to being confused by the overwhelming data on the test and does not understand how the results relate to his recent heart attack and need for a stent. You take a moment to locate his laboratory reports and review his history. The findings are as follows.

R.M. is an active 61-year-old man who works full time for the postal service. He walks 3 miles every other day and admits he doesn't eat a "perfect diet." He enjoys two or three beers every night, uses stick margarine, eats red meat two or three times per week, and is a self-professed "sweet eater." He has tried to quit smoking and is down to one pack per day. Cardiac history includes a recent inferior myocardial infarction (MI) and a heart catheterization revealing three-vessel disease: in the left anterior descending (LAD) coronary artery, a proximal 60% lesion; in the right coronary artery (RCA), proximal 100% occlusion with thrombus; and a circumflex with 40% to 60% diffuse dilated lesions. A stent was deployed to the RCA and reduced the lesion to 0% residual stenosis. He has had no need for sublingual nitroglycerin (NTG). He was discharged on enteric-coated aspirin 325 mg daily, clopidogrel (Plavix) 75 mg daily, atorvastatin (Lipitor) 10 mg at bedtime, and ramipril (Altace) 10 mg/day. Six weeks after his MI and stent placement, he had a fasting advanced lipid profile with other blood work.

Chart View

Six-Week Postprocedure Laboratory Work (Fasting)

Total cholesterol	188 mg/dL
HDL	34 mg/dL
LDL	98 mg/dL
Triglycerides	176 mg/dL
Homocysteine	18 mmol/dL
High-sensitivity C-reactive protein (hsCRP)	8 mg/dL
FBG	99 mg/dL
TSH	1.04 mU/L

1. When you start to discuss R.M.'s laboratory values with him, he is pleased about his results. "My cholesterol level is below 200!—and my 'bad cholesterol' is good! That's good news, right?" What would you say to him?

2. R.M.'s physician adds niacin, a vitamin preparation (folic acid, vitamin B_6, and vitamin B_{12} [Foltx]) daily with food, and omega-3 fatty acids to his list of medications. How do these medications affect lipids? R.M. states, "But I already take Lipitor. What do all these medications do?" How do you answer him?

3. Discuss the significance of R.M.'s hsCRP level.

4. Discuss the significance of the homocysteine test and R.M.'s results.

5. What else in R.M.'s history might be contributing to his elevated homocysteine levels?

6. You are teaching R.M. about the side effects of niacin. Which effects will you include in your teaching? Select all that apply.
   a. Flushed skin
   b. Headache
   c. Gastrointestinal (GI) distress
   d. Pruritus
   e. Dizziness

7. R.M. tells you that he really does not want to "put up with" the side effects of the niacin. Is there an alternative to niacin?

8. You review his other medications, including atorvastatin (Lipitor). Which statement by R.M. indicates a need for further teaching about this medication?
   a. "I will take this drug at night."
   b. "I will try to exercise more each week."
   c. "I like to take my medicines with grapefruit juice."
   d. "I will call the doctor right away if I experience muscle pain."

CASE STUDY PROGRESS

You enter R.M.'s room and hear the physician say, "There are many options for changing your LDL and triglyceride levels. You need to continue modifying your diet and exercise to enhance your medication regimen." The physician asks R.M. whether he has any questions, and the patient responds, "No."

9. After the physician leaves the room, R.M. tells you he really didn't understand what the physician said. Explain the necessary lifestyle changes to R.M.

10. R.M. tells you that he knows that exercise will help him to lose weight, which is good, but he does not understand how exercise helps his cholesterol levels. How do you answer him?

Case Study 11

Name _____ Class/Group _____ Date _____

Group Members _____

▶ Scenario

The wife of C.W., a 70-year-old man, brought him to the emergency department (ED) at 0430. She told the ED triage nurse that he had had diarrhea for the past 3 days and that last night he had a lot of "dark red" diarrhea. When he became very dizzy, disoriented, and weak this morning, she decided to bring him to the hospital. C.W.'s vital signs (VS) in the ED were 70/− (systolic blood pressure [SBP] 70 mm Hg, diastolic blood pressure [DBP] inaudible), pulse rate 110 beats/min, 22 breaths/min, oral temperature 99.1°F (37.3°C). A 16-gauge IV catheter was inserted and a lactated Ringer's (LR) infusion was started. The triage nurse obtained the following history from the patient and his wife. C.W. has had idiopathic dilated cardiomyopathy for several years. The onset was insidious, but the cardiomyopathy is now severe, as evidenced by an ejection fraction of 13% found during a recent cardiac catheterization. He experiences frequent problems with heart failure (HF) because of the cardiomyopathy. Two years ago, he had a cardiac arrest that was attributed to hypokalemia. He has a long history of hypertension and arthritis. He had atrial fibrillation in the past but it has been under control recently. Fifteen years ago he had a peptic ulcer.

Endoscopy showed a 25-×15-mm duodenal ulcer with adherent clot. The ulcer was cauterized and C.W. was admitted to the medical intensive care unit (MICU) for treatment of his volume deficit. You are his admitting nurse. As you are making him comfortable, Mrs. W. gives you a paper sack filled with the bottles of medications he has been taking: enalapril (Vasotec) 5 mg PO bid, warfarin (Coumadin) 5 mg/day PO, digoxin (Lanoxin) 0.125 mg/day PO, potassium chloride 20 mEq PO bid, and diclofenac (Voltaren) 50 mg PO tid. As you connect him to the cardiac monitor, you note he is in sinus tachycardia. Doing a quick assessment, you find a pale man who is sleepy but arousable and slightly disoriented. He states he is still dizzy. His BP is 98/52, pulse is 118, and respiratory rate 26. You hear S_3 and S_4 heart sounds and a grade II/VI systolic murmur. Peripheral pulses are all 2+, and trace pedal edema is present. Lungs are clear. Bowel sounds are present, midepigastric tenderness is noted, and the liver margin is 4 cm below the costal margin. A Swan-Ganz pulmonary artery catheter and a peripheral arterial line are inserted.

1. What may have precipitated C.W.'s gastrointestinal (GI) bleeding?

2. From his history and assessment, identify five signs and symptoms (S/S) of GI bleeding and loss of blood volume.

3. What is the most serious potential complication of C.W.'s bleeding?

4. Calculate C.W.'s mean arterial pressure (MAP) and explain why this measure is important.

CASE STUDY PROGRESS

As soon as you get a chance, you review C.W.'s admission laboratory results.

Chart View

Laboratory Results

Sodium	138 mEq/L
Potassium	6.9 mEq/L
BUN	90 mg/dL
Creatinine	2.1 mg/dL
WBC	16,000/mm³
Hgb	8.4 g/dL
Hct	25%
PT	23.4 seconds
INR	4.8

5. After examination of the lab results, are there any concerns with C.W.'s electrolyte levels? Explain your answer.

6. In view of the previous laboratory results, what diagnostic test will be performed and why?

7. Evaluate this electrocardiogram (ECG) strip and note the effect of any electrolyte imbalances.

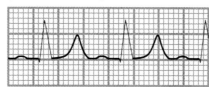

8. Why do you think the BUN and creatinine are elevated?

9. What do the low Hgb and Hct levels indicate about the rapidity of C.W.'s blood loss?

10. What is the explanation for the prolonged PT/INR?

11. What will be your response to the prolonged PT/INR? Select all that apply.
    a. Prepare to administer a STAT dose of protamine sulfate.
    b. Hold the warfarin.
    c. Monitor C.W. for signs and symptoms of bleeding.
    d. Obtain an order for aspirin if needed for pain.
    e. Avoid injections as much as possible.

 12. What safety precautions should be considered in light of his prolonged PT and INR?

13. How do you account for the elevated WBC count?

CASE STUDY PROGRESS

C.W. receives a total of 4 units of packed red blood cells (PRBCs), 5 units of fresh frozen plasma (FFP), and several liters of crystalloids to keep his mean BP above 60 mm Hg. On the second day in the MICU, his total fluid intake is 8.498 L and output is 3.66 L. His hemodynamic parameters after fluid resuscitation are pulmonary capillary wedge pressure (PCWP) 30 mm Hg and cardiac output (CO) 4.5 L/min.

14. Calculate his fluid balance and identify whether it is positive or negative.

15. Why will you want to monitor his fluid status very carefully?

16. List at least six things you will monitor to assess C.W.'s fluid balance.

17. Explain the purpose of the FFP for C.W.

CASE STUDY PROGRESS

Mrs. W. has been with her husband since he arrived at the emergency department and is worried about his condition and his care.

18. List five things you might do to make her more comfortable while her husband is in the MICU.

Case Study 12

Name _____ Class/Group _____ Date _____

Group Members _____

▶ Scenario

J.F. is a 50-year-old married homemaker with a genetic autoimmune deficiency; she has had recurrent infective endocarditis. The most recent episodes were a *Staphylococcus aureus* infection of the mitral valve 16 months ago and a *Streptococcus viridans* infection of the aortic valve 1 month ago. During the latter hospitalization, an echocardiogram showed moderate aortic stenosis, moderate aortic insufficiency, chronic valvular vegetations, and moderate left atrial enlargement. Two years ago, J.F. received an 18-month course of total parenteral nutrition (TPN) for malnutrition caused by idiopathic, relentless nausea and vomiting (N/V). She has had coronary artery disease for several years and, 2 years ago had an acute anterior wall myocardial infarction (MI). In addition, she has a history of chronic joint pain.

Now, after having been home for only a week, J.F. has been readmitted to your floor with endocarditis, N/V, and renal failure. Since yesterday, she has been vomiting and retching constantly; she also has had

Chart View

Admission Orders

STAT blood cultures (aerobic and anaerobic) × 2 30 minutes apart
STAT CMP & CBC
Begin TPN at 85 mL/hr
Penicillin G potassium (Pfizerpen) 2 million units IVPB q4h
Vancomycin (Vancocin), renal dosing per pharmacy, IVPB q12h
Furosemide (Lasix) 80 mg/day PO
Amlodipine (Norvasc) 5 mg/day PO
Potassium chloride (K-Dur) 40 mEq/day PO
Metoprolol (Lopressor) 25 mg PO bid
Ondansetron (Zofran) 4 mg IV every 4-6 hours for N/V
Transesophageal echocardiogram ASAP

Admission Assessment

Blood pressure	152/48 (supine) and 100/40 (sitting)
Pulse rate	116 beats/min
Respiratory rate	22 breaths/min
Temperature	100.2° F (37.9° C)

Oriented × 3 but drowsy
Grade II/VI holosystolic murmur and a grade III/VI diastolic murmur noted on auscultation
Lungs clear bilaterally
Abdomen soft with slight left upper quadrant (LUQ) tenderness
Multiple petechiae on skin of arms, legs, and chest; splinter hemorrhages under the fingernails; hematuria noted in voided urine

chills, fever, fatigue, joint pain, and headache. As you go through the admission process with her, you note that she wears glasses and has a dental bridge. Intravenous (IV) access is obtained with a double lumen peripherally inserted central catheter (PICC) line. Other orders and your assessment are shown in the box.

1. What is the significance of the orthostatic hypotension and tachycardia?

2. What is the significance of the abdominal tenderness, hematuria, joint pain, and petechiae?

3. What are splinter hemorrhages and what is their significance?

4. Mark the area on the accompanying diagram where you would place the stethoscope to auscultate an aortic valve murmur.

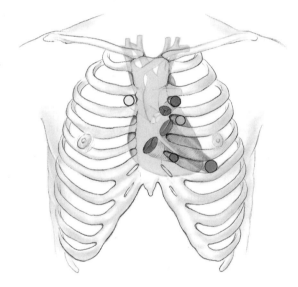

5. As you monitor J.F. throughout the day, what other signs and symptoms of embolization will you watch for?

6. Explain the diagnostic criteria for infectious endocarditis.

CASE STUDY PROGRESS

The next day, you review J.F.'s laboratory test results.

Chart View

Laboratory Test Results

Na	138 mEq/L
K	3.9 mEq/L
Cl	103 mEq/L
BUN	85 mg/dL
Creatinine	3.9 mg/dL
Glucose	165 mg/dL
WBC	6700/mm³
Hct	27%
Hgb	9.0 g/dL

7. Identify the values that are not within normal ranges and explain the reason for each abnormality.

8. You note that a new intern writes an order for "Fasting blood glucose levels daily." Is this order appropriate for J.F.? Explain.

1 Cardiovascular Disorders

9. What is the greatest risk for J.F. during the process of rehydration, and what would you monitor to detect its development?

CASE STUDY PROGRESS

You were aware that as soon as J.F. became stable, she would be going home on TPN and IV antibiotics. As part of the discharge preparations, you contact the home care agency that will be providing her care.

10. List five important questions in assessing her home health care needs.

CASE STUDY PROGRESS

Fortunately, J.F. has a supportive husband and two daughters who live nearby who can function as care-givers when J.F. is discharged. They, along with J.F., will need teaching about endocarditis. Although J.F. has been ill for several years, you discover that she and her family have received little education about the disease. You prepare a teaching plan for the family.

11. List six things you will teach J.F. and her family.

12. After you have taught J.F. about oral hygiene, which statement by J.F. reflects a need for further education?
    a. "I will remove my bridge after every meal and clean it thoroughly before replacing it."
    b. "I will use a water irrigation device to clean my teeth and gums."
    c. "I will use a soft toothbrush to brush my teeth."
    d. "I will rinse my mouth thoroughly with water after brushing my teeth."

CASE STUDY PROGRESS

Your hospital discharge planner facilitates J.F.'s transition to home care. During the initial home visit, the home health nurse evaluates J.F.'s IV site for implementation of the IV therapy program. The nurse interviews the family members to determine their willingness to be caregivers and their level of understanding and enlists the patient's and family's assistance to identify goals.

13. The home health nurse also writes short- and long-term goals for J.F. and her family. Identify two short-term and three long-term goals.

CASE STUDY OUTCOME

Mr. F. and his two daughters learned to administer J.F.'s antibiotic and 8-month treatment of TPN. J.F.'s endocarditis resolves with no worsening of her cardiac condition.

Case Study **13**

Name _____ Class/Group _____ Date _____

Group Members _____

▶ **Scenario**

Your patient, 58-year-old K.Z., has a significant cardiac history. He has long-standing coronary artery disease (CAD) with occasional episodes of heart failure (HF). One year ago, he had an anterior wall myocardial infarction (MI). In addition, he has chronic anemia, hypertension, chronic renal insufficiency, and a recently diagnosed 4-cm suprarenal abdominal aortic aneurysm. Because of his severe CAD, he had to retire from his job as a railroad engineer about 6 months ago. This morning, he is being admitted to your telemetry unit for a same-day cardiac catheterization. As you take his health history, you note that his wife died a year ago (at about the same time that he had his MI) and he does not have any children. He is a current cigarette smoker with a 50–pack-year smoking history. His vital signs (VS) are 158/94, 88, 20, and 97.2° F (36.2° C). As you talk with him, you realize that he has only a minimal understanding of the catheterization procedure.

1. Before he leaves for the catheterization laboratory, you briefly teach him the important things he needs to know before having the procedure. List five priority topics you will address.

2. Look at his past history. What other factors are present that could contribute to his risk for cardiac ischemia?

CASE STUDY PROGRESS

Several hours later, K.Z. returns from his catheterization. The catheterization report shows 90% occlusion of the proximal left anterior descending (LAD) coronary artery, 90% occlusion of the distal LAD, 70% to 80% occlusion of the distal right coronary artery (RCA), an old apical infarct, and an ejection fraction (EF) of 37%. About an hour after the procedure is finished, you perform a brief physical assessment and note a grade III/VI systolic ejection murmur at the cardiac apex, crackles bilaterally in the lung bases, and trace pitting edema of his feet and ankles. Except for the soft systolic murmur, these findings were not present before the catheterization.

3. Using the following diagram, identify the superior vena cava, the aorta, and the left and right ventricles. Identify the main coronary arteries, and circle the areas of the LAD and RCA that have significant occlusion, as identified in the previous report. Lightly shade the area of the heart where K.Z. had the earlier infarct.

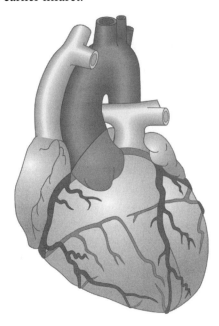

4. What is your evaluation of the catheterization results?

5. Explain the significance of having an EF of 37%.

6. What problem do the changes in assessment findings suggest to you? What led you to your conclusion?

7. List five actions you should take as a result of your evaluation of the assessment, and state your rationales.

CASE STUDY PROGRESS

After assessing K.Z., the physician admits him with a diagnosis of CAD and HF for coronary artery bypass graft (CABG) surgery. Significant laboratory results drawn at this time are Hct 25.3%, Hgb 8.8 g/dL, BUN 33 mg/dL, and creatinine 3.1 mg/dL. K.Z. is given furosemide (Lasix) and 2 units of packed red blood cells (PRBCs).

8. Review K.Z.'s health history. Can you identify a probable explanation for his chronic renal insufficiency and anemia?

9. Why is he receiving 2 units of PRBCs? What is the purpose of the furosemide?

CASE STUDY PROGRESS

Five days later, after his condition is stabilized, K.Z. is taken to surgery for a three-vessel coronary artery bypass graft (CABG × 3 V). When he arrives in the surgical intensive care unit (SICU), he has a Swan-Ganz catheter in place for hemodynamic monitoring and is intubated. He is put on a ventilator at Fio_2 0.70 and positive end-expiratory pressure (PEEP) at 5 cm H_2O. His latest Hgb is 10.3 mg/dL. You review his first hemodynamic readings and arterial blood gases.

Chart View

Hemodynamic Readings

Pulmonary artery pressure (PAP)	38/23 mm Hg
Central venous pressure (CVP)	16 mm Hg
Pulmonary capillary wedge pressure (PCWP)	18 mm Hg
Cardiac index (CI)	1.88 L/min/mm^2

Arterial Blood Gases

pH	7.37
$Paco_2$	46 mm Hg
Pao_2	61 mm Hg
Sao_2	85%

10. Why are arterial blood gases necessary in K.Z.'s case? Explain why it would be inappropriate to use pulse oximetry to assess his O_2 saturation status.

11. What is your interpretation of his arterial blood gases on 70% oxygen?

12. What is your evaluation of K.Z.'s hemodynamic status, based on the results displayed?

13. Do you think the hemodynamic values reported previously reflect poor left ventricular function or fluid overload, and why?

14. K.Z. is receiving continuous IV infusions of norepinephrine (Levophed) and dobutamine. Why is K.Z. receiving these medications?

15. What are your responsibilities when administering norepinephrine and dobutamine to K.Z.?

CASE STUDY PROGRESS

After 3 days in the SICU, K.Z.'s condition was stable, and he was returned to your telemetry floor. Now, 5 days later, he is ready to go home, and you are preparing him for discharge.

16. List at least four general areas related to his CABG surgery in which he should receive instruction before he goes home.

Case Study **14**

Name _____ Class/Group _____ Date _____

Group Members _____

▶ **Scenario**

R.K. is an 85-year-old woman who lives with her husband, who is 87. Two nights before her admission to your cardiac unit, she awoke with heavy substernal pressure accompanied by epigastric distress. The pain was reduced somewhat when she rolled onto her side but did not completely subside for about 6 hours. The next night, she experienced the same chest pressure. The following morning, R.K.'s husband took her to the physician and she was subsequently hospitalized to rule out myocardial infarction (MI). Laboratory specimens were drawn in the emergency department. She was given an intravenous (IV) line, oxygen (O_2) at 2 L via nasal cannula, and 325 mg chewable, non–enteric-coated aspirin.

You obtain the following information from your history and physical examination: R.K. has no history of smoking or alcohol use, and she has been in good general health, with the exception of osteoarthritis of her hands and knees and some osteoarthritis of the spine. Her only medications are simvastatin (Zocor), ibuprofen as needed for bone and joint pain, and "herbs." Her admission vital signs (VS) are blood pressure 132/84 mm Hg, pulse 88 beats/min, respirations 18 breaths/min, and oral temperature 99° F (37.2° C). Her weight is 114 lb and height is 5 ft, 4 in. Moderate edema of both ankles is present; capillary refill is brisk and peripheral pulses are 1+. You hear a soft systolic murmur. She denies any discomfort at present. You place her on telemetry, which shows the rhythm in the following figure.

1. Identify her cardiac rhythm.

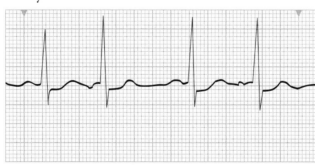

2. Give at least two reasons for inserting an IV line.

3. Explain the purpose of the aspirin tablet. Why is "non–enteric-coated" aspirin specified? What would be a contraindication to administering aspirin?

4. What additional history and physical information should you obtain related to her admitting diagnosis? Name at least four for each.

5. List seven laboratory or diagnostic tests you would expect to be performed; suggest what each might contribute.

6. What other sources, in addition to cardiac ischemia, might be responsible for her chest and abdominal discomfort?

7. Define the concept of *differential diagnosis* and explain how the concept applies to R.K.'s symptoms.

CASE STUDY PROGRESS

After some rest, R.K.'s chest pain has subsided, and she tells you she feels much better now. You review her laboratory results.

Chart View

Laboratory Results

12-lead ECG: Light left-axis deviation, normal sinus rhythm with no ventricular ectopy
Serial CPK tests are 30 units/L at admission, 32 units/L 4 hours after admission
Cardiac troponin T is less than 0.01 ng/mL (at admission) and same result 4 hours after admission
Cardiac troponin T is less than 0.03 ng/mL (at admission) and same result 4 hours after admission
D-dimer test result less than 250 ng/mL

8. On the basis of the information presented so far, do you believe she had an MI? What is your rationale?

9. Do you think she may have a pulmonary embolus?

10. While you care for R.K., you carefully observe her. Identify two possible complications of coronary artery disease (CAD) and the signs and symptoms associated with each.

11. R.K. rings her call bell. When you arrive, she has her hand placed over her heart and tells you she is "having that heavy feeling again." She is not diaphoretic or nauseated, but states she is short of breath. What else do you assess, and what can you do to make her more comfortable?

CASE STUDY PROGRESS

During the episode of chest pain, R.K.'s vital signs were as follows: pulse 110 beats/min; blood pressure 140/92 mm Hg, respirations 20 breaths/min. The rhythm strip shows sinus tachycardia, and she was very anxious. Her chest discomfort subsided in 3 minutes after one nitroglycerin dose, and she is resting quietly with O_2 per nasal cannula at 2 L/min. R.K.'s physician is making rounds.

12. Using SBAR (*Situation, Background, Assessment, Recommendation*), how would you communicate this episode to R.K.'s physician?

CASE STUDY PROGRESS

R.K.'s husband is upset. He tells you they have been married for 62 years and he doesn't know what he would do without his wife. One way to help people deal with their anxieties is to help them focus on concrete issues.

13. What information would be useful to get from him? What other health care professional might be able to help with some of these issues?

R.K. has no further episodes of chest pain, and she is discharged to home the next day. She is to see a cardiologist this week and set up an appointment for outpatient testing. As you present the discharge instructions, you review the proper technique for taking sublingual nitroglycerin for chest pain.

14. Which statement by R.K. indicates that further teaching is needed?
    a. "At the first sign of chest discomfort, I will stop what I'm doing and sit down."
    b. "I will place one nitroglycerin tablet under my tongue."
    c. "If the chest pain does not stop, I can take another tablet in 5 minutes."
    d. "My husband will need to call 911 if the chest pain does not stop after three nitroglycerin tablets."

Case Study **15**

Name _____ Class/Group _____ Date _____

Group Members _____

▶ Scenario

The time is 1900. You are working in a small, rural hospital. It has been snowing heavily all day, and the medical helicopters at the large regional medical center, 4 hours away by car (in good weather), have been grounded by the weather until morning. The roads are barely passable. W.R., a 48-year-old plumber with a 36–pack-year smoking history, is admitted to your floor with a diagnosis of rule out myocardial infarction (R/O MI). He has significant male-pattern obesity ("beer belly," large waist circumference) and a barrel chest and reports a dietary history of high-fat food. His wife brought him to the emergency department after he complained of unrelieved "indigestion." His admission vital signs (VS) were blood pressure (BP) 202/124 mm Hg, pulse (P) 106 beats/min, respirations 18 breaths/min, and oral temperature 98.2° F (36.8° C). W.R. was put on oxygen (O_2) by nasal cannula (NC) titrated to maintain Spo_2 over 92% and started on an IV nitroglycerin (NTG) infusion. He was given aspirin 325 mg to chew and swallow and was admitted to Dr. A.'s service. There are plans to transfer him by helicopter to the regional medical center for a cardiac catheterization in the morning when the weather clears. Meanwhile, you have to deal with limited laboratory and pharmacy resources. The minute W.R. comes through the door of your unit, he announces he's "just fine" in a loud and angry voice and demands a cigarette. He also says he has no time to fool around with hospitals.

1. What is the first priority in his care?

2. Are these VS reasonable for a man of his age? If not, which one(s) concern(s) you? Explain why or why not.

3. Identify five priority problems associated with the care of a patient such as W.R.

4. Which laboratory tests might be ordered to investigate W.R.'s condition? If the order is appropriate, place an *A* in the space provided. If inappropriate, mark with an *I*. Provide rationales for your decisions.

_____1. Complete blood count (CBC)

_____2. Electroencephalogram (EEG) in the morning

_____3. Basal metabolic panel (BMP)

_____4. Prothrombin time (PT) and partial thromboplastin time (PTT)

_____5. Bilirubin

_____6. Urinalysis (UA)

_____7. STAT 12-lead electrocardiogram (ECG) and repeat in the morning

_____8. Type and crossmatch for 2 units of packed red blood cells (PRBCs)

_____9. Chest x-ray on admission and in the morning

5. What significant laboratory tests are missing from the previous list?

6. How are you going to respond to W.R.'s angry demands for a cigarette? He also requests something for his "heartburn." How will you respond?

7. Mrs. R. asks you, "If he can't smoke, why can't you give him one of those nicotine patches?" How will you respond?

8. Are there any alternatives to help him with his nicotine cravings? Would they be helpful now?

CASE STUDY PROGRESS

At 2000, you phone Dr. A.'s partner, who is on call. She prescribes morphine sulfate 4 to 10 mg IV push (IVP) q1h prn for pain (burning, pressure, and angina).

9. Explain two reasons for this order.

10. What special precautions should you follow when administering morphine sulfate via IVP?

11. The pharmacy supplies morphine for injection in vials of 5 mg/mL only. For the first dose, you will be giving 4 mg of morphine. How many milliliters will you give for this dose? Mark the syringe with your answer.

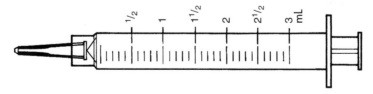

12. What will you do with the rest of the morphine in the vial?
    a. Discard it.
    b. Save it for the next dose.
    c. Return it to the pharmacy.
    d. Discard it with a second witness.

13. Angina is not always experienced as "pain" as many people understand pain. How would you describe symptoms you want him to warn you about? Why is this important?

14. What safety measures or instructions would you give W.R. before you leave his room?

15. Mrs. R. is unable to leave the hospital because of the bad weather. She approaches you and asks, "Did my husband have a heart attack? I'm really scared. His father died of one when he was 51." How are you going to respond to her question?

CASE STUDY PROGRESS

When you come into W.R.'s room at 2230 hours to answer his call light, you see he is holding his left arm and complaining about aching in his left shoulder and arm.

16. What information will you gather? What questions will you ask him?

You titrate the NTG drip up, assess his compliance with the oxygen cannula, and assess his vital signs. In addition, you administer a dose of morphine, but his pain is not relieved. Based on your assessment findings, you decide to call the physician.

17. Using SBAR (*Situation*, *Background*, *Assessment*, *Recommendation*), what information would you provide to the physician when you call?

18. W.R.'s chest pain subsides after the dose of morphine and he settles down for the night. You monitor him closely and watch for side effects of the NTG infusion. Side effects of NTG include which of these? Select all that apply.
    a. Constipation
    b. Headache
    c. Tachycardia
    d. Postural hypotension
    e. Decreased respirations

CASE STUDY PROGRESS

In the morning, W.R. is transferred by helicopter to the medical center, and a cardiac catheterization is performed. It is determined that W.R. has coronary artery disease (CAD). The cardiologist suggests it would be best to treat him medically for now.

19. What does it mean to treat him "medically"? What other approaches might be used to treat CAD?

1 Cardiovascular Disorders

CASE STUDY OUTCOME

The physician orders follow-up counseling regarding risk factor modification, especially smoking cessation, hypertension management, weight loss, and lipid (cholesterol) management. W.R. is discharged with a referral for a follow-up visit to his local internist in 1 week.

Case Study 16

Name _____ Class/Group _____ Date _____

Group Members _____

▶ **Scenario**

You are just getting caught up with your work when you receive the following phone call: "Hi, this is Deb in the emergency department. We're sending you M.M., a 63-year-old Hispanic woman with a past medical history of coronary artery disease (CAD). Her daughter reports that her mom has become increasingly weak over the past couple of weeks and has been unable to do her housework. Apparently, she has had complaints of swelling in her ankles and feet by late afternoon 'she couldn't wear her shoes' and has nocturnal diuresis × 4. Her daughter brought her in because she has had heaviness in her chest off and on over the past few days but denies any discomfort at this time. The daughter took her to see her family physician who immediately sent her here. Vital signs are 146/92, 96, 24, 99° F (37.2° C). She has an IV of D_5W at 50 mL/hr in her right forearm. Her laboratory results are as follows: Na 134 mEq/L, K 3.5 mEq/L, Cl 103 mEq/L, HCO_3 23 mEq/L, BUN 13 mg/dL, creatinine 1.3 mg/dL, glucose 153 mg/dL, WBC 8300/mm³, Hct 33.9%, Hgb 11.7 g/dL, platelets 162,000/mm³. PT/INR, PTT, and urinalysis are pending. She has had her chest x-ray and ECG, and her orders have been written."

1. What additional information do you need from the emergency department (ED) nurse?

2. How are you going to prepare for this patient?

3. M.M. arrives by wheelchair. As she transfers to the bed, what observations will you make? Why?

4. Given the previous information, you can anticipate orders for M.M. Carefully review each order to determine whether it is appropriate or inappropriate as written. If the order is appropriate, mark it as *A*; if the order is inappropriate, mark it as *I* and change the order to make it appropriate. Provide any other orders that might be appropriate for M.M.

    _____ 1. Routine VS
    _____ 2. Serum magnesium (Mg) STAT
    _____ 3. Up ad lib
    _____ 4. 10 g sodium (Na), low-fat diet
    _____ 5. Change IV to a saline lock
    _____ 6. Cardiac enzymes on admission and q8h × 24 hr, then daily every morning
    _____ 7. CBC, BMP, and fasting lipid profile in morning
    _____ 8. Schedule for abdominal CT scan for AM
    _____ 9. Heparin 10,000 units subcut q8h
    _____ 10. Docusate sodium (Colace) 100 mg/day PO
    _____ 11. Ampicillin 250 mg IV piggyback q6h
    _____ 12. Furosemide (Lasix) 200 mg IV push STAT
    _____ 13. Nitroglycerin (NTG) 0.4 mg 1 SL q4h prn for chest pain
    _____ 14. Schedule echocardiogram

5. Which interventions are appropriate for administering subcutaneous heparin? Select all that apply.
   a. Rotate injection sites with each dose.
   b. Monitor activated partial thromboplastin time (aPTT) levels daily.
   c. Massage the area after the injection.
   d. Give the injection at least 2 inches away from the umbilicus.
   e. Do not aspirate the syringe before injecting the heparin.

CASE STUDY PROGRESS

Shortly after admission, M.M.'s call light comes on. When you respond to M.M.'s call light, you observe she is talking rapidly in Spanish and pointing to the bathroom. Her speech pattern indicates she is short of breath; she is having trouble completing a sentence without taking a labored breath. You help her use a bedpan and note that her skin feels clammy. While sitting on the bedpan, she vomits.

6. On a scale of 0 to 10 (0 being no problem, 10 being a code-level emergency), how would you rate this situation, and why?

7. Identify at least four actions you should take next, and state your rationale.

8. M.M.'s physician calls your unit to find out what is happening. Using SBAR, what information would you need to convey at this time?

9. The hospital's staff physician is coming to the floor immediately to evaluate the patient. In the meantime she orders furosemide (Lasix) 40 mg IV push STAT. You have only 20 mg in stock. Should you give the 20 mg now, and then give the additional 20 mg when it comes up from the pharmacy? Explain your answer.

10. M.M. continues to experience vomiting and diaphoresis that are unrelieved by medication and comfort measures. A STAT 12-lead ECG reveals ischemic changes, and she is transferred to the coronary care unit (CCU). As you give the report to the receiving registered nurse, what laboratory value is the most important to report, and why?

11. You are monitoring while a new nurse prepares to administer IV potassium to M.M. Which technique is correct? Explain why the other answers are incorrect.
    a. Give the IV potassium by slow IV push.
    b. Add potassium to a hanging IV bag as needed.
    c. The rate of IV administration should not exceed 10 mEq/hr.
    d. Administer the IV potassium by gravity drip.

CASE STUDY PROGRESS

While recovering in the CCU, M.M. tried to get up out of the bed, fell, and fractured her right humerus. Because of the surgical risks involved, M.M. was treated conservatively and put in a full arm cast. She is transferred back to your floor.

CASE STUDY PROGRESS

A case manager (CM) has been asked to evaluate M.M.'s home to see whether she can be discharged to her own home or will need to stay in a long-term care facility.

12. Identify at least eight things that the CM would assess.

13. M.M.'s nutritional intake over the past few weeks has been poor. She also has increased nutritional needs because of her fractured arm. What are some of the nutritional needs that should be met? What would you recommend to help her with this?

CASE STUDY PROGRESS

Because the case manager determined that M.M. lived in an apartment with poor access, M.M. elects to stay with her daughter and five grandchildren in their small home. A home care nurse comes three times a week to check on her. M.M. is easily fatigued, and the children are quite lively. School is out for the summer.

14. Suggest some ways for M.M.'s daughter to ensure that her mother is not overwhelmed and does not become exhausted in this situation.

Case Study 17

Name _____ Class/Group _____ Date _____

Group Members _____

▶ Scenario

You are in the middle of your shift in the coronary care unit (CCU) of a large urban medical center. Your new admission, C.B., a 47-year-old woman, was just flown to your institution from a small rural community more than 100 miles away. She had a STEMI (ST segment elevation myocardial infarction) last evening. Her current vital signs (VS) are 100/60, 86, 14. After you make C.B. comfortable, you receive this report from the flight nurse: "C.B. is a full-time homemaker with four children. She has had episodes of 'chest tightness' with exertion for the past year, but this is her first known MI. She has a history of hyperlipidemia and has smoked one pack of cigarettes daily for 30 years. Surgical history consists of total abdominal hysterectomy 10 years ago after the birth of her last child. She has no other known medical problems. Yesterday at 8 PM, she began to have severe substernal chest pain that referred into her neck and down both arms. She rated the pain as 9 or 10 on a 0-to-10 scale. She thought it was severe indigestion and began taking Maalox with no relief. Her husband then took her to the local emergency department, where a 12-lead electrocardiogram (ECG) showed hyperacute ST elevation in the inferior leads II, III, aVF and V_5 to V_6. Before tissue plasminogen activator could be given, she went into ventricular fibrillation (V-fib). CPR was started and when the code team arrived, she was successfully defibrillated after two shocks. She then was started on nitroglycerin (NTG), heparin, and amiodarone drips. She was given IV metoprolol and aspirin 325 mg to chew and swallow. This morning her systolic pressure dropped into the 80s, and she was placed on a low-dose norepinephrine drip and urgently flown to your institution for coronary angiography and possible percutaneous transluminal coronary angioplasty. Currently, she has amiodarone infusing at 1 mg/min, heparin at 1200 units/hr, and norepinephrine at 0.5 mcg/kg/min. The NTG has been stopped because of low blood pressure. Laboratory work that was done yesterday showed Na 145 mEq/L, K 3.6 mEq/L, HCO_3 19 mEq/L, BUN 9 mg/dL, creatinine 0.8 mg/dL, WBC 14,500/mm³, Hct 44.3%, and Hgb 14.5 g/dL."

1. Because the 12-lead ECG can tell you the location of the infarction, evaluate the leads that showed ST elevation. What areas of C.B.'s heart have been damaged?

2. Given the diagnosis of acute myocardial infarction (MI), what other laboratory results are you going to look at?

3. Indicate the expected outcome for C.B. associated with each medication she is receiving. For each of the drugs listed, state the purpose.
   a. Intravenous (IV) nitroglycerin (NTG)
   b. IV heparin
   c. IV amiodarone
   d. IV metoprolol
   e. Aspirin, chewed and swallowed
   f. IV norepinephrine

Chart View

Laboratory Test Results

Creatine Phosphokinase (CK) Levels

On ED admission	95 units/L
4 hours	1931 units/L
8 hours	4175 units/L

CK-MB Isoenzymes

On ED admission	5%
4 hours	79%
8 hours	216%
LDL	160 mg/dL
PT	11.9 sec
INR	1.02
aPTT (before heparin)	26.9 sec
Mg	2.2 mg/dL
K	3.3 mEq/L

4. You review the lab work on her chart. For each laboratory value listed previously, interpret the result, and evaluate the meaning for C.B.

5. List at least two complications C.B. is at risk for at this time and the assessments that are needed to identify these risks.

6. You note that C.B.'s Spo$_2$ on oxygen (O$_2$) at 6 L/min by nasal cannula is 92%. How do you interpret this result?

7. What can be done to promote her oxygenation at this time?

1 Cardiovascular Disorders

8. An hour after her admission, you are preparing C.B. for her coronary intervention. Evaluate her readiness for teaching and her learning needs. What would you tell her?

CASE STUDY PROGRESS

The following day, you care for C.B. again. She is now on oral metoprolol, amiodarone, aspirin, and clopidogrel (Plavix). The norepinephrine and heparin have been discontinued. VS are stable.

9. Which laboratory test result should you check before beginning the clopidogrel therapy?
   a. PT/INR
   b. aPTT
   c. Platelet count
   d. Potassium

CASE STUDY PROGRESS

As you work with C.B., you notice that she is extremely anxious. You had observed some anxiety yesterday, which you had attributed to the strange CCU environment, pain, and anticipation of the stenting procedure. The postprocedure test results showed that the stent was performing appropriately. You wonder what is wrong. She tells you that her heart attack occurred right in the middle of a move with her family from her rural community to an even smaller and unfamiliar town some 500 miles away in a neighboring state. She is dreading the move. Her husband "becomes angry easily and starts lashing out" toward her and the children. She is afraid to move to a community where she will have no friends and family to support her.

10. How can you help your patient? Evaluate the situation and describe possible interventions.

CASE STUDY OUTCOME

C.B. agrees to speak with a social worker, and you set up the meeting before she is discharged. As a result, C.B. decides to postpone the move and stay with the children at her sister's home while she recuperates and seeks counseling at a women's support shelter. She tells you she will keep her appointment with the internist in 2 weeks.

Respiratory Disorders

Case Study 18

Name _____ Class/Group _____ Date _____

Group Members _____

▶ **Scenario**

You are a public health nurse working at a county immunization and tuberculosis (TB) clinic. B.A. is a 51-year-old woman who wishes to obtain a food handler's license and is required to show proof of a negative Mantoux (purified protein derivative [PPD]) test result before being hired. She came to your clinic 2 days ago to undergo a PPD test for TB. She has returned to have you evaluate her reaction.

1. What is TB, and what microorganism causes it?

2. What is the route of transmission for TB?

3. The Centers for Disease Control and Prevention (CDC) recommends screening people at high risk for TB. List five populations at high risk for developing active disease.

4. Describe the two methods of TB screening.

5. How do you determine whether a Mantoux test result is positive or negative?

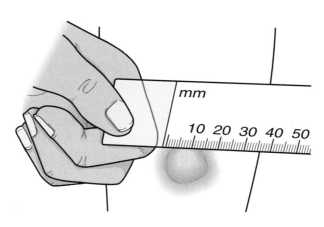

6. Interpret B.A.'s skin test.

7. What additional information do you need to obtain from B.A.?

8. You inform B.A. of the test result. She asks you what the result means. How will you respond?

CASE STUDY PROGRESS

B.A. is a natural-born American and has no risk factors for TB infection according to the CDC guidelines. She has a 6-year history of type II diabetes mellitus that is well controlled with metformin (Glucophage). She admits that her mother had TB when she was a child but says she herself has never tested positive before. She is angry at the proposition that she might have TB and says, "I feel just fine and I don't think anything else is necessary."

9. What steps need to be done to determine whether B.A. has an active TB infection?

CASE STUDY PROGRESS

The physician orders a chest x-ray (CXR) examination and informs B.A. that the image is clear, showing no signs of active TB infection. He tells her that she has class 2 TB, or a latent TB infection (LTBI), and that he will report her condition to the local public health department.

10. What is a LTBI?

11. What parameters determine whether treatment is initiated for LTBI?

12. Is B.A. a candidate for LTBI treatment? State your rationale.

13. Outline the current CDC guidelines for the treatment of LTBI.

CASE STUDY PROGRESS

The physician orders B.A. to begin a 12-dose, once-weekly regimen of isoniazid (INH) and rifapentine (RPT) as directly observed therapy (DOT).

14. How will you describe LTBI and DOT to B.A?

15. The medications used to treat LTBI are associated with different side effects. Identify the test used to monitor each possible side effect listed as follows:

____ A. Peripheral neuropathy	1. Audiogram
____ B. Clinical hepatitis	2. CBC (complete blood count)
____ C. Fever and bleeding problems	3. Blood urea nitrogen (BUN), creatinine, and creatinine clearance
____ D. Nephrotoxicity or renal failure	4. AST (aspartate transaminase) and ALT (alanine transaminase)
____ E. Hyperuricemia	5. Physical examination and monofilament testing
____ F. Optic neuritis	6. Red-green discrimination and visual acuity
____ G. Hearing neuritis	7. Uric acid

16. What additional information does B.A. need to receive before leaving the clinic?

CASE STUDY OUTCOME

B.A. is hired under the condition that she complies with LTBI therapy and will immediately report any signs and symptoms of active disease to the clinic. She reports weekly for her medications and finishes her 12 weeks of therapy without experiencing any significant effects.

Case Study 19

Name _____ Class/Group _____ Date _____

Group Members _____

▶ Scenario

It is 1130 and M.N., age 65, is being admitted to your surgical floor after having undergone an open cholecystectomy for acute cholecystitis. She has a nasogastric tube to continuous low wall suction, one peripheral intravenous (IV) line, and a large abdominal dressing. Her orders are as follows.

Chart View

Physician's Orders

Clear liquid diet; progress low-fat diet as tolerated

D5 ½ NS with 40 mEq KCl at 125 mL/hr

Turn, cough, and deep breathe q2h

Incentive spirometer q2h while awake

Oxygen per protocol to maintain SpO_2 at 95%

Dangle in AM

Morphine sulfate 10 mg IM q4h prn for pain

Ampicillin (Omnipen) 2 g IVPB q6h

Chest x-ray in AM

---

1. Are these orders appropriate for M.N.? State your rationale.

CASE STUDY PROGRESS

At 1530, the nursing assistive personnel (NAP) reports the following:

Chart View

Vital Signs

Blood pressure	148/82 mm Hg
Heart rate	118 beats/min
Respiratory rate	24 breaths/min
Temperature	101° F (38.3° C)
Spo_2	92%

2. Based solely on her vital signs, what could be happening with M.N., and why?

3. You go to assess M. N. What do you need to include in your assessment at this time?

CASE STUDY PROGRESS

Your assessment of M.N. finds her with decreased breath sounds and crackles in the right base posteriorly. Her right middle and lower lobes percuss slightly dull. She splints her right side when attempting to take a deep breath. Her skin is pale, warm, and dry. She does not have a productive cough, chest pain, or any anxiety.

4. What complication do you suspect M.N. is experiencing? State your rationale.

5. Why is M.N. at risk for developing this complication?

6. What is your nursing priority at this time?

7. Describe six interventions you will perform over the next few hours based on this priority.

8. To promote optimal oxygenation with M.N., which action(s) could you delegate to the NAP? Select all that apply.
   a. Reminding M.N. to cough and deep breathe
   b. Instructing M.N. on the use of incentive spirometry
   c. Assisting M.N. in getting up to the chair
   d. Taking M.N.'s temperature and reporting elevations
   e. Encouraging M.N. to splint the incision
   f. Auscultating M.N.'s lung sounds

9. Identify three outcomes that you expect for M.N. as a result of your interventions.

CASE STUDY PROGRESS

At 1830, the NAP reports the following.

Chart View

Vital Signs

Blood pressure	136/72 mm Hg
Heart rate	104 beats/min
Respiratory rate	24 breaths/min
Temperature	100.6° F (38.1° C)
Spo_2	93%

10. Has M.N.'s status improved or not? Defend your response.

11. You need to call the physician regarding M.N.'s status. Using SBAR (*Situation*, *Background*, *Assessment*, *Recommendation*), what would you report to the physician?

12. The physician orders a chest x-ray examination. Afterward, radiology calls with a report, confirming that M.N. has atelectasis. Should this diagnosis change your plan of care for M.N.?

13. If M.N. had pneumonia, what changes might the physician have made to her plan of care?

14. M.N.'s sister questions you, saying, "I don't understand. She came in here with a bad gallbladder. What has happened to her lungs?" How would you respond?

Case Study 20

Name _____ Class/Group _____ Date _____

Group Members _____

▶ **Scenario**

S.R. is a 59-year-old man who comes to the clinic because his wife complains "my snoring is difficult to live with."

1. As the clinic nurse, what routine information would you want to obtain from S.R.?

CASE STUDY PROGRESS

After interviewing S.R., you note the following: S.R. is under considerable stress. He owns his own business. The stress of overseeing his employees, meeting deadlines, and carrying out negotiations has led to poor sleep habits. He sleeps 3 to 4 hours per night. He keeps himself going by drinking 2 quarts of coffee and smoking three to four packs of cigarettes per day. He has gained 50 pounds over the 2 years, leading to a current weight of 250 pounds. He complains of difficulty staying awake, wakes up with headaches on most mornings, and has midmorning somnolence. He states that he is depressed and irritable most of the time and reports difficulty concentrating and learning new things. He has been involved in three auto accidents in the past year.

S.R.'s vital signs are 164/90, 92, 18, and Spo_2 90% on room air. His examination findings are normal, except for a few bruises over the right side of the rib cage. You inquire about the bruises, and S.R. reports that his wife jabs him with her elbow several times every night. In her own defense, the wife states, "Well, he stops breathing and I get worried, so I jab him to make him start breathing again. If I don't jab him, I find myself listening for his next breath and I can't go to sleep." You suspect sleep apnea.

2. Identify two of the main types of apnea, and explain the pathology of each.

3. Based on your findings, which type of sleep apnea do you believe S.R. has?

4. Identify at least five signs or symptoms of this type of sleep apnea, and put a star next to those symptoms that S.R. is experiencing.

5. How does the provider use diagnostic testing to diagnose sleep apnea?

CASE STUDY PROGRESS

The primary care provider examines S.R. and documents a long soft palate, recessed mandible, and medium-sized tonsils. S.R. undergoes an overnight screening oximetry study, which shows 143 episodes of desaturation ranging from 68% to 76% with episodes of apnea. He is tentatively diagnosed with obstructive sleep apnea (OSA), and a full sleep study is ordered.

6. S.R. and his wife ask about a full sleep study. How would you explain a polysomnogram to them?

7. S.R. and his wife ask why they need to be concerned about OSA. You tell them that treating OSA is necessary to prevent which common complications? Select all that apply.
   a. Stroke
   b. Early onset of chronic obstructive pulmonary disease (COPD)
   c. Hypotension
   d. Right-sided heart failure
   e. Cardiac dysrhythmias

8. The provider asks you to teach S.R. about lifestyle changes that he could make immediately to help with his situation. Describe four priority topics you would address with S.R.

CASE STUDY PROGRESS

The polysomnogram confirms S.R.'s diagnosis of OSA. At his 6-week follow-up visit, he reports he has lost 10 pounds, but there has been little improvement in his symptoms. He states that he fell asleep while driving to work and wrecked his car. He wants to discuss further treatment options.

9. What are the treatment options for OSA? Describe each.

CASE STUDY PROGRESS

S.R. and the provider decide to begin S.R. on the least invasive treatment—continuous positive airway pressure (CPAP). The provider writes a prescription for CPAP.

10. List three education topics you need to address with S.R. so he can safely self-manage CPAP therapy.

11. S.R. calls 2 weeks later with complaints of dry nasal membranes, nosebleeds, and sores behind his ears. What instructions would you give S.R.?

12. Describe how you will document the phone call with S.R.

Case Study **21**

Name _____ Class/Group _____ Date _____

Group Members _____

▶ Scenario

B.T., a 31-year-old man who lives in a small mountain town in Colorado, is highly allergic to dust and pollen and has a history of mild asthma. B.T.'s wife drove him to the emergency room when his wheezing was unresponsive to his fluticasone/salmeterol (Advair) inhaler, he was unable to lie down, and he began to use accessory muscles to breathe. B.T. is immediately started on 4 L oxygen by nasal cannula and intravenous (IV) D5W at 75 mL/hr. A set of arterial blood gases is sent to the laboratory. B.T. appears anxious and says that he is short of breath.

Chart View

Vital Signs

Blood pressure (BP)	152/84 mm Hg
Pulse rate	124 beats/min
Respiratory rate	42 breaths/min
Temperature	100.4° F (38.4° C)

1. Are B.T.'s vital signs acceptable? State your rationale.

2. What is the rationale for immediately starting B.T. on O_2?

3. Keeping in mind B.T.'s health history and presenting complaint, what are the most important areas you need to evaluate during your physical assessment?

Chart View

Arterial Blood Gases

pH	7.31
$Paco_2$	48 mm Hg
HCO_3	26 mmol/L
Pao_2	55 mm Hg

4. Interpret B.T.'s arterial blood gas results.

Chart View

Medication Orders

Albuterol 2.5 mg plus ipratropium 250 mcg nebulizer treatment STAT
Albuterol (Ventolin) inhaler 2 puffs q4h
Metaproterenol sulfate (Alupent) 0.4% nebulizer treatment q3h
Fluticasone (Flovent HFA) MDI: 220 mcg, 1 puff twice daily

5. What is the rationale for the albuterol 2.5 mg plus ipratropium 250 mcg nebulizer treatment STAT (immediately)?

6. Indicate the drug classification and expected outcome B.T. should experience with using metaproterenol sulfate (Alupent) and Fluticasone (Flovent).

CASE STUDY PROGRESS

You assess B.T. and find that he has diminished lung sounds with inspiratory and expiratory wheezes in all lung fields with a nonproductive cough and accessory muscle use. His skin is pale, warm and dry. The electrocardiogram (ECG) shows sinus tachycardia without ectopy. He is alert and oriented×4 spheres. He appears anxious and is sitting upright, leaning over the bedside table, and continuing to complain of shortness of breath.

7. What is your primary nursing goal at this time?

8. Describe six actions you must implement based on this priority.

9. You will need to monitor B.T. closely for the next few hours. What is the most serious complication to anticipate?

10. Identify four signs and symptoms of this complication you will assess for in B.T.

11. When combination inhalation aerosols are prescribed without specific instructions for the sequence of administration, you need to be aware of the recommendations for safe drug administration. Describe the correct sequence for administering B.T.'s treatments.

12. What are your responsibilities while administering aerosol therapy?

2 Respiratory Disorders

After several hours of rehydration and aerosol treatments, B.T.'s wheezing and dyspnea resolve, and he is able to expectorate his secretions. The physician discusses B.T.'s asthma management with him; B.T. says he has had several asthma attacks over the last few weeks. The physician discharges B.T. with a prescription for oral steroid "burst" (prednisone 40 mg/day × 5 days), fluticasone/salmeterol (Advair HFA 230/21) two inhalations every morning and evening, albuterol (Proventil) metered-dose inhaler (MDI) two puffs q6h as needed using a spacer, and montelukast (Singulair) 10 mg daily each evening. He instructs B.T. to call the pulmonary clinic for follow-up with a pulmonary specialist.

13. What is the rationale for B.T. being on the oral steroid burst?

14. How does montelukast (Singulair) differ from other asthma medications?

15. B.T. states he had taken his Advair that morning, then again when he started to feel short of breath. He states, "It did not help," and wants to know why he has to remain on it. Is fluticasone/salmeterol (Advair) appropriate for use during an acute asthma attack? Explain.

16. Based on this information, what specific issue do you need to address in discharge teaching with B.T.?

CASE STUDY PROGRESS

You ask B.T. to demonstrate the use of his MDI. He vigorously shakes the canister, holds the aerosolizer at an angle (pointing toward his cheek) in front of his mouth, and squeezes the canister as he takes a quick, deep breath.

17. What common mistakes has B.T. made when using the inhaler?

18. You review the proper use of an MDI with B.T and possible side effects he may experience, including hoarseness, dry mouth, white spots in the oral cavity, coughing, and headaches. What actions can you teach him to prevent or diminish the incidence of these effects? Select all that apply.
    a. Decrease his fluid intake.
    b. Use a spacer on the inhaler.
    c. Use the inhaler only as prescribed.
    d. Rinse out his mouth immediately after using the inhaler
    e. Clean the spacer in the dishwasher on "hot cycle with heated dry" daily.

19. B.T.'s wife asks about the possibility of B.T. having another attack. How would you respond?

20. B.T. states that he would like to read more about asthma on the Internet. List three credible websites to which you could direct him.

Case Study **22**

Name _____   Class/Group _____   Date _____

Group Members _____

▶ Scenario

L.B. is a 40-year-old woman who is being seen in the clinic with complaints of a dry, hacking cough for the past 6 weeks.

1. As the intake nurse, what routine information do you want to obtain from L.B.?

2. L.B.'s chief complaint is a cough. What are the main causes of chronic cough, and what questions should you ask to elicit information about each cause?

CASE STUDY PROGRESS

L.B. says that the cough is worse at night and is associated with shortness of breath. The cough began approximately 6 weeks ago after she recovered from bronchitis. She runs 3 miles four times a week and reports occasionally experiencing a "coughing spell" after running. She has hay fever that seems to be year-round and has eczema in the winter. Both of her children and her maternal grandmother have asthma. She does not smoke and is not taking any medication other than a multivitamin.

3. What would you include in your physical examination, and why?

CASE STUDY PROGRESS

L.B. is not in any acute distress. Vital signs (VS) are 110/60, 55, 18. She has no sinus tenderness, ear examination findings are negative, nasal mucosa is pale and boggy, mouth examination findings are negative, there is no cervical adenopathy, and lungs are clear to auscultation. Forced expiration using the peak flow meter (PFM) generates a cough. Her peak flow is 350 L/min with good effort. Expected peak flow for her height and age is 512 L/min, giving a response of 68% of predicted.

4. The provider orders predilator and postdilator pulmonary function tests (PFTs). What is the purpose of completing predilator and postdilator PFTs?

5. After the PFT, L.B. is diagnosed with mild persistent asthma. She returns to the clinic so that a plan for managing her asthma can be established. What priority topics need addressed?

6. How will you describe mild persistent asthma to L.B.?

7. The provider orders triamcinolone (Azmacort) two puffs bid and albuterol (Ventolin) two puffs every 6 hours as needed. What points will you include when teaching L.B. about these medications?

8. L.B. asks, "Why do I have to use this inhaler? Can't I just take some pills?" Your response to L.B. is based on the knowledge that the inhalation route is:
   a. Safer and more effective than pills
   b. Less expensive than combination therapy
   c. Easier to master than oral therapy
   d. More likely to assist in curing her asthma

9. The provider gives L.B. a prescription for a peak flow meter (PFM). What is a PFM? Give L.B. precise instructions to perform the PFM maneuver.

10. L.B. asks why she has to use the PFM. Explain the purpose of the peak expiratory flow rate (PEFR) measurement, what an asthma action plan is, and the role the PEFR plays in an asthma action plan.

11. You set up an asthma action plan for L.B. What will you teach L.B. to do if her PEFR value falls into the yellow or red zone?

12. You instruct L.B. in the proper use of a metered-dose inhaler (MDI) using a spacer. How would you explain proper MDI use?

13. Because L.B. is taking two puffs twice daily of triamcinolone (Azmacort), how long should the inhaler last? The canister label states that it contains 200 inhalations.

14. As you are concluding your session, L.B. looks at you and says, "This is absolutely, utterly overwhelming." What should you tell her to reassure her?

15. You would recognize the need for additional teaching if L.B. says which of the following? Select all that apply.
   a. "I will use the albuterol inhaler 30 minutes before exercising."
   b. "My husband needs to know what to do in case I have an attack."
   c. "If the reading is in the yellow zone, I need to use rescue drugs and seek help immediately."
   d. "I will keep a diary of all of my PEFR measures."
   e. "I will place a plastic cover on our mattress and my pillows."
   f. "The bed linens need to be washed in cold water to reduce dust mites."

CASE STUDY OUTCOME

At the next follow-up visit, L.B.'s peak flow on the albuterol (Ventolin) and triamcinolone (Azmacort) has increased to 450 L/min, which is 88% of the predicted; her cough has subsided, and she has been running without any problems. There have been no nighttime awakenings, no loss of work, and no emergency department visits. She can demonstrate appropriate inhaler technique and has her completed peak flow diary on her smartphone.

Case Study **23**

Name _____ Class/Group _____ Date _____

Group Members _____

▶ Scenario

C.K.'s sister has brought her 71-year-old brother to the primary care clinic; he came down with a fever 2 days ago. She says he has shaking chills and a productive cough and he cannot lie down to sleep because "he can't stop coughing." After C.K. is examined, he is diagnosed with community-acquired pneumonia (CAP) and admitted to your floor at 1130. The intern is busy and asks you to complete your routine admission assessment and call her with your findings.

1. Identify four priority areas to include in your assessment.

CASE STUDY PROGRESS

Your assessment findings are as follows: CK's vital signs (VS) are 154/82, 105, 32, 103° F (39.4° C), SpO_2 84% on room air. You auscultate decreased breath sounds and coarse crackles in the left lower lobe anteriorly and posteriorly. His nail beds are dusky on fingers and toes. He has cough productive of rust-colored sputum and complains of pain in the left side of his chest when he coughs. He is a lifetime nonsmoker. Past medical history includes coronary artery disease and myocardial infarction with a stent. He is currently on metoprolol (Lopressor), amlodipine (Norvasc), lisinopril (Zestril), and furosemide (Lasix); for his type 2 diabetes mellitus, he is taking metformin (Glucophage) and glipizide (Glucotrol). He has never gotten the Pneumovax or flu shot. He does report getting "hives" when he took "an antibiotic pill" a few years ago, but does not remember the name of the antibiotic.

2. Which of these assessment findings are significant? State your rationale.

2 Respiratory Disorders

Chart View

Physician's Orders

2100-Calorie diabetic diet
VS q2h
IV of D5 ½ NS at 125 mL/hr
Ceftriaxone (Rocephin) 1 g IV every 12 hours
Metaproterenol sulfate (Alupent) 0.4% nebulizer treatment q3h
Titrate O_2 to maintain Spo_2 over 90%
Obtain sputum for C&S
STAT Blood cultures & sensitivity
CBC with differential and basic metabolic panel
Chest x-ray (CXR) now and in the morning
Continue home medications

3. You obtain orders from the physician. Outline a plan of what you need to do in the next 2 to 3 hours.

4. Is the IV fluid D5 ½ NS appropriate for C.K.? State your rationale.

5. What is the rationale for ordering O_2 to maintain Spo_2 over 90%?

6. What is a C&S test, and what role will blood and sputum cultures play in C.K.'s care?

7. What would you expect the CXR results to reveal?

8. You need to follow a specific protocol when obtaining peripheral blood cultures. Place in order the steps you will perform.
    _____ 1. Select venipuncture site. Cleanse and allow to dry.
    _____ 2. Inject 10 mL of blood into the aerobic bottle.
    _____ 3. Perform venipuncture and collect 20 mL of venous blood.
    _____ 4. Verify patient's identity and perform hand hygiene.
    _____ 5. Attach identification to specimens and send to laboratory within 30 minutes.
    _____ 6. Inject 10 mL of blood into the anaerobic bottle.

9. The pharmacy sends the ceftriaxone (Rocephin) IV 1 g in 100 mL 0.9% NaCl with instructions to infuse over 40 minutes. At how many milliliters per hour will you regulate the IV infusion pump?

10. How will you ensure that the home medication list is accurate?

CASE STUDY PROGRESS

The next morning you are again assigned to care for C.K. Your assessment findings are as follows: VS 154/82, 92, 26, 100° F (37.8° C), Spo_2 94% on 2 L oxygen per nasal cannula. He appears to be in no apparent distress and denies any dyspnea. You auscultate decreased breath sounds and coarse crackles in the left lower lobe anteriorly. His skin is pale, warm, and dry. He has a cough productive of yellow-colored sputum and complains of pain in the left side of his chest when he coughs.

11. Is C.K. recovering as expected? Defend your response.

12. Based on your evaluation of C.K., write an outcome to achieve by the end of your shift, then list six priority interventions you will perform toward achieving this goal.

13. By the end of your shift, which of the following assessment findings would best indicate that C.K. is responding to therapy?
    a. Cough productive of yellow sputum; lung sounds clear; Spo_2 96% on room air
    b. Complaints of dyspnea; respiratory rate of 26 on 2 L oxygen; clear lung sounds
    c. Coarse crackles in posterior lower lobes; respiratory rate 22; no complaints of chills
    d. Cough productive of white sputum; temperature 100.0° F (37.8° C); Spo_2 98% on 2 L oxygen

CASE STUDY PROGRESS

After continuing the plan of care for 2 more days, C.K. recovers from his pneumonia and is preparing for discharge.

14. You know that C.K. is at increased risk for contracting another CAP infection. Describe four strategies for preventing CAP infections you will include in C.K.'s discharge teaching plan.

15. C.K. confides in you, "You know, my wife died a year ago, and I live alone now. I've been thinking … this pneumonia stuff has been a little scary." How will you respond?

16. What are some community resources from which C.K. may benefit?

Case Study **24**

Name _____ Class/Group _____ Date _____

Group Members _____

▶ **Scenario**

A.B., a 68-year-old man, is admitted to your medical floor with a diagnosis of pleural effusion. He complains of shortness of breath; pain in his chest; weakness; and a dry, irritating cough. His vital signs (VS) are 142/82, 118, respirations 38 and labored and shallow, 102.1° F (38.9° C), and Spo_2 85% on room air. Chest x-ray examination reveals a large pleural effusion and pulmonary infiltrates in the right lower lobe consistent with pneumonia.

1. Given his diagnosis, are A.B.'s admission VS expected? Explain.

2. How does the underlying pathophysiology relate to A.B.'s presenting signs and symptoms?

CASE STUDY PROGRESS

The physician performs a thoracentesis and drains 1500 mL of fluid. A specimen for culture and sensitivity (C&S) is sent to the laboratory, and A.B. is started on cefuroxime (Ceftin) 1 g intravenously (IV) every 8 hours.

3. What is a thoracentesis?

4. The order for the cefuroxime (Ceftin) reads to infuse 1 g in 100 mL 0.9% NaCl over 30 minutes. You have IV tubing that supplies 20 gtt/mL. At how many drops per minute will you regulate the infusion?

5. What interventions will you implement to promote A.B.'s clearing pulmonary secretions?

CASE STUDY PROGRESS

The pleural C&S results indicate a large amount of *Klebsiella* organism growth that is not sensitive to cefuroxime (Ceftin).

 6. What action will you take next?

7. Because fluid continues to collect in the pleural space, the physician decides to insert a pleural chest tube under nonemergent conditions. What is your responsibility as A.B.'s nurse regarding this procedure?

8. What interventions will you implement afterward to maintain A.B.'s chest tube system?

9. Evaluate each of the following statements about chest tube drainage systems. Enter *T* for true or *F* for false. State why false statements are incorrect.
   _____ 1. The height of the water in the suction control mechanism limits the amount of suction transmitted to the pleural cavity.
   _____ 2. A suction pressure of +20 cm H_2O is usually recommended for adults.
   _____ 3. Bubbling in the water-seal chamber usually means that air is leaking from the lungs, the tubing, or the insertion site.
   _____ 4. The rise and fall of the water level with the patient's respirations reflect normal pressure changes in the pleural cavity with respirations.
   _____ 5. Because the chamber is a closed system, water cannot evaporate from the system.

_____ 6. To declot the drainage tubing, put lotion on your hands, compress the tubing, and vigorously strip long segments of the tubing before releasing.

_____ 7. You lower the bed on top of the drainage system and break it. You immediately clamp the chest tube, leaving it clamped until you can reestablish the drainage system.

_____ 8. The collection chamber is full, so you need to connect a new drainage system to the chest tube. It is fine to momentarily clamp the chest tube while you disconnect the old system and reconnect the new.

CASE STUDY PROGRESS

The next day you are again assigned to care for A.B. At the beginning of the shift, you assess A.B. and find that his condition is stable. His lung sounds remain diminished in the right lower lobe and his Spo_2 is 95% on oxygen at 2 L per nasal cannula. The chest drainage system is attached to suction at 20 mm Hg; there is still an air leak present. His morning chest x-ray examination showed some residual pleural effusion. Four hours into your shift, he pages you through the call system and tells you he feels "short of breath." You immediately go to his room. A.B. is sitting in the chair.

10. Describe the priority assessment you must perform at this time.

11. You determine that the chest tube has become disconnected from the drainage system and is contaminated. What do you need to do?

12. After the chest drainage system has been reestablished, A.B.'s complaints of dyspnea resolve and you need to document what happened. Write an example of a documentation entry describing this event.

CASE STUDY PROGRESS

The remainder of A.B.'s admission is uneventful. After 6 days of aggressive antibiotic and pulmonary therapy, the chest tube is discontinued and A.B. is ready to be discharged.

13. What type of discharge instructions do you need to give to A.B.?

2 Respiratory Disorders

Case Study 25

Name _____ Class/Group _____ Date _____

Group Members _____

▶ Scenario

A.W., a 72-year-old woman with severe emphysema, was walking at a mall when she suddenly grabbed her right side and gasped, "Oh, something just popped." A.W. whispered to her walking companion, "I can't get any air." Her companion yelled for someone to call 911 and helped her to the nearest bench. By the time the rescue unit arrived, A.W. was stuporous and in severe respiratory distress. She was intubated, started on intravenous lactated Ringer's at KVO (keep vein open), and transported to the nearest emergency department (ED).

On A.W.'s arrival at the ED, the physician auscultates muffled heart tones, no breath sounds on the right, and faint sounds on the left. A.W. is stuporous, tachycardic, and cyanotic. The paramedics inform the physician that it was difficult to ventilate A.W. A portable chest x-ray (CXR) examination shows an 80% pneumothorax on the right.

Chart View

Arterial Blood Gases (ABGs; 100% O_2)

pH	7.25
$Paco_2$	92 mm Hg
Pao_2	32 mm Hg
HCO_3	27 mmol/L
Spo_2	53%

1. Given the diagnosis of pneumothorax, explain why the paramedics had difficulty ventilating A.W.

2. Interpret A.W.'s ABGs.

3. What is the reason for A.W.'s ABG results?

4. The physician needs to insert a chest tube. What are your responsibilities as A.W.'s nurse?

5. As the nurse, it is your responsibility to ensure pain control. In A.W.'s case, would you administer pain medication before the chest tube insertion?

6. The ED physician inserts a size 32 Fr chest tube in the sixth intercostal space, midaxillary line. Would you expect to observe an air leak when A.W.'s chest drainage system is in place and functioning?

7. Would you expect A.W.'s lung to reexpand immediately after the chest tube insertion and initiation of underwater suction? Explain.

8. Part of your responsibilities after the chest tube has been inserted is to assess for fluctuation in the water-seal chamber and bubbling in the suction-control chamber. Label the areas on the chest drainage system that you would be monitoring.

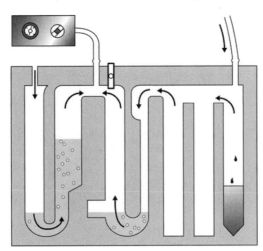

9. What do you need to document regarding A.W.'s chest drainage system?

10. While A.W. has a chest drainage system, what instructions do you need to give to the nursing assistive personnel (NAP) who is working with A.W.?

11. The secretary tells you A.W.'s husband has just arrived. What will you discuss with him about A.W.'s status and her hospital admission?

12. You approach A.W.'s bedside and ask about what look like two healed chest tube sites on her right chest. A.W.'s husband informs you that this is the third time she has had a collapsed lung. He asks whether this will continue to happen. How will you respond?

13. It is now the end of your shift and A.W.'s condition has stabilized. Using the SBAR framework, describe the bedside change-of-shift report you will give the oncoming nurse.

2 Respiratory Disorders

2 Respiratory Disorders

CASE STUDY PROGRESS

Because A.W. has a history of spontaneous pneumothoraces on the right side, the physician elects to perform chemical pleurodesis on A.W. after her condition stabilizes.

14. A.W. asks what a pleurodesis is. How would you describe this procedure and what will happen?

CASE STUDY PROGRESS

A.W. recovers uneventfully and is discharged home 4 days later with a chest tube and Heimlich valve. The physician connects the one-way (Heimlich) valve between the distal end of the chest tube and a drainage pouch.

15. Discuss the purpose of this device.

16. You teach A.W. and her husband about the care of the chest tube and Heimlich valve. Which of these statements would indicate that further teaching is necessary? Select all that apply.
    a. "I will maintain a water-tight dressing around the chest tube site."
    b. "I can shower if the device is completely covered in plastic."
    c. "When I am moving around I must keep the collection system below the insertion site."
    d. "I will notify the physician if there is a change in the color or amount of drainage."
    e. "The arrow on the flutter valve should always point toward me."
    f. "I will check the insertion site twice daily for swelling, redness, and drainage."

Case Study **26**

Name _____   Class/Group _____   Date _____

Group Members _____

▶ Scenario

P.R., a 66-year-old woman who has no history of respiratory disease, is being admitted to your intensive care unit (ICU) from the emergency department (ED) with a diagnosis of pneumonia and acute respiratory failure (ARF). The ED nurse tells you that P.R. was stuporous and cyanotic on her arrival to the ED. Her initial vital signs were 90/68, 134, 38, 101° F (38.3° C) with an Spo_2 of 53%. She was endotracheally intubated orally and placed on mechanical ventilation and has equal breath sounds. Her ventilator settings are synchronized intermittent mandatory ventilation of 12/min, tidal volume (V_T) 700 mL, Fio_2 0.50, positive end-expiratory pressure (PEEP) 5 cm H_2O. The nurse tells you P.R. had an initial chest x-ray (CXR) examination that confirmed the diagnosis of pneumonia, but she needs an additional CXR examination stat.

1. Describe the pathophysiology of ARF.

2. How does the underlying pathophysiology relate to P.R.'s presenting signs and symptoms?

3. Describe each of P.R.'s ventilator settings and the rationale for the selection of each.

4. Why does P.R. need a second CXR examination?

Chart View

Arterial Blood Gases (ABGs)

pH	7.28
$Paco_2$	62 mm Hg
HCO_3	26 mmol/L
Pao_2	48 mm Hg
Spo_2	53%

5. The ABG results from the sample drawn in the ED before intubation are sent to you. Interpret P.R.'s ABG results.

6. List eight collaborative care interventions that would be implemented for P.R. and the rationale for each.

7. What is your priority nursing goal at this time?

8. Describe six interventions you will perform over the next two hour based on this priority.

9. P.R. is not heavily sedated and seems anxious about all that is going on. Describe how you can help her.

Chart View

Arterial Blood Gases

pH	7.30
$Paco_2$	52 mm Hg
HCO_3	22 mmol/L
Pao_2	70 mm Hg
Spo_2	88%

10. ABGs are redrawn after P.R. has been on mechanical ventilation for 2 hours. What ventilator setting changes do you anticipate based on your interpretation of these values? Select all that apply, and explain your rationale.
   a. Increasing the PEEP to 10 cm
   b. Increasing the rate on the ventilator to 16/min
   c. Increasing the V_T to 850 mL
   d. Changing to continuous mandatory ventilation

11. Evaluate each of the following statements about caring for P.R. or a similar patient receiving mechanical ventilation with an endotracheal tube (ETT). Enter *T* for true or *F* for false. Discuss why the false statements are incorrect.

_____ 1. Administer muscle-paralyzing agents to keep P.R. from "fighting the vent."

_____ 2. Check ventilator settings at the beginning of each shift and then hourly.

_____ 3. When suctioning the ETT, each pass should not exceed 15 seconds.

_____ 4. Assign experienced nursing assistive personnel (NAP) to take vital signs every 2 to 4 hours.

_____ 5. Perform a respiratory assessment once per shift.

_____ 6. Empty excess water as it collects in the ventilation tubing back into the humidifier.

_____ 7. Keep a resuscitation bag at the bedside.

_____ 8. Monitor the cuff pressure of the ETT every 8 hours.

_____ 9. Keep ventilator alarms silenced when in the room to maintain a quiet environment.

_____10. Change the ventilator tubing every 12 hours.

12. You hear the high pressure alarm sounding on the mechanical ventilator and see that P.R.'s Sao$_2$ is 80%. What are the potential causes of this problem?

13. You determine that P.R. needs to be suctioned. Place in order the steps for safely performing in-line or closed suctioning.

_____ 1. Hyperoxygenate patient.

_____ 2. Use 5 to 10 mL of saline to rinse the catheter clear of secretions.

_____ 3. Insert catheter until resistance is met or patient coughs.

_____ 4. Assess patient's status and document procedure.

_____ 5. Put on clean gloves and face shield; attach suction.

_____ 6. Apply suction as you withdraw the catheter, not exceeding 10 seconds.

_____ 7. Reassess patient status and suction again as needed.

CASE STUDY PROGRESS

As P.R.'s primary nurse, you are responsible for her nursing care plan. Although the primary concern is her respiratory status, you are concerned about hydration, nutrition, oral hygiene, and skin integrity and decide to address each of these areas in P.R.'s plan of care.

14. Discuss five indicators you can use to assess her fluid status.

15. Write a nutrition-related outcome for P.R.

16. Describe five interventions that could assist in meeting P.R.'s nutrition goals.

17. The goals for P.R.'s mouth care are to preserve the oral mucosa and dentition and prevent P.R. from developing a secondary ventilator-assisted pneumonia. Identify three strategies for providing oral hygiene with an ETT in place.

18. Identify three treatment goals related to skin and positioning.

19. You plan to assess P.R.'s skin every 4 hours. What are four other strategies that will facilitate the expected outcome of maintaining skin integrity?

Case Study **27**

Name _____   Class/Group _____   Date _____

Group Members _____

▶ **Scenario**

P.W., a 33-year-old woman diagnosed with Guillain-Barré syndrome (GBS), is being cared for on a special ventilator unit of an extended care facility because she requires 24-hour-a-day nursing coverage. She has been intubated and mechanically ventilated for 2 weeks and has shown no signs of improvement in respiratory muscle strength. Her ventilator settings are assist-control (A/C) of 12/min, tidal volume (V_T) 700 mL, Fio_2 0.50, and positive end-expiratory pressure (PEEP) 5 cm H_2O. She is receiving enteral nutrition with Ensure Plus by PEG (percutaneous endoscopic gastrostomy [with a transjejunal limb]) tube (2800 kcal/24 hr). The NAP (nursing assistive personnel) reports that P.W.'s morning vital signs are 108/64, 118, 12, 100.6° F (38.1° C) and that P.W. may have diarrhea.

1. Do any of P.W.'s vital signs concern you and why?

2. Why is P.W.'s respiratory rate 12 breaths per minute?

3. What are common causes of enteral nutrition diarrhea?

4. Describe the assessment you need to perform at this time.

5. While you are assessing P.W., she has an explosive, watery stool. Because her other assessment findings are unremarkable, you believe a gastrointestinal infection, possibly *Clostridium difficile,* is responsible for the onset of the fever and the diarrhea. Based on this premise, what actions do you need to take?

6. Because she had diarrhea, you decide to give P.W. a bath. You note that her cheeks are billowing slightly outward each time the ventilator delivers a breath. What could cause this phenomenon?

7. Describe how you can determine the cause of the problem.

CASE STUDY PROGRESS

You believe that P.W. has developed an air leak, and you insert more air in the cuff to seal the leak. This temporarily corrects the problem, but over the next 24 hours, the leak returns and becomes worse, and the ventilator's low exhaled volume alarm begins to sound frequently.

8. What action will you take?

9. The physician elects to insert a No. 8 Shiley tracheostomy ("trach") tube with a disposable inner cannula. P.W. becomes increasingly anxious after receiving the news. How would you prepare P.W. and her husband for the tracheostomy?

10. What are three evidence-based practices you will need to continue or implement to prevent ventilator-assisted pneumonia after she has the tracheostomy?

CASE STUDY PROGRESS

P.W. undergoes the tracheostomy procedure without complications. In the interim, the cultures come back confirming the presence of a *C. difficile* infection and she is started on antibiotic therapy. When you return the morning after the tracheostomy procedure and assess the new tracheostomy, you note that the trach tape looks tight. You are unable to insert one finger between P.W.'s neck and the trach tape. You note that the tissue surrounding the incision is edematous. As you palpate the area, your fingers sink into the skin, and you auscultate a popping sound through your stethoscope.

11. Discuss the significance of these assessment findings.

12. What should be your next actions?

13. P.W.'s husband arrives and you speak with him about her having developed subcutaneous emphysema. He collapses into the nearest chair, tears begin to roll down his cheeks, and he says, "It's been almost a month now, and all these things keep happening. Are you sure she'll recover?" How would you respond?

14. P.W. has been receiving lorazepam (Ativan) 1 mg IV every 4 hours to reduce her anxiety. Given her current situation and her husband's distress, describe six nonpharmacologic options you could use to promote the well-being of P.W. and her husband.

CASE STUDY PROGRESS

Over the next several weeks, P.W. progressively regains neurologic functioning.

15. What factors would be considered in determining when P.W. is ready to be weaned from mechanical ventilation?

16. What are your responsibilities during the weaning process?

17. Which assessment finding during the weaning process would indicate P.W. should be placed back on the ventilator?
    a. Heart rate 92 beats/min
    b. Temperature 99.3° F (37.4° C)
    c. Respiratory rate 34 breaths/min
    d. Sao_2 of 94%

Case Study 28

Name _____ Class/Group _____ Date _____

Group Members _____

▶ Scenario

C.E., a 73-year-old married man and retired railroad engineer, visited his internist, complaining, "Whenever I try to do anything, I get so out of breath I can't go on. I think I'm just getting older, but my wife told me I had to come see you about it." His resting Spo$_2$ registered 83%. He was sent to the local hospital for a chest x-ray examination and arterial blood gases (ABGs) after resting 20 minutes on room air. C.E. returned to the office. After evaluating the results, the physician told C.E. he had severe emphysema and must start on continuous oxygen (O$_2$) therapy at a 2 L flow rate. The physician completed a prescription for the oxygen therapy, including on the prescription C.E.'s pulse oximetry and ABG results.

1. What is the rationale for starting C.E. on oxygen at a 2 L flow rate?

2. What criteria need to be fulfilled for Medicare to pay for C.E.'s home oxygen therapy?

3. Based on the most common cause of emphysema, what assessment regarding health behaviors is needed?

CASE STUDY PROGRESS

C.E. affirmed he has been a half-pack-per-day smoker for 50 years. The physician counseled C.E. on smoking cessation and C.E. agreed to stop smoking. The physician told C.E. his office would have a home equipment company call him to arrange delivery of the oxygen equipment and educate him on its use. As a registered nurse (RN) working for the company, you are assigned to be C.E's case manager.

4. How would you prepare for the initial home visit?

5. What would you address with C.E. and his wife at the first visit?

6. What assessment do you need to do at each follow-up visit with C.E.?

CASE STUDY PROGRESS

The next time you visit, C.E. complains of sores behind his ears. He explains, "That long oxygen tubing seems to take on a life of its own. It twists around and gets caught under doors, chairs, everything. It darn near rips the ears off my head."

7. What can you tell him that could help?

8. You auscultate C.E.'s breath sounds and detect the odor of Vicks VapoRub. When you question C.E. about the use of Vicks, he tells you that he started to apply it in and around his nose to prevent his nose from becoming dry and sore. What specific teaching do you need to reinforce with C.E. and his wife?

9. After you have finished, his wife seems upset and tells you that C.E. is still "'smoking a couple of cigarettes" a day. How do you handle this situation?

CASE STUDY PROGRESS

At your next visit 2 weeks later, C.E. tells you that he has not smoked since your previous visit. He is upset, though, over an episode a week ago. He says he walked to the kitchen for a snack and became increasingly short of breath. Per your instructions, C.E. removed the nasal cannula (NC), tested the flow against his check, and felt no O_2 flowing from the catheter. He lacked the force and volume required to yell for help and was too short of breath to return to the living room to check his O_2 tank. He bent forward with his elbows on the countertop and struggled to breathe. He became more frightened with each passing second, and his breathing became increasingly more difficult. A minute later, C.E.'s wife found him and reconnected his O_2 tubing. C.E. sat at the table for 20 minutes before he could walk back to the living room.

10. Why did C.E. assume the peculiar position at the countertop?

11. C.E.'s wife states that since the incident, C.E. "doesn't want her out of his sight." She asks you to "talk some sense into him." She further elaborates, saying that since then "All he does is sit in a chair all day. He won't even get up to get himself a glass of water. I've got a bad hip and this is all very hard on me." What will you do to help C.E. and his wife cope with his condition?

2 Respiratory Disorders

12. What referrals could you consider at this time and why?

CASE STUDY PROGRESS

The next few visits are uneventful. C.E. has continued to not smoke and is doing better with managing episodes of dyspnea. At your next visit, you greet C.E., immediately note that he sounds congested, and comment that he sounds like he has a cold. He replies, "Oh, our great-grandchildren were over to visit several days ago and they all had snotty noses."

13. What is your immediate concern and why?

14. What assessment do you need to perform?

15. You do not find any signs of an infection. What information would you want to review with C.E. and his wife about the signs and symptoms of infection and when to seek treatment?

16. What basic hygiene measures would you include in a teaching plan for C.E. and his wife to prevent his developing an infection? Select all that apply.
    a. Practice good hand washing technique, and wash hands often.
    b. Avoid people with cold and flu infections, and screen visitors.
    c. Avoid enclosed, public areas at all times.
    d. Get pneumonia and flu vaccines every year.
    e. Use the dishwasher to wash eating utensils, glasses, and plates.
    f. Use antibacterial wipes daily to clean frequently touched surfaces.

17. C.E.'s wife says she would like to read more about emphysema on the Internet. List two credible resources to which you could direct her.

Case Study 29

Name _____ Class/Group _____ Date _____

Group Members _____

▶ Scenario

D.Z., a 68-year-old man, is admitted at 1600 to a medical floor with a diagnosis of acute exacerbation of chronic obstructive pulmonary disease (COPD). His other past medical history includes hypertension and type 2 diabetes. He has had pneumonia yearly for the past 3 years and has been a two-pack-a-day smoker for 38 years. His current medications include enalapril (Vasotec), hydrochlorothiazide (HCTZ), metformin (Glucophage), and fluticasone/salmeterol (Advair). He appears a cachectic man who is experiencing difficulty breathing at rest. D.Z. seems irritable and anxious; he complains of sleeping poorly and states that lately he feels tired most of the time. He reports cough productive of thick yellow-green sputum. You auscultate decreased breath sounds, expiratory wheezes, and coarse crackles in both lower lobes anteriorly and posteriorly. His vital signs (VS) are 162/84, 124, 36, 102° F (38.9° C), and Spo_2 88%.

Chart View

Physician's Orders

Diet as tolerated
Out of bed with assistance
Oxygen (O_2) to maintain Spo_2 of 90%
IV of D5W at 50 mL/hr
ECG monitoring
Arterial blood gases (ABGs) in AM
CBC with differential now
Basic metabolic panel (BMP) now
Chest x-ray (CXR) daily
Sputum culture
Albuterol 2.5 mg plus ipratropium 250 mcg nebulizer treatment STAT

1. Are D.Z.'s VS and Spo_2 acceptable? If not, explain why.

2. Describe a plan for implementing these physician's orders.

3. What is the primary nursing goal at this time?

4. Based on this priority, identify three independent nursing actions you would implement.

5. Identify three expected outcomes for D.Z. as a result of your interventions.

Chart View

Medication Administration Record

Methylprednisolone (Solu-Medrol) 125 mg IVP every 8 hours
Azithromycin (Zithromax) 500 mg IVPB q24h×2 days then 500 mg PO×7 days
Fluticasone/salmeterol (Advair) 100/50 mcg 2 puffs twice daily
Heparin 4000 units subcut every 12 hours
Enalapril (Vasotec) 10 mg PO daily
Albuterol 2.5 mg/ipratropium 250 mcg nebulizer treatment every 6 hours
Metformin (Glucophage) 500 mg PO twice daily

6. Indicate the expected outcome for D.Z. that is associated with each medication he is receiving.

7. Because D.Z. is on azithromycin (Zithromax), what interventions need to be included in his plan of care? Select all that apply.
   a. Monitor intravenous (IV) site for inflammation or extravasation.
   b. Assess liver function study results and bilirubin levels.
   c. Request a hearing test before initiating therapy.
   d. Carefully dilute the medication in the proper amount of solution.
   e. Place D.Z. on intake and output.
   f. Administer the medication over 30 minutes.

8. D.Z is ordered heparin 4000 units subcutaneous q12h. The following vial is available. How many milliliters will D.Z. receive? Shade in the dose on the tuberculin syringe.

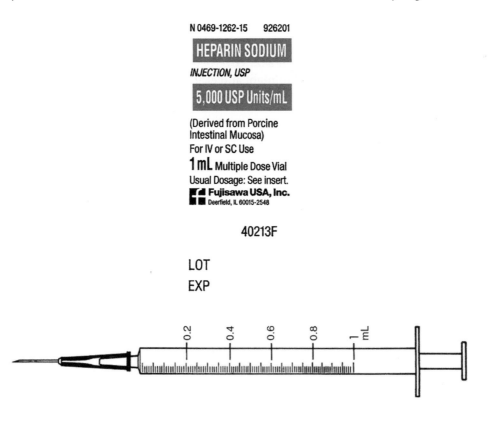

9. What are two common side effects of bronchodilators that you need to assess for?

10. You deliver D.Z.'s dietary tray, and he comments on how hungry he is. As you leave the room, he is rapidly consuming the mashed potatoes. When you pick up the tray, you notice that he has not touched anything else. When you question him, he states, "I don't understand it. I can be so hungry, but when I start to eat, I have trouble breathing and I have to stop." One theory for the increased work of breathing is based on carbohydrate (CHO) loading. Explain this phenomenon.

11. Identify four interventions that might improve his caloric intake.

12. You notice a box of dark chocolate on D.Z.'s overbed table. He tells you that his wife brought him those because he always wakes at night and eats four or five pieces. What is thought to be the basis for this craving for chocolate?

13. After speaking with D.Z. about his diet and reviewing his medications, you are now concerned about his glycemic control. Hospital policy allows you to obtain as-needed blood glucose levels for diabetic patients, so you direct the nursing assistive personnel (NAP) to obtain D.Z.'s blood glucose level at 2100. What is your responsibility in delegating this task to the NAP?

14. The NAP reports that D.Z.'s blood glucose level is 366 mg/dL. What action do you need to take and why?

15. What other health care professional would probably be involved in D.Z.'s treatments and how?

CASE STUDY PROGRESS

The next morning, D.Z. is sitting in the bedside chair and appears to be experiencing less difficulty breathing. He states his cough remains productive of yellow-green sputum, although it is "easier to cough up" than it was the previous day. You auscultate decreased breath sounds and a few coarse crackles in both lower lobes posteriorly. His VS are 150/78, 94, 24, 99.7° F (37.6° C). His Spo_2 is 92% with oxygen on at 2 L per nasal cannula.

Chart View

Arterial Blood Gases (ABGs)

pH	7.34
$Paco_2$	58 mm Hg
HCO_3	32 mmol/L
Pao_2	65 mm Hg
Sao_2	92%

---

16. Interpret D.Z.'s ABG values.

17. Has D.Z.'s status improved or not? Defend your response.

18. What interventions would you include in your plan of care for D.Z. today?

CASE STUDY PROGRESS

D.Z.'s wife approaches you in the hallway and says, "I don't know what to do. My husband used to be so active before he retired 6 months ago. Since then he's lost 35 pounds. He is afraid to take a bath, and it takes him hours to dress—that's if he gets dressed at all. He has gone downhill so fast that it scares me. He's afraid to do anything for himself. He wants me in the room with him all the time, but if I try to talk with him, he snarls and does things to irritate me. I have to keep working. His medical bills are draining all of our savings, and I have to be able to support myself when he's gone. Sometimes I go to work just to get away from the house and his constant demands. He calls me several times a day asking me to come home, but I can't go home. You may not think I'm much of a wife, but quite honestly, I don't want to come home anymore. I just don't know what to do."

19. How would you respond to her statement?

Case Study **30**

Name _____ Class/Group _____ Date _____

Group Members _____

▶ Scenario

The intensive care unit (ICU) nurse calls to give you the following report: "D.S. is a 66-year-old man with a past medical history of chronic bronchitis. He quit smoking 12 years ago and exercises regularly. He went to see his physician with complaints of increasing exertional dyspnea; a large mass was found in his right lung. Three days ago, he underwent a right middle and lower lobe lobectomy; the pathology report showed adenocarcinoma. He has no neurologic deficits. His vital signs run 120/70, 110, about 30, with a fever around 100.2° F. His heart tones are clear, all peripheral pulses are palpable, and he is receiving IV D5 ½ NS at 50 mL/hr in his right forearm. He has a right midaxillary chest tube to Pleur-evac drain; there is no air leak, and it is draining small amounts of serosanguineous fluid. He has complaints of pain at the insertion site, but the site looks good, and the dressing is dry and intact. He is on 5 L oxygen by nasal cannula. He refuses pain medication. He is a real nervous person and has not slept since surgery. He'll be there in about 20 minutes."

1. What additional information would you ask the nurse to provide at this time?

CASE STUDY PROGRESS

D.S. is transported by wheelchair past the nurses' station to a room at the far end of the hall. You enter his room for the first time to find him sitting on the edge of the bed with his left leg in bed and his right foot on the floor. You introduce yourself and tell him that you are going to be his nurse for the rest of the shift. You note that he keeps rubbing his left hand over the right side of his chest.

2. What issues or problems can you already identify?

3. Describe four things you need to do right now for D.S.

CASE STUDY PROGRESS

D.S. states, "I have a nephew who rolled his Jeep and busted himself up real bad. He got hooked on those drugs, and I don't want any part of them."

4. How would you respond to D.S.'s statement?

5. Which of the following nonpharmacologic methods of pain relief would most likely help D.S. at this time? Select all that apply.
   a. Distraction
   b. Hypnosis
   c. Positioning
   d. Acupuncture
   e. Biofeedback

6. D.S. is experiencing difficulty using his right arm. Given the type of surgery he underwent, is this expected and why?

7. You administer morphine sulfate 4 mg IV and tell D.S. that you will return in 30 minutes; 15 minutes later, he turns on his call light. When you enter the room, D.S. says, "I think I'm going to throw up." What are the next three things you would do?

8. D.S. states, "I started to feel sick a couple minutes ago. It just kept getting worse until I knew I was going to throw up." What do you think is responsible for the sudden onset of nausea?

9. Would it be appropriate to give D.S. a second dose of morphine? State your rationale.

10. You decide to call the physician to report the reaction. Using SBAR, what would you report to the physician?

11. The physician changes D.S.'s pain medication to fentanyl and orders ondansetron (Zofran) 4 mg IV every 6 hours as needed for nausea. You use a floor-stocked multidose vial to administer the first dose. How many milliliters of Zofran will you administer?

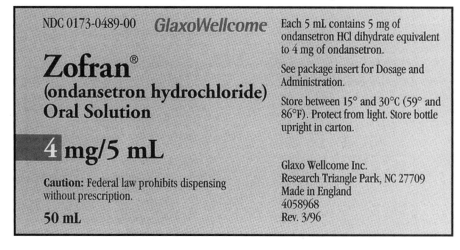

12. D.S.'s pain and nausea are under control an hour later. You remove the chest tube dressing and note that the area around the insertion site looks slightly inflamed, the tissue immediately around the tube looks white and moist, and there is a scant amount of brown drainage. What action would you take next?

CASE STUDY PROGRESS

The next afternoon, the nurse giving you D.S.'s report says that he has been driving her crazy all morning. She tells you that he is fine but has been paranoid and demanding. You enter D.S.'s room to see how he is doing and to tell him you are going to be his nurse again today. He is sitting on the side of the bed with his arms hunched up on the overbed table. You note that his head bobs up and his mouth opens, like a fish taking in water, every time he inhales. He says, "I just can't [breath] seem to [breath] get enough [breath] air."

13. Identify six possible problems that D.S. could have that would account for his behavior.

14. What actions will you take next? Give your rationale.

CASE STUDY PROGRESS

D.S.'s respiratory rate is 46. You auscultate slight air movement over the large airways and no breath sounds distal to the third intercostal space. The chest drainage system is intact. His gown is in his lap, he is diaphoretic, you note intercostal retractions with inspiration, and all muscles of the upper torso are engaged in respiration.

15. What will you do next?

16. The rapid response team stabilizes D.S. and you accompany him during transfer to the ICU. Why do you do this, and what information would you provide to the ICU nurse?

2 Respiratory Disorders

CASE STUDY PROGRESS

After stabilizing D.S. in the ICU, the physician returns to your floor and compliments you on your clear thinking and fast action. The next day the nurse who gave you his report comes to you to apologize. She is relatively new and asks you to explain how you know when a patient is in the early and late stages of respiratory difficulty. She states that she wants to learn from her mistakes so that she does not put another patient through what D.S. experienced.

17. How do you distinguish between early and late stages of respiratory failure?

CASE STUDY OUTCOME

D.S. experiences no further complications and completely recovers from the lobectomy after 2 months. He receives 6 months of external beam radiation therapy to the chest. His chest x-ray examination at 5 years shows no recurrence.

Case Study **31**

Name _____ Class/Group _____ Date _____

Group Members _____

▶ **Scenario**

G.S., a 56-year-old secretary, was involved in a motor vehicle accident; a car drifted left of the centerline and struck G.S. head-on, pinning her behind the steering wheel. She was intubated immediately after extrication and flown to your trauma center. Her injuries were found to be extensive: bilateral flail chest, right hemothorax and pneumothorax, fractured spleen, multiple small liver lacerations, open fractures of both legs, and probable cardiac contusion. She was taken to the operating room (OR) for repair of her injuries. In the OR she received 36 units of packed red blood cells (RBCs), 20 units of platelets, 12 units of fresh frozen plasma, and 18 L of lactated Ringer's solution. G.S. was admitted to the intensive care unit (ICU) postoperatively, where she developed acute respiratory distress syndrome (ARDS).

1. What is ARDS?

2. What are the risk factors for developing ARDS? Which does G.S. have?

CASE STUDY PROGRESS

G.S. was in the ICU for 4 weeks, and her ARDS is almost resolved. She is being transferred to your unit. The ICU nurse gives you the following report: "She is awake, alert, and oriented to person and place. Both legs remain casted from hip to toe. She can wiggle her toes on both feet. Heart tones are clear, last vital signs were 138/90, 88, 26, 99.3° F (37.4° C); bilateral radial pulses 3+. All of her surgical incisions are healed. She has bilateral chest tubes to water suction with closed drainage, both dressings are dry and intact. She has a duodenal feeding tube, a Foley catheter to down drain, and a left double-lumen peripherally inserted central catheter (PICC) line. Her morning labs are still pending."

2 Respiratory Disorders

3. What additional information do you need from the ICU nurse?

CASE STUDY PROGRESS

You complete your assessment of G.S. You note she is dyspneic and has fine crackles throughout all lung fields posteriorly and in both lower lobes anteriorly, and coarse crackles over the large airways. She has oxygen on at 2 L per nasal cannula and her Spo_2 is 94%.

4. What is the significance of the fine and coarse crackles?

5. The nurse from the previous shift charted the following statement: "Fine and coarse crackles that clear with vigorous coughing." Based on your knowledge of pathophysiology, determine the accuracy of this statement.

6. It is time to administer scheduled furosemide (Lasix) 60 mg intravenous push (IVP). What effect, if any, should furosemide have on G.S.'s breath sounds?

7. What action do you need to take before giving the furosemide?

Chart View

Laboratory Results

Sodium	129 mmol/L
Potassium	3.0 mmol/L
Chloride	92 mmol/L
HCO_3	26 mmol/L
BUN	37 mg/dL
Creatinine	2 mg/dL
Glucose	128 mg/dL
Calcium	7.1 mg/dL

8. Which laboratory values concern you, and why?

 9. Given G.S.'s laboratory values, what action do you need to take and why?

CASE STUDY PROGRESS

The physician wants you to administer the furosemide and prescribes the following.

Chart View

Physician's Orders

STAT magnesium (Mg) level
Potassium chloride (KCl) 40 mEq IVPB
Calcium gluconate 2 g in 100 mL NS IVPB over 3 hr

10. Why did the physician order a magnesium level?

11. G.S. has one available port to use on the PICC line. Outline a plan for administering the potassium chloride and the calcium gluconate.

12. What interventions do you need to perform to safely administer intravenous (IV) potassium chloride? Select all that apply.
   a. Place G.S. on continuous electrocardiogram (ECG) monitoring.
   b. Administer the infusion using an intravenous pump.
   c. Assess the patency of the PICC line before initiating the infusion.
   d. Administer the potassium infusion over a time period of at least 2 hours.
   e. Invert the potassium-containing IV bag several times before and during the infusion.

13. You go to prepare G.S.'s furosemide dose and find only one 20-mg vial in the medication-dispensing system. The floor stock is empty. The pharmacist tells you that it will be at least an hour before he can send the drug to you. What are your options?

14. While you are administering the furosemide, G.S. says, "This is so weird. A couple times this morning, I felt like my heart flipped upside down in my chest, but now I feel like there's a bird flopping around in there." What are the first two actions you should take next?

15. G.S.'s pulse is 66 beats/min and irregular. Her blood pressure is 92/70 and respirations are 26. She admits to being "a little lightheaded" but denies having pain or nausea. Your co-worker connects G.S. to the code cart monitor for a "quick look." Interpret what you see.

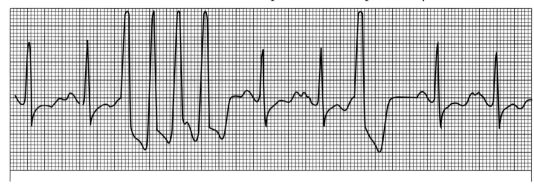

16. Why is G.S. likely experiencing a dysrhythmia?

17. What will your next actions be?

Chart View

Arterial Blood Gases (ABGs) on 6 L O$_2$ by Nasal Cannula (NC)

pH	7.30
Paco$_2$	59 mm Hg
Pao$_2$	82 mm Hg
HCO$_3$	36 mmol/L
Spo$_2$	91%

---

18. You increase her oxygen to 6 L and the physician orders a stat set of ABGs. How would you interpret G.S.'s ABGs?

19. What are your nursing priorities at this time?

20. Describe four interventions you will perform over the next few hours based on this priority.

21. You notice that G.S. looks frightened and is lying stiff as a board. How would you respond to this situation?

CASE STUDY OUTCOME

G.S.'s pulmonary status does not improve after administration of the furosemide and she continues to have frequent ventricular dysrhythmias despite the administration of the electrolytes. The physician transfers G.S. back to the ICU, where she is found to have a pulmonary embolus. Unfortunately, 1 week later she throws another embolus and all attempts at resuscitation fail.

Musculoskeletal Disorders

Case Study 32

Name _____ Class/Group _____ Date _____

Group Members _____

▶ **Scenario**

M.S., a 72-year-old white woman, comes to your clinic for a complete physical examination. She has not been to a provider for 11 years because "I don't like doctors." Her only complaint today is "pain in my upper back." She describes the pain as sharp and knifelike. The pain began approximately 3 weeks ago when she was getting out of bed in the morning and hasn't changed at all. M.S. rates her pain as 6 on a 0- to 10-point pain scale and says the pain decreases to 3 or 4 after taking "a couple of ibuprofen." She denies recent falls or trauma.

M.S. admits she needs to quit smoking and start exercising but states, "I don't have the energy to exercise, and besides, I've always been thin." She has smoked one to two packs of cigarettes per day since she was 17 years old. Her last blood work was 11 years ago, and she can't remember the results. She went through menopause at the age of 47 and has never taken hormone replacement therapy. The physical examination findings are unremarkable other than moderate tenderness to deep palpation over the spinous process at T7. No masses or tenderness to the tissue surround the tender spot. No visible masses, skin changes, or erythema are noted. Her neurologic findings are intact, and no muscle wasting is noted.

1. An x-ray examination of the thoracic spine reveals a collapsed vertebra at T7 and bone density changes in the spine. What could this result indicate?

2. The physician suspects osteoporosis. List seven risk factors associated with osteoporosis.

3. Place a star or asterisk next to those risk factors specific to M.S.

CASE STUDY PROGRESS

M.S. has never had an osteoporosis screening. She confides that her mother and grandmother were diagnosed with osteoporosis when they were in their early 50s.

4. What diagnostic test is most commonly used to diagnose osteoporosis?

5. M.S.'s diagnostic test revealed a bone density T-score of −2.7. How will this be interpreted?

6. M.S. receives a prescription for alendronate (Fosamax) 70 mg/wk. Which instructions are appropriate as you provide patient teaching to M.S. about this drug? Select all that apply.
   a. "Take the medication with 8 ounces of water immediately on arising."
   b. "You can take this medication with your morning coffee or orange juice."
   c. "You can eat your breakfast along with this medication."
   d. "You need to sit or stand upright for at least 30 minutes after taking the medication."
   e. "If you experience any severe abdominal pain, vomiting, or jaw pain, notify your doctor immediately."

7. M.S. asks whether she needs to take a calcium supplement. How do you answer her?

8. What nonpharmacologic interventions will you teach M.S. to prevent further bone loss?

CASE STUDY PROGRESS

M.S. asks you about foods that contain calcium. "I'd rather eat than take all these pills," she states. You review food sources of calcium with her.

9. Which of these foods are considered good sources of dietary calcium? Select all that apply.
   a. Chicken salad
   b. Banana
   c. 8 ounces of yogurt
   d. 1 cup of cooked spinach
   e. Baked potato with margarine

CASE STUDY PROGRESS

M.S. begins to cry and says, "I cannot possibly stop smoking, change my diet, and exercise all at the same time."

10. You encourage M.S. to start working on one problem at a time. How should it be decided which problem M.S. should attempt first?

Case Study **33**

Name _____ Class/Group _____ Date _____

Group Members _____

▶ Scenario

J.C. is a 41-year-old man who comes to the emergency department with complaints of acute low back pain. He states that he did some heavy lifting yesterday, went to bed with a mild backache, and awoke this morning with terrible back pain, which he rates as a 10 on a 1-to-10 scale. He admits to having had a similar episode of back pain years ago "after I lifted something heavy at work." J.C. has a past medical history of peptic ulcer disease (PUD) related to nonsteroidal anti-inflammatory drug (NSAID) use. He is 6 feet tall, weighs 265 pounds, and has a prominent "potbelly."

1. What questions would be appropriate to ask J.C. in evaluating the extent of his back pain and injury?

2. What observable characteristic does J.C. have that makes him highly susceptible to low back injury?

3. J.C. used to take piroxicam (Feldene) 20 mg until he developed his duodenal ulcer. What is the relationship between the two? What signs and symptoms (S/S) would you expect if an ulcer developed?

CASE STUDY PROGRESS

All serious medical conditions are ruled out, and J.C. is diagnosed with lumbar strain. The nurse practitioner (NP) orders a physical therapy consultation to develop a home stretching and back-strengthening exercise program and a dietary consultation for weight reduction. J.C. is given prescriptions for cyclobenzaprine (Flexeril) 10 mg tid × 3 days only, and celecoxib (Celebrex) 100 mg/day for 3 months. He receives the following instructions: heat applications to the lower back for 20 to 30 minutes four times a day (using moist heat from heat packs or hot towels), no twisting or unnecessary bending, and no lifting more than 10 pounds. J.C. is instructed to rest his back for 1 or 2 days, getting up only now and then to move around to relieve muscle spasms in his back and strengthen his back muscles. He is given a written excuse to stay off work for 5 days and, when he returns to work, specifying the limitation of lifting no more than 10 pounds for 3 months. He is instructed to contact his primary care provider if the pain gets worse.

4. J.C. looks at the prescription for cyclobenzaprine (Flexeril) and states, "I'm glad you didn't give me that Valium. They gave me Valium last time and that stuff knocked me out." How would you respond to J.C.?

5. Why do you think that cyclobenzaprine was prescribed instead of diazepam (Valium)?

6. J.C. states, "Well, I'm glad I'll still be able to take my sleeping pill." True or False? Explain.

CASE STUDY PROGRESS

J.C. asks, "What is Celebrex? I hope it won't do what that Feldene did to me years ago."

7. Why do you think it was prescribed for J.C., considering his gastrointestinal (GI) history?

8. It has been over 5 years since his last episode of GI bleeding. Are there any other conditions that you need to assess for before J.C. begins to take the celecoxib? Explain.

9. Why would the NP prescribe an NSAID rather than acetaminophen for J.C.'s pain?

10. A physical therapist teaches J.C. maintenance exercises he can do on his own to promote back health. Identify two common exercises that would be included.

11. In addition to learning exercises, J.C. needs to learn proper body mechanics for lifting and performing day-to-day activities. Which statement by J.C. indicates a need for further instruction?
    a. "I will bend my knees when I lean forward."
    b. "When lifting heavy boxes, I will bend at the waist."
    c. "I will not lift anything above the level of my elbows."
    d. "I will avoid standing in one position for a long period of time."

Case Study **34**

Name _____ Class/Group _____ Date _____

Group Members _____

▶ **Scenario**

D.M., a 25-year-old man, hops into the emergency department (ED) with complaints of right ankle pain. He states that he was playing basketball and stepped on another player's foot, inverting his ankle. You note swelling over the lateral malleolus down to the area of the fourth and fifth metatarsals, and pedal pulses are 3+ bilaterally. His vital signs (VS) are 124/76, 82, 18. He has no allergies and takes no medication. He states he has had no prior surgeries or medical problems.

1. In assessing D.M.'s injured ankle, what should be evaluated?

2. What will initial management of the ankle involve to prevent further swelling and injury?

3. You note significant swelling over the fourth and fifth metatarsals. How would you further evaluate this finding?

CASE STUDY PROGRESS

X-ray results are negative for fracture, and a second-degree sprain is diagnosed. The physician orders immobilization with an elastic bandage and an air stirrup brace, with instructions for crutches. The physician instructs D.M. not to bear weight on his ankle for 2 days, then to use only partial weight bearing until the ankle heals.

4. Describe the technique for applying an elastic wrap. Give the rationale.

5. When instructing D.M. to use crutches, D.M. states that he "likes it better" when the crutches rest under his arms while he walks with the crutches. Is this correct? Explain.

6. You instruct D.M. on using the three-point gait with the crutches. Which would be the correct first step for the three-point gait?
   a. Step first with the affected leg.
   b. Step first with the unaffected leg.
   c. Step first with both crutches and the affected leg.
   d. Step first with the affected leg and the crutch opposite of the affected leg.

7. You are to instruct D.M. on application of cold, activity, and care of the ankle. What would be appropriate instructions in these areas?

8. D.M. is given a prescription for Lortab 2.5/500. Explain the meaning of the numbers.

9. What instructions concerning the Lortab are needed?

CASE STUDY PROGRESS

Four days later, D.M. hobbles into the ED and boldly informs you that he "did it again, only this time it was touch football." He states that the pain pills worked so well, he thought it would be okay. You detect the odor of beer on his breath.

10. What are you going to do?

11. D.M.'s blood alcohol concentration (BAC) result is 0.06 mg%. Interpret this result. Does this level reflect legal intoxication?

12. You remove his sock and find a large hematoma forming on the lateral aspect of an already swollen ankle. The ankle also shows the color of a bruise that is several days old. You inquire about D.M.'s pain perception. He states, "It doesn't feel too bad now, but I sure saw stars when it popped." What is the significance of his statement?

Case Study 35

Name _____   Class/Group _____   Date _____

Group Members _____

▶ Scenario

S.P. is admitted to the orthopedic ward. She fell at home and sustained an intracapsular fracture of the hip at the femoral neck. The following history is obtained from her: She is a 75-year-old widow with three children living nearby. Her father died of cancer at age 62; her mother died of heart failure at age 79. Her height is 5 ft 3 in; weight is 118 lb. She has a 50–pack-year smoking history and denies alcohol use. She has severe rheumatoid arthritis (RA) and gastroesophageal reflux disease (GERD) and had coronary artery disease with a coronary artery bypass graft 9 months ago. Since then she has engaged in "very mild exercises at home." Vital signs (VS) are 128/60, 98, 14, 99° F (37.2° C), SpO_2 94% on 2 L oxygen by nasal cannula. Her oral medications are rabeprazole (Aciphex) 20 mg/day, prednisone (Deltasone) 5 mg/day, and methotrexate (Rheumatrex) 2.5 mg/wk.

1. List at least four risk factors for hip fractures.

2. Place a star or asterisk next to each of the responses in question 1 that represent S.P.'s risk factors.

CASE STUDY PROGRESS

S.P. is taken to surgery for a total hip replacement. Because of the intracapsular location of the fracture, the surgeon chooses to perform an arthroplasty rather than internal fixation. The postoperative orders include the following.

Chart View

Physician's Orders

Cefazolin (Kefzol) 1000 mg IV q8h×3 doses. Give last dose no later than 24 hours after anesthesia end time.

Enoxaparin (Lovenox) 30 mg subcut q12h, begin at 2200.

Warfarin (Coumadin) 2.5 mg PO, starting postoperative day 1, then titrated to international normalized ratio (INR) per pharmacy dosing

Docusate and senna (Peri-Colace) 1 capsule PO bid

Multivitamin with iron 1 capsule/day PO with meals

Complete blood count (CBC) in morning after blood reinfusion

Hydromorphone (Dilaudid) by IV patient-controlled analgesia, intermittent with 0.1 mg dosing, lockout 10 minutes

Physical therapist (PT) and occupational therapist (OT) to evaluate on postoperative day 1 and start therapy

Ketorolac (Toradol) 15 mg IV q6h prn pain×5 days only

Hip precautions per protocol

Ondansetron (Zofran) 4 mg IV q6h prn for nausea

Toilet seat extension

Straight catheterization if no void by 8 hours postoperatively

3. Why is S.P. receiving enoxaparin (Lovenox) and warfarin (Coumadin)?

4. Why is the antibiotic to be stopped before the anesthesia end time?

5. S.P. had an arthroplasty. For each characteristic listed, mark *A* for arthroplasty or *O* for open reduction and internal fixation (ORIF) of the hip.

_____a. Also known as *total hip replacement*.

_____b. Metal pins, screws, rods, and plates are used to immobilize the fracture.

_____c. Replacement of the entire hip joint with a prosthetic (artificial) joint system.

6. S.P. receives reinfused blood as an intraoperative blood salvage. Which statements about this procedure are true? Select all that apply.
   a. The blood lost from surgery is immediately readministered to the patient.
   b. The blood lost from surgery is collected into a cell saver.
   c. One hundred percent of the red blood cells are saved for reinfusion.
   d. This procedure has the same risks as blood transfusions from donors.
   e. The salvaged blood must be reinfused within 6 hours of collection.

7. List four critical potential postoperative problems for S.P.

8. How will you monitor for excessive postoperative blood loss?

9. According to the posterior surgical approach, there are two main goals for maintaining proper alignment of S.P.'s operative leg. What are they, and how are they achieved?

10. Postoperative wound infection is a concern for S.P. Describe what you would do to monitor her for a wound infection.

11. Taking S.P.'s RA into consideration, what is the reason for the PT and OT consultations?

12. What predisposing factors, identified in S.P.'s medical history, increase her risk for respiratory complications?

13. What predisposing factors, identified in S.P.'s medical history, place her at risk for infection, bleeding, and anemia?

14. Briefly discuss S.P.'s nutritional needs. Why is she receiving an iron supplement?

CASE STUDY PROGRESS

Discharge planning began when S.P. was admitted. The case manager who has been working with S.P. and her family is initiating S.P.'s placement in a rehabilitation facility after discharge. She would like to be near her children but realizes that they work and cannot be with her 24 hours a day.

15. What factors need to be taken into consideration by the patient, family, and case manager when choosing a rehabilitation facility?

CASE STUDY OUTCOME

S.P.'s daughters visit several facilities. S.P. is admitted to the rehabilitation facility close to one daughter's home. After 2 weeks, she completes rehabilitation and is discharged to home. Her children check on her every day.

Case Study 36

Name _____ Class/Group _____ Date _____

Group Members _____

▶ Scenario

H.K. is a 26-year-old man who tried to light a cigarette while driving and lost control of his truck. The truck flipped and landed on the passenger side. H.K. was transported to the emergency department with a deformed, edematous right lower leg and a deep puncture wound approximately 5 cm long over the deformity. Blood continues to ooze from the wound.

1. What further assessment will you make of the leg injury and what precautions will you take in making this assessment?

2. What is the most appropriate method for controlling bleeding at this wound site?

3. What is the best way to immobilize the leg injury before surgery?

4. From the information given, it is clear that H.K. is a smoker. List at least three issues related to his smoking that can complicate his care and recovery. What interventions could be instituted to counter these complications?

CASE STUDY PROGRESS

H.K. is taken to surgery for open reduction and internal fixation (ORIF) of the tibia and fibula fractures. He returns with a full-leg fiberglass cast with windows over the areas of surgery.

5. Describe the assessment of a patient with a long leg cast involving trauma and surgery.

6. In assessing H.K.'s cast on the third day postoperatively, you notice a strong foul odor. Drainage on the cast is extending, and H.K. is complaining of pain more often and seems considerably more uncomfortable. Vital signs are 123/78, 102, 18, 102.2° F (39° C). What is your analysis of these findings?

CASE STUDY PROGRESS

H.K. returns to surgery. The wound over H.K.'s fracture site has become necrotic with purulent drainage. The wound is debrided and cultured and a posterior splint is applied. H.K. returns to his room with orders for wet-to-moist dressing changes. The physician suspects osteomyelitis and orders nafcillin (Unipen) and ciprofloxacin (Cipro). Contact precautions are implemented.

7. Why are two antibiotics ordered?

8. H.K. asks you about the isolation precautions. "Does this mean I have something bad?" What is your best answer?
   a. "These are precautions that we use for every patient who has surgery."
   b. "These precautions prevent the spread of the infection to other patients and to health care personnel."
   c. "These are precautions we are taking to help your infection get better."
   d. "This is an extremely serious infection; these precautions will keep the infection from getting worse."

9. As you continue to assess H.K. over the following days, what evidence will you look for that antibiotics are effectively treating the infection?

10. What will H.K. be taught concerning the care of his cast?

11. What nutritional needs will H.K. have and why?

CASE STUDY PROGRESS

To ensure pain management, H.K. is given a fentanyl (Duragesic) 75 mcg/hr transdermal patch. You prepare to give him the first dose.

12. Name this drug's therapeutic category.

13. What signs and symptoms would you see if he were to have a toxic or overdose reaction to the fentanyl? Select all that apply.
    a. Dilated pupils
    b. Respiratory depression
    c. Nausea
    d. Central nervous system (CNS) depression
    e. Pruritus

14. What is the first thing you will need to do if you note a toxic or overdose reaction to the fentanyl transdermal patch?

15. What is the antidote for toxic opioid reactions and how is it administered?

CASE STUDY PROGRESS

H.K. has no further complications with his leg wound and responds well to physical therapy. The discharge planner meets with him to discuss his posthospital care.

16. What issues would the discharge planner need to address with H.K.?

CASE STUDY OUTCOME

H.K. stayed in his apartment with a loan from his parents. Friends drove him to physical therapy on their way to class at the university and took him back on their way home. He managed well and went back to work while still in his cast.

Case Study 37

Name _____ Class/Group _____ Date _____

Group Members _____

▶ Scenario

M.M., a 76-year-old retired schoolteacher, is postoperative day 2 after an open reduction and internal fixation (ORIF) for a fracture of his right femur. His preoperative control prothrombin time/international normalized ratio (PT/INR) was 11 sec/1.0 and his activated partial thromboplastin time (aPTT) was 35 seconds. He has been on bed rest since surgery. At 0800, his vital signs (VS) are 132/84, 80 with regular rhythm, 18 unlabored, and 99° F (37.2° C). He is awake, alert, and oriented with no adventitious heart sounds. Breath sounds are clear but diminished in the bases bilaterally. Bowel sounds are present and he is taking sips of clear liquids. He is receiving an intravenous (IV) infusion of D5 ½ NS at 75 mL/hr in his left hand, and orders are to change it to a saline lock this morning if he is able to maintain adequate oral fluid intake. He has orders for oxygen (O_2) to maintain Spo_2 over 92%, but he has been refusing to wear the nasal cannula. His laboratory work shows Hct, 34%; Hgb, 11.3 mg/dL; K, 4.1 mEq/L; aPTT, 44 sec. Pain is controlled with morphine sulfate 4 mg IV as needed every 4 hours, and he has promethazine (Phenergan) 25 mg IV q4h if needed for nausea. He is receiving heparin 5000 units subcutaneously bid, taking docusate sodium (Colace) PO once daily, and wearing a nitroglycerin patch.

At 1830 you answer M.M.'s call light and find him lying in bed breathing rapidly and rubbing the right side of his chest. He is complaining of right-sided chest pain and appears to be restless.

1. What will you do?

CASE STUDY PROGRESS

You check his VS, with these results: blood pressure (BP) 98/60; P 120; R 24. You note he is restless and slightly confused. The pulse oximeter reads 86%, so you start him on 6 L O_2 by nasal cannula (NC). You identify faint crackles in the posterior bases bilaterally. The heart monitor on lead II shows nonspecific T wave changes.

2. Using SBAR, what information, based on the findings, would you provide to the physician when you call?

3. The physician orders that the patient be transferred to the intensive care unit (ICU) and undergo blood coagulation studies, arterial blood gases (ABGs) on room air, continuous pulse oximetry, STAT chest x-ray (CXR), and STAT 12-lead electrocardiogram (ECG). What information will the physician gain from each of these?

4. Why would the physician order ABGs on room air as opposed to with supplemental O_2?

CASE STUDY PROGRESS

You evaluate the room air ABG results.

Chart View

Arterial Blood Gases

pH	7.55
$Paco_2$	24 mm Hg
HCO_3	24 mEq/L
Pao_2	56 mm Hg
Sao_2	86% (room air)

Vital Signs

BP	150/92 mm Hg
Heart rate	110 beats/min
Respiratory rate	28 breaths/min
Temperature	99° F (37.2° C)

5. What is your interpretation of the ABGs, and what do you think the physician will order next, and why?

CASE STUDY PROGRESS

The CXR image shows a small right infiltrate. The physician suspects an embolism, either fat or pulmonary, and orders a STAT spiral CT scan of the lungs. The interpretation of the results reads "strongly suggestive of a pulmonary embolus (PE)."

6. What are the most likely sources of the embolus?

7. For each characteristic listed in the following, note whether it is a characteristic of a fat embolus *(F)*, a blood clot embolus *(BC)* in the lungs, or both *(B)*.
    _____a. Altered mental status
    _____b. Decreased Spo$_2$
    _____c. Petechiae
    _____d. Chest pain
    _____e. Crackles
    _____f. Increased respirations and pulse

8. Before the latest PT/INR results are back, the physician orders a heparin bolus of 5000 units IV followed by an infusion of 1200 units/hr. The laboratory calls with a critical value—the aPTT is 120 seconds. Based on this result, what action will you take?

9. The physician is considering administering an antidote to the heparin. Which generic drug is considered an antidote to heparin therapy?
    a. Potassium chloride
    b. Vitamin K
    c. Protamine sulfate
    d. Atropine

CASE STUDY PROGRESS

The physician decides not to administer an antidote, and M.M. is monitored closely. Four hours later, the aPTT is 40 seconds.

10. The next day the physician's orders read, "Warfarin (Coumadin) 2.5 mg PO, PT/INR in AM; D/C heparin." What is wrong with these orders?

11. Some thrombolytics, such as alteplase (Activase), have been beneficial in the treatment of PE. Would M.M. be a candidate for treatment with thrombolytics? Why or why not?

12. List three priority problems related to the care of M.M. in his current situation.

13. Several days later you hear M.M. asking his son to bring in a "decent razor" because he is tired of having beard stubble. How would you address this issue?

14. Before M.M. goes home, you provide education about warfarin therapy. You inform him that he will be on this medication for several months to prevent another occurrence of VTE. Which of these statements will be included in the teaching? Select all that apply, and correct the ones that are wrong.
    a. "Take the warfarin at the same time every day."
    b. "You will need to have blood work done on a regular basis while on this drug."
    c. "There are no dietary restrictions while on this drug."
    d. "Watch for bleeding from your gums, nose, and bowels."
    e. "It's a good idea to wear a medical alert bracelet or necklace while on this drug."

Case Study 38

Name _____ Class/Group _____ Date _____

Group Members _____

▶ Scenario

J.F., a 67-year-old woman, was involved in an auto accident and flown by emergency helicopter to your facility. She sustained a ruptured spleen, fractured pelvis, and compound fractures of the left femur. On admission (5 days ago) she underwent a splenectomy. Her pelvis was stabilized with an external fixation device 3 days ago, and, yesterday, her left femur was stabilized using balanced suspension with skeletal traction. She has a Thomas splint with a Pearson attachment on her left leg. She has 20 pounds of skeletal traction and 5 pounds applied to the balanced suspension. Her left femur is elevated off the bed at approximately 45 degrees. The lower leg is parallel to the bed and lies in a sling that the nurse adjusts on the frame, and the foot hangs freely. This morning, J.F. was transferred to your orthopedic unit for specialized care. You are the nurse assigned to care for her on the night shift.

1. You enter J.F.'s room for the first time. What aspects of the traction will you inspect?

2. When inspecting the skeletal pin sites, you note that the skin is reddened for an inch around the pin on both the medial and lateral left leg. What does this finding indicate, and what action will you take?

CASE STUDY PROGRESS

You perform a neurovascular assessment and note the following findings: Left foot pale, temperature slightly cooler than right foot. Right foot color pink. Capillary refill less than 3 seconds on both sides. Edema +1 on left foot and lower leg; no edema on right leg. Dorsalis pedis palpable on both feet. Sensation equal on both sides. Able to dorsiflex feet and rotate ankles freely. Rates pain in left femur as a 5 out of 10.

3. Your institution uses electronic charting. Based on the assessment in the previous paragraph, which of the following systems would you mark as "abnormal" as you document the neurovascular assessment? For abnormal findings provide a brief narrative note.
   X Abnormal

   ☐ Skin color:
   ☐ Skin temperature:
   ☐ Capillary refill:
   ☐ Edema:
   ☐ Peripheral pulses:
   ☐ Sensation:
   ☐ Motor function:
   ☐ Pain:

4. What other key points of the assessment will you document in the patient's record?

5. You find J.F.'s body in the lower 75% of the bed and her left upper leg at an exaggerated angle (more than 45 degrees). The knot at the end of the bed is caught in the pulley and the 20-pound weight is dangling just above the floor. What are you going to do?

6. When you lift J.F., you notice that her sheets are wet. You decide to change J.F.'s linen. How would you accomplish this task?

7. J.F. tells you that she feels like she needs to have a bowel movement (BM) but it is too painful to sit on the bedpan. How would you respond?

8. J.F. expels a few small, hard, round pieces of stool. What could be done to promote normal elimination?

CASE STUDY PROGRESS

You ask J.F. whether she is ready for her bath and she responds positively. You let her bathe the parts she can reach and engage her in a conversation as you attend to the rest of her body. While performing perineal care, you notice that the folds of skin around her perineal area are reddened and excoriated.

9. What is the likely cause of the problem and what needs to be done to encourage healing?

10. You ask J.F. what she is doing to exercise while she is confined to the bed. She looks surprised and states that she isn't doing anything. What activities can J.F. engage in while on bed rest?

11. You realize that maintaining skin integrity is a challenge in J.F.'s case. What measures will you take to prevent skin breakdown?

12. Although J.F. is recovering nicely, she is becoming increasingly withdrawn. You enter her room and find her crying. She tells you that she is all alone here, that she misses her family terribly. You know that her son is flying into town tomorrow but will only be able to stay a few days. What can be done so that J.F. benefits from her family support system?

Case Study **39**

Name _____ Class/Group _____ Date _____

Group Members _____

▶ **Scenario**

You are working in the emergency department when M.C., an 82-year-old widow, arrives by ambulance. Because M.C. had not answered her phone since noon yesterday, her daughter went to her home to check on her. She found M.C. lying on the kitchen floor, incontinent of urine and stool, with complaints of pain in her right hip. Her daughter reports a past medical history of hypertension, angina, and osteoporosis. M.C. takes propranolol (Inderal), a nitroglycerin patch, indapamide (Lozol), and conjugated estrogen (Premarin) daily. M.C.'s daughter reports that her mother is normally very alert and lives independently. On examination, you see an elderly woman, approximately 100 pounds, holding her right thigh. You note shortening of the right leg with external rotation and a large amount of swelling at the proximal thigh and right hip. M.C. is oriented to person only and is confused about place and time, but she is able to say that her "leg hurts so bad." M.C.'s vital signs (VS) are 90/65, 120, 24, 97.5° F (36.4° C); her Spo_2 is 89%. She is profoundly dehydrated. Preliminary diagnosis is a fracture of the right hip.

1. Considering her medical history and that she has been without her medications for at least 24 hours, explain her current VS.

2. Based on her history and your initial assessment, what three priority interventions would you expect to be initiated?

3. M.C.'s daughter states, "Mother is always so clear and alert. I have never seen her act so confused. What's wrong with her?" What are three possible causes for M.C.'s disorientation that should be considered and evaluated?

CASE STUDY PROGRESS

X-ray films confirm the diagnosis of intertrochanteric femoral fracture. Knowing that M.C. is going to be admitted, you draw admission labs and call for the orthopedic consultation.

4. What laboratory and diagnostic studies will be ordered to evaluate M.C.'s condition, and what critical information will each give you?

5. You insert a Foley catheter and take careful note of the amount and appearance of M.C.'s urine. Why?

6. What are the five Ps that should guide the assessment of M.C.'s right leg before and after surgery?

7. In evaluating M.C.'s pulses, you find her posterior tibial pulse and dorsalis pedis pulse to be weaker on her right foot than on her left. What could be a possible cause of this finding?

8. You carefully monitor M.C.'s right extremity for compartment syndrome. Which of these is a characteristic of compartment syndrome? Select all that apply.
   a. Warmth of the extremity
   b. Pain distal to the injury that is not relieved by opioid analgesics
   c. Numbness and tingling of the extremity
   d. Pallor of the extremity
   e. Petechiae over the extremity

9. In planning further care for M.C., list four potential complications for which M.C. should be monitored.

10. M.C. keeps asking about "Peaches." No one seems to be paying attention. You ask her what she means. She says Peaches is her little dog, and she's worried about who is taking care of it. How will you answer?

CASE STUDY PROGRESS

M.C. is placed in Buck's traction and sent to the orthopedic unit until an open reduction and internal fixation (ORIF) can be scheduled. Hydrocodone-acetaminophen (Lortab 2.2/500) q4h prn is ordered for severe pain with orders for acetaminophen (Tylenol) 650 mg q4h prn, and tramadol (Ultram) 100 mg q6h prn, for mild and moderate pain, respectively. She is placed on enoxaparin (Lovenox) 30 mg subcut bid. M.C.'s cardiovascular, pulmonary, and renal status is closely monitored.

11. As you assess the traction, you check the setup and M.C.'s comfort. Which of these are characteristics of Buck's traction? Select all that apply.
    a. The weights can be lifted manually as needed for comfort.
    b. Weights need to be freely hanging at all times.
    c. Pin site care is an essential part of nursing management for Buck's traction.
    d. A Velcro boot is used to immobilize the affected leg and connect to the weights.
    e. Weights used for Buck's traction are limited to 5 to 10 pounds.

12. Ultram and Lortab are both constipating. What will you do to prevent constipation?

13. Between her admission at 1500 and the next day, she receives four doses of Lortab and one dose of acetaminophen (Tylenol). At 1300, she develops a fever of 101° F (38.3° C), and the physician writes an order to give acetaminophen (Tylenol), 650 mg PO every 4 hours for temperature over 100.5° F (38.1° C). Is there a concern with this order?

CASE STUDY OUTCOME

After an uneventful postoperative course, M.C. is transferred to a skilled-care facility for physical and occupational therapy rehabilitation.

Case Study **40**

Name _____ Class/Group _____ Date _____

Group Members _____

▶ Scenario

E.B., a 69-year-old man with type 1 diabetes mellitus (DM), is admitted to a large regional medical center complaining of severe pain in his right foot and lower leg. The right foot and lower leg are cool and without pulses (absent by Doppler). Arteriogram demonstrates severe atherosclerosis of the right popliteal artery with complete obstruction of blood flow. Despite attempts at percutaneous catheter-directed thrombolytic therapy with alteplase (tissue plasminogen activator [TPA]) over 48 hours and surgical thrombectomy, the foot and lower leg become necrotic. Finally, the decision is made to perform an above-the-knee amputation (AKA) on E.B.'s right leg. E.B. is recently widowed and has a son and daughter who live nearby. In preparation for E.B.'s surgery, the surgeons wish to spare as much viable tissue as possible. Hence, an order is written for E.B. to undergo 5 days of hyperbaric therapy for 20 minutes bid.

1. What is the purpose of hyperbaric therapy?

CASE STUDY PROGRESS

As you prepare E.B. for surgery, he is quiet and withdrawn. He follows instructions quietly and slowly without asking questions. His son and daughter are at his bedside, and they also are very quiet. Finally, E.B. tells his family, "I don't want to go like your mother did. She lingered on and had so much pain. I don't want them to bring me back."

2. You look at his chart and find no advance directives. What is your responsibility?

3. What is your assessment of E.B.'s behavior at this time?

4. What are some appropriate interventions and responses to E.B.'s anticipatory grief?

CASE STUDY PROGRESS

E.B. returns from surgery with the right residual limb dressed with gauze and an elastic wrap. The dressing is dry and intact, without drainage. He is drowsy with the following vital signs: 142/80, 96, 14, 97.9° F (36.6° C), SpO_2 92%. He is receiving a maintenance intravenous (IV) infusion of D5NS at 125 mL/hr in his right forearm.

5. The surgeon has written to keep E.B.'s residual limb elevated on pillows for 48 hours; after that, have him lie in a prone position for 15 minutes, four times a day. In teaching E.B. about his care, how will you explain the rationale for these orders?

6. In reviewing E.B.'s medical history, what factors do you notice that might affect the condition of his residual limb and ultimate rehabilitation potential?

CASE STUDY PROGRESS

You have just returned from a 2-day workshop on guidelines for the care of surgical patients with type 1 DM. You notice that E.B.'s daily fasting blood glucose has been running between 130 and 180 mg/dL. The sliding scale insulin intervention does not begin until blood glucose values equal to or greater than 200 mg/dL are reported. You recognize that patients with blood glucose values even slightly above normal levels experience impaired wound healing. However, you also recognize that the risks related to hypoglycemia, such as falls, might outweigh the risk of impaired healing from elevated glucose levels.

7. Identify four interventions that would facilitate timely healing of E.B.'s residual limb.

8. What should the postoperative assessment of E.B.'s residual limb dressing include?

9. You are reviewing the plan of care for E.B. Which of these care activities can be safely delegated to the nursing assistive personnel (NAP)? Select all that apply.
   a. Rewrapping the residual limb bandage
   b. Checking E.B.'s vital signs
   c. Assessing E.B.'s IV insertion site
   d. Assisting E.B. with repositioning in the bed
   e. Asking E.B. to report his level of pain on a 1-to-10 scale

10. On the evening of the first postoperative day, E.B. becomes more awake and begins to complain of pain. He states, "My right leg is really hurting; how can it hurt so bad if it's gone?" What is your best response?
    a. "That is a side effect of the medication."
    b. "You can't be feeling that because your leg was amputated."
    c. "Don't worry, that sensation will go away in a few days."
    d. "Are you able to rate that pain on a scale of 1 to 10?"

11. What is causing E.B.'s pain?

3 Musculoskeletal Disorders

CASE STUDY PROGRESS

The case manager is contacted for discharge planning. E.B. will be discharged to an extended care facility for strength training. Once the patient receives his prosthesis, he will receive balance training. After that, he will be discharged to his daughter's home. A physical therapy and occupational therapy home evaluation should be ordered. You have provided several sessions of teaching to E.B. and his daughter about care of the residual limb.

12. Which of these statements by E.B. reflects a need for further instruction?
    a. "I will inspect my limb daily for signs of skin irritation and infection, such as redness, drainage, and odor."
    b. "I will wash my limb every night with warm water and a bacteriostatic soap and dry it gently, allowing it to air dry for 20 minutes."
    c. "I will apply a mild lotion to my limb twice a day."
    d. "I will perform range-of-motion exercises to all my joints daily."

 13. What instructions should be given to E.B.'s daughter concerning safety around the home?

CASE STUDY OUTCOME

E.B. makes a smooth transition from the hospital to the rehabilitation facility and then to the daughter's home. He was never able to adapt to independent living, so he eventually moved into his daughter's home.

Case Study **41**

Name _____   Class/Group _____   Date _____

Group Members _____

▶ Scenario

J.T. has injured his hand at work and is accompanied to the emergency department (ED) by a co-worker. You examine his left hand and find a piece of a drill bit sticking out of the skin between the third and fourth knuckles. There is another puncture site about an inch below and toward the center of the hand. Bleeding is minimal. J.T. is 41 years old and has no significant medical history. He states the accident occurred when a mill at work malfunctioned and knocked his hand onto a rack of drill bits. His last tetanus booster was 12 years ago. It is your job to provide the initial care for J.T.'s injury.

1. You examine J.T.'s hand. What is the priority action? What should you include in your initial assessment, and why?

CASE STUDY PROGRESS

You record that J.T.'s fingers are warm with capillary refill in less than 2 seconds. Sensory perception is intact. He is able to flex and extend the distal joints but not the proximal joints of the third and fourth fingers. He rates his pain as a 5 out of 10.

2. You notice J.T.'s wedding band and promptly ask him to remove it. Why is this important?

3. J.T. asks you why the doctor can't just pull the bit out and then he can go home. How should you respond to his question?

4. What common diagnostic test will identify fractures and the location of metal fragments in J.T.'s hand?

3 Musculoskeletal Disorders

CASE STUDY PROGRESS

The drill bit is impaled ½ inch below the surface of the skin, and there are no fractures. Because the hand contains so many blood vessels, nerves, ligaments, and tendons, the ED physician decides to consult a surgical hand specialist. A neurologic consultation reveals that there is no nerve damage. The surgeon suspects tendon damage and decides to operate immediately.

5. You accompany the surgeon to J.T.'s bedside and listen to the explanation of the surgery, and then you witness J.T. signing the surgical consent form. List at least eight interventions needed to prepare J.T. for immediate surgery.

6. How will you verify that he understands about the surgical procedure?

7. You record that J.T. has had no food "since 8:00 PM yesterday" and drank "some water" this morning. Based on this information, do you anticipate problems during surgery, and why?

8. Does J.T. need a tetanus booster? If so, will he receive a Td or Tdap? Explain your answer, based on the latest Centers for Disease Control and Prevention (CDC) guidelines.

CASE STUDY PROGRESS

The surgeon repairs two partially severed tendons and wraps the hand in a large padded dressing. The distal ½ inch of each digit protrudes from the bulky dressing.

9. While in the short-stay recovery area, J.T. asks the nurse why his fingers look yellowish brown. How should the nurse respond to his question?

10. How will you assess his hand after the surgery?

CASE STUDY PROGRESS

The surgeon tells J.T. that he had to repair tendons in his third and fourth fingers and instructs J.T. that he is not to work until approval is given after he has been reevaluated. He gives J.T. prescriptions for ceftazidime (Ceptaz) and naproxen (Naprosyn). He instructs J.T. to make an appointment to see him in the surgery clinic in 2 days. The nurse provides patient teaching about the purpose of these medications, as well as how to take them and possible side effects.

11. Which statement by J.T. indicates that further teaching about the medications is needed?
    a. "I need to take these pills on an empty stomach."
    b. "I won't stop taking these until the prescription is finished."
    c. "I will not drink alcohol or take over-the-counter medicines while on these drugs."
    d. "I will call my doctor if I notice a rash, diarrhea, or increased bruising."

12. What additional instructions should the nurse in the short-stay area discuss with J.T. and his wife before releasing him?

13. J.T. says, "How in the world is the ice supposed to keep my hand cold with this big bandage on it?" How will the nurse reply?

3 Musculoskeletal Disorders

14. J.T. says, "I'll be able to keep my hand up when I'm awake, but what about when I go to sleep?" What suggestion can the nurse make to help J.T. comply with the instructions?

CASE STUDY OUTCOME

J.T.'s recovery is uncomplicated; he receives follow-up physical and occupational therapy as an outpatient and regains the full use of his hand.

Gastrointestinal Disorders

Case Study 42

Name _____ Class/Group _____ Date _____

Group Members _____

▶ Scenario

T.H., a 57-year-old stockbroker, has come to the gastroenterologist for treatment of recurrent mild to severe cramping in his abdomen and blood-streaked stool. You are the registered nurse doing his initial workup. Your findings include a mildly obese man who demonstrates moderate guarding of his abdomen with both direct and rebound tenderness, especially in the left lower quadrant (LLQ). His vital signs are 168/98, 110, 24, 100.4° F (38° C); he is slightly diaphoretic. T.H. reports that he has periodic constipation. He has had previous episodes of abdominal cramping, but this time the pain is getting worse.

Past medical history reveals that T.H. has a "sedentary job with lots of emotional moments," he has smoked a pack of cigarettes a day for 30 years, and he had "two or three mixed drinks in the evening" until 2 months ago. He states, "I haven't had anything to drink in 2 months." He denies having regular exercise: "just no time." His diet consists mostly of "white bread, meat, potatoes, and ice cream with fruit and nuts over it." He denies having a history of cardiac or pulmonary problems and has no personal history of cancer, although his father and older brother died of colon cancer. He takes no medications and denies the use of any other drugs or herbal products.

1. Identify four general health risk problems that T.H. exhibits.

2. Identify a key factor in his family history that might have profound implications for his health and present state of mind.

3. Identify three key findings on his physical examination, and indicate their significance.

CASE STUDY PROGRESS

The physician ordered a KUB (x-ray study of the kidneys, ureters, and bladder), complete blood count (CBC), and complete metabolic profile. Based on x-ray and laboratory findings, physical examination findings, and history, the physician diagnoses T.H. as having acute diverticulitis and discusses an outpatient treatment plan with him.

4. What is diverticulitis? What are the consequences of untreated diverticulitis?

5. While the patient is experiencing the severe crampy pain of acute diverticulitis, what interventions would you perform to help him feel more comfortable?

6. What is the rationale for ordering bed rest?

CASE STUDY PROGRESS

T.H. is being sent home with prescriptions for metronidazole (Flagyl) 500 mg PO q6h, ciprofloxacin (Cipro) 500 mg PO q12h, and dicyclomine (Bentyl) 20 mg qid PO×5 days.

7. For each medication, state the drug class and the purpose for T.H.

8. Given his history, what questions must you ask T.H. before he takes the initial dose of metronidazole? State your rationale.

- Stop all aspirin (ASA) and over-the-counter (OTC) or herbal pain relief medications (ibuprofen, naproxen, and so on).
- Stop or limit alcohol intake and smoking.

13. Why does the patient need to take the pantoprazole first thing in the morning?

14. After discussing lifestyle modifications for controlling acid reflux with M.R., which statement by M.R. indicates a further need for teaching?
   a. "I will try to stop smoking."
   b. "I will wait 30 minutes before lying down or sitting in my recliner after meals."
   c. "I will avoid fatty foods, caffeine, and chocolate."
   d. "I will avoid eating 2 to 3 hours before my bedtime."

CASE STUDY OUTCOME

M.R. goes home and vows to stop smoking and take better care of himself. He calls his primary care physician to schedule a sleep study because of his snoring and cuts back his working hours.

4 Gastrointestinal Disorders

Case Study 45

Name _____ Class/Group _____ Date _____

Group Members _____

▶ Scenario

While as a nurse on a gastrointestinal (GI) unit, you receive a call from an affiliate outpatient clinic notifying you of a direct admission with an estimated time of arrival of 60 minutes. The clinic nurse gives you the following information: A.G. is an 82-year-old woman with a 3-day history of intermittent abdominal pain, abdominal bloating, and nausea and vomiting (N/V). A.G. moved from Italy to join her grandson and his family only 2 months ago, and she speaks very little English. All information was obtained through her grandson. Past medical history includes colectomy for colon cancer 6 years ago and ventral hernia repair 2 years ago. She has no history of coronary artery disease, diabetes mellitus, or pulmonary disease. She takes only ibuprofen (Motrin) occasionally for mild arthritis. Allergies include sulfa drugs and meperidine. A.G.'s tentative diagnosis is small bowel obstruction (SBO) secondary to adhesions. A.G. is being admitted to your floor for diagnostic workup. Her vital signs (VS) are stable, she is receiving an intravenous (IV) infusion of D5 ½ NS with 20 mEq KCl at 100 mL/hr, and 2 L oxygen by nasal cannula.

1. Based on the nurse's report, what signs of bowel obstruction does A.G. manifest?

2. Are there other signs and symptoms that you should observe for while A.G. is in your care?

3. While A.G. is on the way, you secure the hospital's interpreter service on the telephone. A.G. arrives on your unit with her grandson. You admit A.G. to her room and introduce yourself as her nurse. As her grandson introduces her, she pats your hand. You know that you need to complete a physical examination and take a history. What will you do first?

4. Before you begin your examination, the grandson, an attorney, tells you that elderly Italian women are extremely modest and might not answer questions completely. He indicates that he'd like to stay in the room during the examination. How will you proceed?

5. What key questions must you ask this patient while you have the use of an interpreter?

6. For each characteristic listed, specify whether it is a characteristic of small-bowel obstruction (SBO), large bowel obstruction (LBO), or both (B).

_____ a. Intermittent lower abdominal cramping

_____ b. Abdominal discomfort or pain accompanied by visible peristaltic waves in the upper and middle abdomen

_____ c. Upper or epigastric abdominal distention

_____ d. Distention in the lower abdomen

_____ e. Obstipation

_____ f. Ribbon-like stools

_____ g. Nausea and early, profuse vomiting, which may contain fecal material

_____ h. Minimal or no vomiting

_____ i. Severe fluid and electrolyte imbalances

7. What is obstipation?

8. During your examination, you note that she does not have muscle guarding and rebound tenderness on palpation. Is this important? Explain your answer.

CASE STUDY PROGRESS

The physician orders the insertion of a Salem Sump nasogastric tube (NGT). You insert the NGT into A.G. and connect it to intermittent low wall suction.

 9. How will you check for placement of the NGT?

10. List, in order, the structures through which the NGT must pass as it is inserted.

11. A.G.'s grandson asks you, "What is that blue thing at the end of the tube? Shouldn't it be connected to something?" How do you answer?

12. What comfort measures are important for A.G. while she has an NGT?

13. You note that A.G.'s NGT has not drained in the last 3 hours. What can you do to facilitate drainage?

14. The NGT suddenly drains 575 mL; then drainage slows down to about 250 mL over 2 hours. Is this an expected amount?

15. You enter A.G.'s room to initiate your shift assessment. A.G.'s abdomen seems to be more distended than yesterday. How would you determine whether A.G.'s abdominal distention has changed?

CASE STUDY PROGRESS

After 24 hours, A.G.'s symptoms are unrelieved. She reports continued nausea, cramps, and sometimes strong abdominal pain; her hand grips are weaker; and she seems to be increasingly lethargic. You look up her latest laboratory values and compare them with the admission data.

Chart View

Laboratory Test Results

Test	Admission	Hospital Day 3
Sodium	136 mEq/L	130 mEq/L
Potassium	3.7 mEq/L	2.5 mEq/L
Chloride	108 mEq/L	97 mEq/L
Carbon dioxide	25 mEq/L	31 mEq/L
BUN	19 mg/dL	38 mg/dL
Creatinine	1 mg/dL	2.2 mg/dL
Glucose	126 mg/dL	65 mg/dL
Albumin	3.0 g/dL	3.1 g/dL
Protein	6.8 g/dL	4.9 g/dL

16. Which laboratory values are of concern to you? Why?

17. What measures do you anticipate to correct in each of the imbalances described in Question 16?

CASE STUDY OUTCOME

In view of A.G.'s continued deterioration, the surgeon meets with the patient and her family and they agree to surgery. The surgeon releases an 18-inch section of proximal ileum that had been constricted by adhesions. Several areas look ischemic, so these are excised, and an end-to-end anastomosis is done. A.G. tolerates the procedure well. Her recovery is slow but steady. A.G. goes home in the care of her grandson and his wife on the seventh postoperative day. Discharge plans include a home health nurse, home health aide, in-home physical therapy, and dietitian consultation. The grandson is included in the plans.

4 Gastrointestinal Disorders

Case Study 46

Name _____ Class/Group _____ Date _____

Group Members _____

▶ Scenario

P.M., a 24-year-old house painter, has been too ill to work for the past 3 days. When he arrives at your outpatient clinic with his girlfriend, he seems alert but acutely ill, with an average build and a deep tan over the exposed areas of skin. He reports headaches, joint pain, a low-grade fever, cough, anorexia, and nausea and vomiting (N/V), especially after eating any fatty food. P.M. describes vague abdominal pain that started about the same time as the other problems. He states that he has been using "a lot of Tylenol" for his pain. His past medical history reveals he has no health problems, is a nonsmoker, and drinks "a few" beers each evening to relax. Vital signs are 128/84, 88, 26, 100.6°F (38.1°C); awake, alert, and oriented×3; moves all extremities well with complaints of aching pain in his muscles; very slight scleral jaundice present; heart and breath sounds clear and without adventitious sounds; bowel sounds clear throughout abdomen and pelvis; and abdomen soft and palpable without distinct masses. You note moderate hepatomegaly measured at the midclavicular line; liver edge is easily palpated and tender to palpation. P.M. mentions that his urine has been getting darker over the past 2 days.

1. Your institution uses electronic charting. Based on the health history and assessment described in the scenario, which of the following systems would you mark as "abnormal" as you document your findings? Mark abnormal findings with an X and provide a brief narrative.
   X Abnormal

   ☐ Neurologic:
   ☐ Respiratory:
   ☐ Cardiovascular:
   ☐ Gastrointestinal:
   ☐ Genitourinary:
   ☐ Musculoskeletal:
   ☐ Skin:
   ☐ Pain:

CASE STUDY PROGRESS

P.M. is manifesting key signs of hepatitis. Laboratory work is requested for identification of his precise problem.

2. Which key diagnostic tests will determine exactly what type of hepatitis is present?

Chart View

Laboratory Test Results

Sodium	140 mEq/L
Potassium	3.9 mEq/L
Chloride	102 mEq/L
CO_2	26 mEq/L
BUN	10 mg/dL
Creatinine	1.0 mg/dL
Platelets	210,000/mm³
Indirect bilirubin	1.6 mg/dL
Total bilirubin	2.3 mg/dL
Albumin	3.8 g/dL
Total protein	6.5 g/dL
ALT	66 units/L
AST	52 units/L
LDH	245 units/L
ALP	176 units/L
PT/INR	12 sec/1.06
aPTT	32 sec
Urine urobilinogen	1.6 IU/L
Anti-HAV	Negative
IgM	Negative
HBsAg	Positive

3. Which of P.M.'s laboratory results specifically indicates liver disease?

4. What is the difference between the hepatitis B surface antigen (HBsAg) and the hepatitis B surface antibody (HBsAb)?

5. What factors in his history could have compounded the increased ALT levels?

6. Considering the basic pathology of hepatitis, what type of diet will you strongly encourage P.M. to follow?

7. For each characteristic below, identify whether it describes hepatitis A *(A)* or hepatitis B *(B).*
   _____ a. Fecal-oral transmission.
   _____ b. Transmitted by sharing needles.
   _____ c. Transmitted by blood transfusions.
   _____ d. Vaccination is a three-shot series.
   _____ e. Illness is usually mild, similar to a flulike infection.
   _____ f. Symptoms include anorexia, nausea, vomiting, fever, fatigue, and jaundice.

8. In P.M.'s case, the HBsAg is positive. This result indicates that P.M. is infected with hepatitis B and is in the acute period of the disease. Is this disease contagious? What precautions would you take while he is in the hospital?

9. Pruritus is usually associated with jaundice. What will you do to ease this problem for P.M.? Name five interventions.

10. How will you explain to P.M. the likely progression of his disease?

11. P.M. is living at home with his parents and four younger siblings. The youngest is 4 years old. His parents ask how to prevent the rest of the family from getting hepatitis. What specific instructions will you give?

12. How will you know that these instructions are understood?

13. Given P.M.'s lifestyle, what specific patient teaching points must you emphasize?

CASE STUDY PROGRESS

P.M. is ready for discharge in a few days, and he confides to you that he feels so "guilty" about having hepatitis and endangering his girlfriend and family. He tells you he was at a party and did not think the one-time needle use could hurt him. He has lost his job because he is not able to go back to work and he hopes his family is not too afraid to have him return home.

14. What action will you take?

Case Study 47

Name _____   Class/Group _____   Date _____

Group Members _____

▶ Scenario

John Doe, approximately 50 years old, is admitted to your unit for observation from the emergency department (ED) with the diagnosis of rule out hepatic encephalopathy with acute alcohol (ETOH) intoxication. This man was sent to the ED by local police, who found him lying unresponsive along a rural road.

Examination and x-ray studies are negative for any injury and you are awaiting the results of the blood alcohol level (BAL) and toxicology tests. He has no identification and is not awake or coherent enough to give any history or to answer questions. He is lethargic, has a cachectic appearance, does not follow commands consistently, and is mildly combative when aroused. He smells strongly of ETOH and has a notably distended abdomen and edematous lower extremities. He has a Foley catheter and is receiving an intravenous (IV) infusion of D5 ½ NS with 20 mEq KCl and 1 ampule of multivitamins at 75 mL/hr.

Admitting orders are shown in the chart.

Chart View

Admission Orders

IV D5 ½ NS with 20 mEq KCl at 75 mL/hr; add 1 ampule multivitamins to 1 L of IV fluid per day

Insert Salem Sump nasogastric tube and attach to low continuous suction

Insert Foley catheter to gravity drainage

Elevate HOB at 30 to 45 degrees at all times

Check all stools for occult blood

Lactulose (Cephulac) 45 mL PO qid. Call if diarrhea develops

Abdominal ultrasound in AM

Vitamin K (AquaMEPHYTON) 10 mg/day IV × 3 doses; change to PO when alert and able to swallow

Vitamin B_1/thiamine 100 mg/day IV; change to PO when alert and able to swallow

Vitamin B_9/folic acid 0.4 mg/day IM

Vitamin B_6/pyridoxine 100 mg/day PO

Labs: CBC with differential, BMP, liver function tests (LFTs), PT/INR and aPTT, serum ammonia (NH_3) now and in AM

Once patient is alert and able to swallow, may have low-protein diet. Observe for any difficulty swallowing, and offer assistance with meals if needed.

Call house officer for any sign of gastrointestinal (GI) bleed; delirium tremens (DTs); systolic blood pressure (BP) over 140 or less than 100 mm Hg; diastolic BP less than 50 mm Hg; or pulse over 120 beats/min.

1. What do you need to do for John Doe, and what can you delegate to the nursing assistive personnel (NAP)?

2. Of all the vitamins ordered, which should be given immediately? Explain your answer.

3. Some of the lab work drawn in the ED has come back. The BAL is 320 mg/dL, and the blood ammonia (NH_3) level is 155 mcg/dL. His total protein is 5.2 g/dL and albumin is 2.1 g/dL. What do these values indicate?

4. Which of the ordered medications will alter the ammonia levels, and how?

5. Why are so many different vitamins ordered for John Doe?

CASE STUDY PROGRESS

While you are getting John Doe settled, you continue your assessment.

Neurologic findings: PERRL (*Pupils Equal, Round, Reactive to Light*), moves all extremities, but patient is sluggish, pulling away during assessment, and follows commands sporadically.

Cerebrovascular findings: Pulse is regular without adventitious sounds. All peripheral pulses are palpable at 3+ bilaterally; 3+ pitting edema in lower extremities.

Respiratory assessment: Breath sounds decreased to all lobes, no adventitious sounds audible, patient not cooperating with cough and deep breathing, and Spo$_2$ at 90% on room air.

Gastrointestinal (GI) assessment: Tongue and gums are beefy red and swollen, abdomen is enlarged and protuberant, and abdominal skin is taut and slightly tender to palpation. Salem Sump NGT is patent, connected to LCS with small to moderate greenish drainage; bowel sounds positive with NGT clamped.

Genitourinary (GU) assessment: Foley to gravity drainage, with 75 mL dark amber urine past 2 hours.

Skin: Pale on torso and lower extremities; heavily sunburned on upper extremities and head. Skin appears thin and dry. Numerous spider angiomas are found on the upper abdomen with several dilated veins across abdomen.

Vital signs: 120/60, 104, 32, 99.1° F (37.3° C).

6. What is the significance of the spider angiomas, dilated abdominal veins, peripheral edema, and distended abdomen?

7. How would you further assess the distended abdomen, and what is the clinical name for your findings?

8. Name at least three concerns you have about John Doe's nutritional status.

9. What are your objective findings regarding his nutritional assessment?

10. If his protein levels are so low, why isn't John Doe on a high-protein diet?

4 Gastrointestinal Disorders

11. What is a priority intervention regarding his nutritional status?

CASE STUDY PROGRESS

You continue your assessment and implementation of the admission orders. Another nurse comes to help you and states, "Why are we wasting time with this wino? He isn't worth the time or money. Why don't they let him die?"

12. How might you respond to this nurse's remarks?

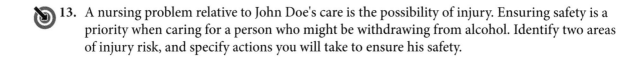 **13.** A nursing problem relative to John Doe's care is the possibility of injury. Ensuring safety is a priority when caring for a person who might be withdrawing from alcohol. Identify two areas of injury risk, and specify actions you will take to ensure his safety.

14. You monitor John Doe for signs and symptoms of alcohol withdrawal and DTs. So far he is restless, has tremors, and has a low-grade fever. Which of the symptoms listed are symptoms of the more severe DTs? Select all that apply.
a. GI bleeding
b. Hallucinations
c. Hypotension
d. Somnolence
e. Extreme diaphoresis
f. Tachycardia
g. Vomiting

15. Falls are particularly dangerous for someone in this patient's situation. Why?

CASE STUDY PROGRESS

During John Doe's hospitalization, a staff psychiatrist evaluates him for mental decline associated with alcohol abuse and dependence, including Korsakoff's psychosis.

16. For each effect of chronic alcohol abuse listed, mark *W* if it is associated with Wernicke's encephalopathy and *K* if it is associated with Korsakoff's psychosis.

_____a. Confusion

_____b. Nystagmus

_____c. Confabulation

_____d. Ataxia

_____e. Inability to learn

_____f. Short-term memory loss

CASE STUDY PROGRESS

John Doe survives a rocky course of hepatic encephalopathy and near–renal failure. After 27 days, including a week in the intensive care unit (ICU), he is discharged to a drug and alcohol rehabilitation facility. He is employed as a longshoreman; fortunately, his insurance covers his month of in-house intense rehabilitation.

Case Study **48**

Name _____ Class/Group _____ Date _____

Group Members _____

▶ Scenario

C.W., a 36-year-old woman, was admitted several days ago with a diagnosis of recurrent inflammatory bowel disease (IBD) and possible small bowel obstruction (SBO). C.W. is married, and her husband and 11-year-old son are supportive, but she has no extended family in the state. She has had IBD for 15 years and has been taking mesalamine (Asacol) for 15 years and prednisone 40 mg/day for the past 5 years. She is very thin; at 5 feet 2 inches, she weighs 86 pounds and has lost 40 pounds over the past 10 years. She averages 5 to 10 loose stools per day. C.W.'s life has gradually become dominated by her disease, with anorexia, lactase deficiency, profound fatigue, frequent nausea and diarrhea, frequent hospitalizations for dehydration, and recurring, crippling abdominal pain that often strikes unexpectedly. The pain is incapacitating and relieved only by a small dose of diazepam (Valium), oral electrolyte solution (Pedialyte), and total bed rest. She confides in you that sexual activity is difficult: "It always causes diarrhea, nausea, and lots of pain. It's difficult for both of us." She is so weak she cannot stand without help. You indicate complete bed rest on the nursing care plan.

1. Identify six priority problems for C.W.

2. Considering C.W.'s weakness, chronic diarrhea, and lower-than-desired body weight, what nursing interventions need to be implemented to minimize skin breakdown? Name at least six.

3. What is the mechanism of action of the mesalamine (Asacol) in relation to the IBD?
   a. It increases bulk and moisture content in the stool.
   b. It blocks prostaglandin production, thus diminishing inflammation in the colon.
   c. It slows intestinal motility, prolonging transit time of intestinal contents.
   d. It relaxes the smooth muscle of the intestines, thus reducing motility.

CASE STUDY PROGRESS

C.W.'s condition deteriorates; on the third day after admission she experiences intractable abdominal pain and unrelenting nausea and vomiting. C.W. is taken to the operating room because of probable SBO and is readmitted to your unit from the postanesthesia care unit. During surgery, 38 inches of her small bowel were found to be severely stenosed with two areas of visible perforation. Much of the remaining bowel is severely inflamed and friable. A total of 5 feet of distal ileum and 2 feet of colon have been removed, and a temporary ileostomy was established. She has a Jackson-Pratt (JP) drain to bulb suction in her right lower quadrant (RLQ), and her wound was packed and left open. She has two peripheral IVs, a Salem Sump nasogastric tube (NGT), and a Foley catheter. Her vital signs (VS) are 112/72, 86, 24, 100.8° F (38.2° C) (tympanic). You attach her NGT to low-continuous wall suction per the postoperative orders.

4. You begin a thorough postoperative assessment of C.W.'s abdomen. What does your assessment include? List the steps in the order in which the assessment should be completed.

5. A nursing student enters C.W.'s room and auscultates her abdomen. She looks at you and excitedly announces that she hears good bowel sounds. You take the opportunity to teach her the proper method of auscultating bowel sounds on a patient who has NGT to low-continuous wall suction. How would you correct her error?

6. Four hours later, you measure the drainage from the JP tube. Look at the following figure and state how much drainage you obtained.

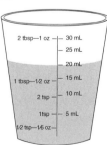

7. What else will you note about the drainage?

8. Describe the proper method for reestablishing suction on the JP drain after you have emptied the bulb container.

9. C.W. asks you, "I know why I have the pouch. Why do I have to have this other little tube?" How will you explain the purpose of the JP drain?

CASE STUDY PROGRESS

It is 4 days after C.W.'s surgery. During the routine dressing change, you note a small pool of yellow-green drainage in the deepest part of the wound. You obtain an order for a wound culture.

10. How will you obtain a culture specimen from C.W.'s wound?

11. What information do you need to send to the laboratory with the wound culture specimen?

12. You obtain a wound culture specimen, complete the dressing change, obtain a full set of VS, note a temperature of 100.4° F (38° C), and assess increased tenderness in C.W.'s abdomen. What orders do you anticipate receiving once you notify the physician of C.W.'s condition?

13. The physician calls back and asks you to describe C.W.'s wound. What key aspects of the wound should be included?

14. As you assess C.W.'s stoma and drainage, what would indicate that they are healthy? Select all that apply.
    a. The stoma will be in the shape of a donut.
    b. The stoma will be level with the skin.
    c. The stoma will be a uniform medium cherry red in color.
    d. The stoma will be light pink, and an occasional dark spot might appear.
    e. The skin around the stoma should be intact.
    f. The drainage will be thick and dark brown in color.

15. Will any aspect of C.W.'s history significantly affect the wound healing process? If so, how?

16. With a fairly significant wound infection developing, why is C.W.'s temperature relatively low?

17. The physician tells you she will be over to examine C.W. As you tell C.W. that her doctor is coming to talk to her, C.W. says that she feels something wet running down her side. You find some leakage of intestinal drainage onto the skin. What should you do?

CASE STUDY OUTCOME

You change the ileostomy appliance before the physician arrives. C.W. is evaluated, and it is determined that she needs to return to surgery for exploratory laparotomy.

Case Study 49

Name _____   Class/Group _____   Date _____

Group Members _____

▶ Scenario (Continuation of Case Study 48)

C.W. is a 36-year-old woman admitted 7 days ago with inflammatory bowel disease (IBD) with small bowel obstruction (SBO). She underwent surgery 3 days after admission for a colectomy and ileostomy. She developed peritonitis and, 4 days later, returned to the operating room (OR) for an exploratory laparotomy, which revealed another area of perforated bowel, generalized peritonitis, and a fistula tract to the abdominal surface. Another 12 inches of ileum were resected (total of 7 feet of ileum and 2 feet of colon). The peritoneal cavity was irrigated with normal saline (NS), and three drainage tubes were placed: a Jackson-Pratt (JP) drain to bulb suction, a rubber catheter to irrigate the wound bed with NS, and a sump drain to remove the irrigation. The initial JP drain remains in place. A right subclavian triple-lumen catheter was inserted.

1. You have received report from the postanesthesia recovery unit (PACU) nurse, and C.W. returns during your shift. What do you do when she is in the bed in her room?

2. You pull the covers back to inspect the abdominal dressing and find that the original surgical dressing is saturated with fresh bloody drainage. What are the priority actions?

3. C.W. has a total of four tubes in her abdomen, as well as a nasogastric tube (NGT). What information do you want to know about each tube?

4. The sump irrigation fluid bag is nearly empty. You close the roller clamp, thread the IV tubing through the infusion pump, check the irrigation catheter connection site to make certain it is snug, and then discover that the nearly empty liter bag infusing into C.W.'s abdomen is D5W, not NS. Does this require any action? If so, give a rationale for actions, and explain the overall situation.

CASE STUDY PROGRESS

The surgeon arrives on the unit and removes C.W.'s surgical dressing. There is a small "bleeder" at the edge of the incision, so the surgeon calls for a suture and ties off the bleeder. C.W. is waking up and complaining of pain. You take the opportunity to ask the surgeon about an opioid via a patient-controlled analgesia (PCA) pump for C.W.; she says she will write the orders.

5. Postoperative pain will be a problem for C.W. after the anesthesia wears off. How do you plan to address this?

6. C.W. is still experiencing pain from the peritonitis as well as from the surgical incision. Which position may help to make her more comfortable?
   a. Supine with legs extended
   b. Head of bed slightly elevated, with knees flexed
   c. Lying on her left side
   d. Lying on her right side

CASE STUDY PROGRESS

C.W. has been on nothing by mouth (NPO) status since the surgery. The attending physician orders total parenteral nutrition (TPN) at a rate of 50 mL/hr.

7. What is the purpose of these orders?

8. Pharmacy delivers C.W.'s first bag of TPN. You have an order to stop the maintenance IV infusion after starting the TPN. What is the purpose of this order?

9. The attending physician orders glucose monitoring every 6 hours with sliding scale insulin coverage. What is the rationale for this order?

10. During the night shift the TPN solution bag becomes nearly empty, and the night nurse discovers that the next bag of TPN has not been prepared. The hospital pharmacy does not prepare TPN during the night shift. What does the nurse need to do next?
    a. Convert the line to a saline lock until the TPN solution is ready.
    b. Slow the TPN rate to 10 mL/hr until the next TPN bag can be prepared.
    c. Hang a bag of D5W when the TPN is finished.
    d. Hang a bag of D10W when the TPN is finished.

4 Gastrointestinal Disorders

CASE STUDY PROGRESS

You discuss your concerns about C.W.'s nutritional status with C.W.'s surgeon and she agrees to request a consultation from a registered dietitian (RD). After gathering data and making several calculations, the RD makes recommendations to the attending physician. The TPN orders are adjusted, C.W. begins to gain weight slowly, and her wound shows signs of healing.

11. You and a co-worker read the following in C.W.'s progress notes: "Wound healing by secondary closure. Formation of granular tissue with epithelialization noted around edges. Have requested dietitian consult on ongoing basis. Will continue to follow." Your co-worker turns to you and asks whether you know what that means. How would you explain?

12. Both of you start to discuss what specific digestive difficulties C.W. is likely to face in the future. What problems might C.W. be prone to develop after having so much of her bowel removed?

13. The RD consults with C.W. about dietary needs. You attend the session so that you will be able to reinforce the information. What basic information is the RD likely to discuss with C.W.?

14. After 3 days of dressing changes, C.W.'s skin is irritated, and a small skin tear has appeared where tape was removed. How can you minimize this type of skin breakdown and help this area heal?

15. What specifics of ostomy teaching do you plan to do?

CASE STUDY OUTCOME

C.W. is successful in her battle with peritonitis. Gradually tubes are removed as she grows stronger with TPN and time. C.W. learns how to change her ostomy appliance and is discharged to home.

Case Study **50**

Name _____ Class/Group _____ Date _____

Group Members _____

▶ Scenario

You are a nurse working on a surgical unit and take the following report from the registered nurse in the emergency department. "We are sending you a patient with rule out small bowel obstruction and/or food blockage. Dr. N., the gastrointestinal specialist, is on his way in to see the patient. D.S. is a 78-year-old obese man with complaints of sudden onset of severe abdominal cramping, distention, and nausea and vomiting; he denies passing of flatus or stool within the past 12 hours. Past medical history includes heart failure, hypertension, colon cancer, and ulcerative colitis. He underwent a total colectomy 16 years ago and had an enterocutaneous fistula 12 years ago. Laboratory samples have been drawn, and the results will be sent to your floor. We started an IV and placed a Salem Sump nasogastric tube (NGT). His vital signs are 143/76, 82, respirations 26 and slightly labored, and 101.1° F (38.4° C). He is on his way up."

1. Given that D.S. had had a total colectomy, would he have a colostomy or an ileostomy? Explain your answer.

2. What would you expect to see if D.S.'s ostomy has normal function?

CASE STUDY PROGRESS

After D.S. is settled into his room, the NGT and IV line are functioning well, and he receives pain medication, you begin your admission assessment. His abdomen is extremely large, firm to touch, with multiple scars and an ileostomy pouching system in his right lower quadrant (RLQ).

3. Describe the common complications of an ileostomy.

4. D.S.'s past medical history (PMH) of fistula, combined with the probability of blockage or obstruction, places him at an increased risk for which problems?

5. As you assess the stoma, you look for signs that it is healthy. Which of these assessment findings are the characteristics of a healthy stoma? Select all that apply.
   a. The stoma is cherry-red to dark pink in color.
   b. The stoma is pale pink in color.
   c. The stoma is moist.
   d. The stoma is dry.
   e. The stoma is flat against the skin.

6. What stoma changes would you report immediately to the physician? Name at least four.

7. Why are transparent ostomy pouches recommended for postoperative patients or for patients who are hospitalized?

8. Will the stoma present visual clues of D.S.'s bowel blockage or obstruction?

CASE STUDY PROGRESS

D.S. continues to complain of abdominal pain and cramping and becomes increasingly restless. You notice that the abdomen behind and around his stoma and pouch appears larger when compared with the other side of his abdomen.

9. How would you assess for a possible peristomal hernia?

10. Why is a peristomal hernia a problem?

CASE STUDY PROGRESS

You note the ostomy pouch has liquid brown effluent along the lateral edge of the wafer. You check to see that the pouch is properly attached to the wafer and discover that stool is indeed leaking from under the barrier. D.S. apologizes for not bringing any supplies with him, stating, "My ostomy nurse told me to always carry extra supplies for times like this." D.S. does not remember what size he needs; you note he is wearing a two-piece system with a plastic ring-flange that attaches to the pouch with a matching ring.

11. How will you determine the correct pouching size and system?

CASE STUDY PROGRESS

You finish your general head-to-toe assessment and order the appropriate pouching products for D.S. You take clean towels, washcloths, and underpads into his room, along with a hamper to receive dirty, used laundry. You gather scissors, Skin-Prep, and adhesive remover to assist with the pouching change.

12. As you return to his room, you review the steps for changing an ostomy pouch. What are the steps you will need to follow?

CASE STUDY PROGRESS

You have gathered all needed supplies, and D.S. is as comfortable as possible. You begin the pouching change. Using the adhesive remover, with the push-pull method, you gently remove the wafer. As you lift the wafer, you note that the peristomal skin has severe erythema directly encircling the stoma. There is denudation (partial-thickness breakdown) at the medial stoma-skin edge.

13. How should the skin around the stoma look?

14. In general, there are four different causes of erythema or skin breakdown. Identify two.

15. After you discover the reddened skin, how will you proceed with the ostomy care?

16. As you clean the site, D.S. tells you, "You need to scrub that with strong soap! It's dirty!" How do you reply to D.S.?

CASE STUDY PROGRESS

The next day, D.S.'s vital signs return to normal and his abdomen is less distended. The ileostomy is steadily draining greenish-brown liquid stool. The NGT is removed and D.S. is started on sips of clear liquids. When you go to check his ileostomy pouch, D.S. tells you, "I know I've had this a long time, but I still can't stand to look at this thing. My wife usually helps me with it, and I hate that."

17. What will you suggest for D.S. at this time?

Case Study **51**

Name _____ Class/Group _____ Date _____

Group Members _____

4 Gastrointestinal Disorders

▶ **Scenario**

B.K. is a 63-year-old woman who is admitted to the step-down unit from the emergency department (ED) with nausea and vomiting (N/V) and epigastric and left upper quadrant (LUQ) abdominal pain that is severe, sharp, and boring and radiates through to her mid back. The pain started 24 hours ago and awoke her in the middle of the night. B.K. is a divorced, retired sales manager who smokes a half-pack of cigarettes daily. The ED nurse reports that B.K. is anxious and demanding. B.K. denies using alcohol. Her vital signs (VS) are as follows: 100/70, 97, 30, 100.2° F (37.9° C) (tympanic), Spo$_2$ 88% on room air and 92% on 2 L of oxygen by nasal cannula (NC). She is in normal sinus rhythm. She will be admitted to the hospitalist service. She has no primary care provider (PCP) and has not seen a physician "in years."

The ED nurse giving you the report states that the admitting diagnosis is acute pancreatitis of unknown etiology. A computed tomography (CT) scan has been ordered, but unfortunately the CT scanner is down and will not be fixed until morning. However, an ultrasound of the abdomen was performed, and "no cholelithiasis, gallbladder wall thickening, or choledocholithiasis was seen. The pancreas was not well visualized due to overlying bowel gas." Admission labs have been drawn; a clean-catch urine specimen was sent to the lab, and the urine was dark in color.

1. What are the possible causes of pancreatitis?

2. What other information do you need from the ED nurse before you assume responsibility for the patient?

3. What preparation is needed for B.K.'s CT scan?

CASE STUDY PROGRESS

You complete your admission assessment and note the following abnormalities: B.K. is restless and alert, lying on her right side in a semifetal position. Assessment findings are as follows: Skin is cool, diaphoretic, and pale with poor skin turgor; mucous membranes are dry. Heart rhythm is regular, rate 96, without murmurs or rubs. Peripheral pulses are faintly palpable in four extremities. Respiration rate 24, but unlabored on 2 L O_2/NC with Spo_2 90%. Breath sounds are absent in lower left lobe (LLL) posteriorly—otherwise, clear to auscultation throughout. She complains of nausea and is having dry heaves. Bowel sounds are hypoactive. Abdomen is distended, firm, and tender in a diffuse fashion to light palpation, with guarding noted.

4. Your institution uses electronic charting. Based on the assessment given, which of the following systems would you mark as "abnormal" as you document your findings? Mark abnormal findings with an X and provide a brief narrative.
   X Abnormal

   ☐ Neurologic
   ☐ Respiratory
   ☐ Cardiovascular
   ☐ Gastrointestinal
   ☐ Genitourinary
   ☐ Musculoskeletal
   ☐ Skin
   ☐ Psychosocial
   ☐ Pain

Chart View

Admission Laboratory Test Results

Lipase	3000 units/L
Amylase	2000 units/L
ALP	350 units/L
ALT	90 units/L
AST	150 units/L
Total bilirubin	2.0 mg/dL
Albumin	3.0 g/dL
BUN	24 mg/dL
Creatinine	1.4 mg/dL
WBC count	17,500/mm^3

5. Which specific laboratory results point to a diagnosis of pancreatitis?

6. Which laboratory results are the most important to monitor in acute pancreatitis? Why are they significant?

7. What do the BUN and creatinine tell you about her renal function and volume status?

8. Why are the WBCs elevated?

CASE STUDY PROGRESS

During your physical examination of B.K., you noted "respirations rapid, rate 24, but unlabored on 2 L O_2 per nasal cannula with Spo_2 90%. Breath sounds are absent in LLL posteriorly—otherwise, clear to auscultation throughout." The admission chest x-ray report reads, "small pleural effusion in the left lower lobe."

9. Identify three actions you could initiate to help correct this situation.

10. B.K. turns on her call light. She complains of thirst and demands something to drink. Her orders indicate "NPO, except sips and chips." What is your response to her request? What nursing action would help her complaints?

CASE STUDY PROGRESS

B.K. eventually falls asleep and seems to be sleeping peacefully. Several hours later, you hear an alarm on her pulse oximeter and enter her room to investigate. You find B.K. moaning softly; her oximeter reads 87%.

11. What will you do next?

12. B.K.'s respirations become increasingly labored, and you call the rapid response team. While waiting for the team to arrive, you continue a quick assessment, with findings as follows: Lung sounds absent in the LLL and very diminished in the right lower lobe (RLL). You percuss a dull thud over the left middle lobe (LML) and LLL up to the scapula tip. On percussion, you hear resonance over the entire right lung and left upper lobe (LUL). What is the significance of your findings?

CASE STUDY PROGRESS

The physician orders a STAT CXR examination, which shows a significant pleural effusion developing in the LLL, with extension into the RLL.

13. Based on the evolving pleural effusion with evidence of decompensation (hypoxia) by the patient, what treatment would the physician likely pursue, and what preparations would you be responsible for?

CASE STUDY PROGRESS

The physician removed 200 mL of slightly cloudy serous fluid. Antibiotics were adjusted to provide broad-spectrum coverage for an upper respiratory tract infection until culture and sensitivity results are returned. B.K. is resting quietly with oxygen at 3 L per NC, and her respirations are unlabored and regular. Her Spo_2 reads 96%.

It is now 72 hours after B.K.'s admission, and her laboratory test results show improvement. An abdominal CT scan is completed and shows "a moderately severe pancreatitis, but no local fluid collection or pseudocysts. No ileus or evidence of neoplasia was noted." BUN is 9.0 mg/dL, and creatinine is 1.0 mg/dL. She has adequate urinary output. Her IV fluids are decreased to 75 mL/hr. Her amylase and lipase levels are decreasing toward normal levels. The physician writes an order to advance B.K.'s diet to full liquids.

14. How would you know if B.K. was not able to tolerate the advancement in diet?

15. If B.K. does not tolerate the advancement in diet, what physiologic need should be addressed at 72 hours?

CASE STUDY PROGRESS

After 72 hours of hospitalization, B.K. becomes agitated with tremors, some disorientation, and auditory hallucinations. Her pulse and blood pressure are elevated, although her pain has not increased, and the pain medication schedule has not changed. B.K. has had no visitors since being admitted.

16. What is B.K. most likely experiencing, and what actions will you take?

CASE STUDY OUTCOME

You contact the physician with your observations, and he orders scheduled chlordiazepoxide (Librium) and a social services consultation to evaluate and treat for possible alcohol abuse. Three days later, B.K. is lucid and tolerating clear liquids, and her pain is controlled with oral pain medications. As she becomes oriented and calmer, B.K. eventually admits to drinking "three or four Scotch-on-the-rocks" daily. You also discover that B.K. is estranged from her family because of her drinking. The physician advances her diet to "low-fat/low-cholesterol" and writes orders to discharge that evening if she tolerates the advancement in diet, which she does.

17. What will you include in your discharge teaching with B.K.?

Genitourinary Disorders

5

Case Study 52

Name _____ Class/Group _____ Date _____

Group Members _____

▶ Scenario

You are working in an extended care facility when M.Z.'s daughter brings her mother in for a week's stay while she goes on a planned vacation. M.Z. is an 89-year-old widow with a 4-day history of nonlocalized abdominal pain, incontinence, new-onset mental confusion, and loose stools. Her most current vital signs are 118/60, 88, 18, 98.4° F (37.4° C). The medical director ordered a postvoid catheterization, which yielded 100 mL of cloudy urine that had a strong odor, and several lab tests on admission. Urine culture and sensitivity results are pending; the other results are shown in the chart.

Chart View

Laboratory Test Results

Complete metabolic panel: Within normal limits except for the following results:

BUN	25 mg/dL
Sodium	131 mEq/L
Potassium	3.2 mEq/L
White blood cell count	11,000/mm^3

Urinalysis

Appearance	Cloudy
Odor	Foul
pH	6.9
Protein	Negative
Nitrites	Positive
Crystals	Negative
WBCs	6 per low-power field
RBCs	3

1. What condition do the lab reports point toward?

2. Which assessment findings are typical of an older adult with the condition in Question 1?

3. Considering her history and laboratory results, what other condition is a possibility?

4. The medical director makes rounds and writes orders to start an IV of D$_5$½NS at 75 mL/hr and insert a Foley catheter to gravity drainage. Because M.Z. is unable to take oral medications, the medical director orders ciprofloxacin (Cipro) 400 mg q12h IV piggyback (IVPB). Are the type of fluid and rate appropriate for M.Z.'s age and condition? Explain.

5. While the IVPB ciprofloxacin is being administered, which adverse effects might occur? Select all that apply.
   a. Hypotension
   b. Headache
   c. Drowsiness
   d. Restlessness
   e. Nausea
   f. Tendon rupture

6. You enter the room to start the IV infusion and insert the Foley catheter and find that the nursing assistive personnel (NAP) has taken M.Z. to the bathroom for a bowel movement. M.Z. asks you to help her, and, as you open the door, you observe her wiping herself from back to front. What do you need to do at this time?

7. Because M.Z. has been having diarrhea, what special instructions should you give the NAP assigned to give basic care to M.Z.?

CASE STUDY PROGRESS

The next day, you are the nurse assigned to M.Z.'s care. You notice that the NAP emptying the gravity drain is not wearing personal protection devices. You also observe that the drainage port of the drainage bag was contaminated during the process because the NAP allowed it to touch the floor.

 8. What issues need to be considered in protecting M.Z.'s safety? Describe your actions in working with the nursing assistant.

9. As you assess M.Z., you notice that her catheter tubing is not secured. Why does the tubing need to be secured, and where is the correct place for the catheter tubing?

CASE STUDY PROGRESS

On the third day after M.Z.'s admission, the urinary culture and sensitivity (C&S) results are as follows: *Escherichia coli*, more than 100,000 colonies, sensitive to ciprofloxacin, trimethoprim-sulfamethoxazole, and nitrofurantoin.

10. What changes, if any, will be made to the antibiotic therapy?

11. The NAP reports that M.Z.'s 8-hour intake is 520 mL and the output is 140 mL. Identify two possible reasons that could account for the difference, and explain how you would assess each.

CASE STUDY PROGRESS

M.Z. has completed her antibiotic therapy. Her mental status has cleared, the Foley catheter has been discontinued, and she is ready for discharge.

12. What instructions should you discuss with the daughter?

13. She needs to notify the primary care physician if her mother develops which problems? Name at least six.

Case Study **53**

Name _____ Class/Group _____ Date _____

Group Members _____

5 Genitourinary Disorders

▶ **Scenario**

You are working in the emergency department when M.B., a 72-year-old man, enters with a chief complaint of the inability to void. His initial vital signs (VS) are 168/92, 88, 20, 98.2° F (36.8° C).

1. Are M.B.'s VS appropriate for a man of his age? If not, offer a rationale for the abnormal readings.

2. Given M.B.'s chief complaint, what would you expect to find during your initial assessment?

CASE STUDY PROGRESS

While you are taking M.B.'s history, he tells you he is generally in good health and leads an active life. His current medications include finasteride (Proscar) 5 mg/day and vitamin supplements. He reports that he has been unable to void for 12 hours and is very uncomfortable. He asks you to help him.

3. What do you need to know about his use of the finasteride?

4. If you are going to administer the finasteride, what precautions are necessary?

5. What are your priorities for this patient?

6. After examining M.B., the ED physician asks you to insert an indwelling urethral Foley catheter. What will you include in M.B.'s teaching before placing the Foley?

7. Put in order the steps to follow when inserting a Foley catheter, with 1 being the first step:
   _____ a. Apply sterile gloves.
   _____ b. Anchor the catheter to the patient's inner thigh.
   _____ c. Ensure that the drainage bag is secured to the bed, below the level of the bladder.
   _____ d. Position and drape the patient.
   _____ e. Cleanse the urethral meatus, following the proper procedure for a male.
   _____ f. Open lubricant container, antiseptic container. Test balloon with the fluid from the prefilled syringe if recommended by the manufacturer.
   _____ g. Inflate the balloon fully with the amount of fluid recommended for the catheter.
   _____ h. Gently insert the catheter 7 to 9 inches (17 to 22,5 cm) or until urine flows into the catheter tubing.
   _____ i. Perform hand hygiene.
   _____ j. Lubricate catheter.
   _____ k. Open the catheterization kit and place the underpad, if present, under the patient.

8. After two unsuccessful attempts to advance the catheter into the bladder, you stop. What is your next intervention? Why? What could be causing this problem?

9. The ED physician successfully inserts the indwelling catheter with the use of the type of catheter illustrated in the accompanying figure. What type of catheter is this, what is its advantage in this situation, and how is it inserted?

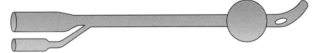

10. As the physician begins to inflate the catheter balloon, M.B. winces in pain and states, "*Ouch, you're hurting me!*" What happened, and what will the physician do?

11. You watch the urine drain into the bag and note that the amount is approaching 500 mL. What do you do at this time?

12. After the catheter is in place, the ED physician writes orders to discharge M.B. with instructions to see his primary care provider (PCP) on the following day. It is your responsibility to give discharge instructions. Outline your care plan.

13. The next day, M.B. is seen by his PCP, who changes M.B.'s medication to alfuzosin (Uroxatral). The catheter will be discontinued 2 days later. What teaching is essential regarding this new medication?
   a. Alfuzosin needs to be taken in the morning.
   b. This medication might cause fainting when he first starts taking it.
   c. M.B. needs to take each dose on an empty stomach.
   d. M.B. can stop taking the alfuzosin once the urinary symptoms subside.

5 Genitourinary Disorders

Case Study **54**

Name _____ Class/Group _____ Date _____

Group Members _____

▶ **Scenario**

You are working on a postoperative surgical floor and are assigned to A.T., a 65-year-old woman with a 30-year smoking history who has recently had a radical cystectomy with ileal conduit for invasive bladder cancer.

1. You begin your assessment and look at the transparent urostomy pouch covering the ileal conduit. The stomal opening is red and is draining urine with mucus. Is this normal? Explain your answer.

2. A nursing student who is working with you asks you to explain the difference between an ileal conduit and an ileostomy. How do you answer?

3. The student replies, "So eventually A.T.'s ileal conduit will become continent, and she won't need to wear a pouch, right?" How do you answer?

4. What is the proper size for an appliance for an ileal conduit?

5 Genitourinary Disorders

CASE STUDY PROGRESS

A.T. is quiet and sullen. You ask her if something is wrong, and she confides she is concerned about whether her husband will find her attractive after he sees her "pee hanging in that smelly bag."

5. What is the underlying problem?

CASE STUDY PROGRESS

You ask A.T. whether she would love her husband or children any less if they had a physical problem that required surgical repair. She quickly tells you, "No, of course not." You suggest that her family will likely respond the same way to her surgery. You suggest that someone from the ostomate program come and talk to her.

6. What is the ostomate program?

7. A.T. is well enough to begin self-care but asks you if you will change her pouch because she doesn't "want to look at it." Is there anyone on the hospital staff who could help teach A.T. ostomy self-care and offer more support?

CASE STUDY PROGRESS

It is now the fourth postoperative day and A.T. is now willing to learn how to change her appliance. She tells you the stoma feels wet, and it has no feeling when she touches it.

8. Which statements about the stoma are true? Select all that apply.
   a. "The lining of the stoma is the same type of tissue as the inside of your mouth."
   b. "It has touch receptors, just like your skin, and you should have feeling in it."
   c. "The color should be a beefy red, and the stoma should feel wet."
   d. "Normally the stoma is dry. Feeling moisture is a problem."
   e. "The tissue is tough and rarely bleeds."

9. A.T. asks you, "How will I know when to empty it? What about at night? Do I have to get up at night to empty this little pouch?" How do you answer her?

10. What other topics need to be addressed when teaching A.T. regarding the ileal conduit?

CASE STUDY PROGRESS

A.T.'s urine looks cloudy, and another nurse suggests that you send a specimen from her pouch to the laboratory for analysis. Her urine does not smell foul, and she has no fever or flank pain.

11. Should you follow through on this suggestion? Why or why not?

12. What are the signs and symptoms of a urinary tract infection (UTI) in a patient with an ileal conduit?

13. A.T. asks you, "How will they collect a urine specimen when it just dribbles out all the time?" How will you answer her?

14. As you make rounds, you notice that A.T.'s pouch has sprung a urine leak and she has placed a washcloth over the pouch to absorb the urine. She asks you for tape to attach the washcloth to the bag. How will you respond to her request?

CASE STUDY PROGRESS

A.T. eventually masters the pouch application and is discharged to home. She returns to the urology clinic in 1 month for a follow-up visit. She has lost 8 pounds and is seen with a smaller stoma which is surrounded by a crusty material and reddened skin. A.T. asks you if it is normal for the stoma to shrink, and what can be done about the crusty material around the stoma.

15. How will you answer A.T.'s questions?

CASE STUDY OUTCOME

A.T. mastered her ileal conduit and became a popular ostomate.

Case Study 55

Name _____ Class/Group _____ Date _____

Group Members _____

▶ Scenario

S.M. is a 68-year-old man who is being seen at your clinic for routine health maintenance and health promotion. He reports that he has been feeling well and has no specific complaints, except for some trouble "emptying my bladder." Vital signs at this visit are 148/88, 82, 16, 96.9° F (36.1° C). He had a complete blood count and complete metabolic panel completed 1 week before his visit, and the results are listed in the chart.

Chart View

Laboratory Test Results

Sodium	140 mEq/L
Potassium	4.2 mEq/L
Chloride	100 mEq/L
Bicarbonate	26 mEq/L
BUN	19 mg/dL
Creatinine	0.8 mg/dL
Glucose	94 mg/dL
RBC	5.2 million/mm^3
WBC	7400/mm^3
Hgb	15.2 g/dL
Hct	46%
Platelets	348,000/mm^3
Prostate-specific antigen (PSA)	4.23 ng/mL
Urinalysis	Within normal limits

1. What can you tell S.M. about his lab work?

2. What is the significance of the PSA result?

3. What other specific examination will S.M. need to have along with the PSA test?

5 Genitourinary Disorders

CASE STUDY PROGRESS

While obtaining your nursing history, you record no family history of cancer or other genitourinary problems. S.M. reports frequency, urgency, and nocturia×4; he has a weak stream and has to sit to void. These symptoms have been progressive over the past 6 months. He reports he was diagnosed with a "large prostate" a number of years ago. Last month, he began taking saw palmetto capsules but had to stop taking them because "they made me sick."

   4. Why did S.M. try taking the saw palmetto, and why do you think he stopped taking it?

   5. S.M. is curious why his enlarged prostate would affect his urination. He is concerned that he has prostate cancer. What would you teach him?

CASE STUDY PROGRESS

The primary care provider (PCP) performs a digital rectal examination (DRE) and asks for a post-void residual (PVR) urine test.

   6. Which of these findings from the digital rectal examination indicate BPH? Select all that apply.
   a. Prostate is symmetrically enlarged.
   b. Prostate feels firm.
   c. Prostate feels hard.
   d. Prostate is nodular.
   e. Prostate feels smooth.

   7. You use a bedside bladder scanner and document that S.M. voided 60 mL and his PVR is 110 mL. You report the PVR to the PCP. What is the significance of his PVR?

   8. Commonly used medications for BPH are 5-alpha -reductase inhibitors, such as finasteride (Proscar), and alpha-blocking drugs, such as tamsulosin (Flomax). How do these drugs differ?

9. The PCP orders tamsulosin (Flomax) 0.4 mg/day PO. You enter S.M.'s room to teach him about this medication. What side effects will you tell S.M. about? Select all that apply.
   a. Dizziness
   b. Diarrhea
   c. Dry mouth
   d. Headache
   e. Heartburn
   f. Orthostatic hypotension

10. S. M. asks, "Will this condition affect my relationship with my wife?" What should you tell him?

11. What would you expect S.M. to report if the medication was successful?

CASE STUDY PROGRESS

S.M. returns in 8 months to report that his symptoms are worse than ever. He has tried several different medications, but medication management failed and he is told that surgical intervention is necessary.

12. What surgical options are available to S.M.? Name at least three.

CASE STUDY OUTCOME

S.M. chose an outpatient procedure. He did well postoperatively and was discharged to home.

5 Genitourinary Disorders

Case Study **56**

Name _____ Class/Group _____ Date _____

Group Members _____

5 Genitourinary Disorders

▶ **Scenario**

K.B. is a 32-year-old woman being admitted to the medical floor for complaints of fatigue and dehydration. While taking her history, you discover that she has diabetes mellitus (DM) and has been insulin dependent since the age of 8. She has undergone hemodialysis (HD) for the past 2 years because of end-stage renal disease (ESRD). Your initial assessment of K.B. reveals a pale, thin, slightly drowsy woman. Her skin is warm and dry to the touch with poor skin turgor, and her mucous membranes are dry. Her vital signs are 140/88, 116, 18, 99.9° F (37.7° C). She tells you she has been nauseated for 2 days so she has not been eating or drinking. She reports severe diarrhea. The following blood chemistry results are back.

Chart View

Laboratory Test Results	
Sodium	145 mEq/L
Potassium	6.0 mEq/L
Chloride	93 mEq/L
Bicarbonate	27 mEq/L
BUN	48 mg/dL
Creatinine	5.0 mg/dL
Glucose	238 mg/dL

1. What aspects of your assessment support her admitting diagnosis of dehydration?

2. Explain any laboratory results that might be of concern.

3. Identify two possible causes for K.B.'s low-grade fever.

CASE STUDY PROGRESS

The rest of K.B.'s physical assessment is within normal limits. You note that she has an arteriovenous (AV) fistula in her left arm.

4. What is an AV fistula? Why does K.B. have one?

5. What steps do you take to assess K.B.'s AV fistula, and what physical findings are expected? Explain.

6. As you continue the assessment, you notice that a nursing assistive personnel (NAP) comes in to take K.B.'s blood pressure (BP). The NAP places the BP cuff on K.B.'s left arm. What, if anything, do you do?

CASE STUDY PROGRESS

K.B.'s admission CBC yields the following results:

Chart View

Laboratory Test Results

WBC	7600/mm^3
RBC	3.2 million/mm^3
Hgb	8.1 g/dL
Hct	24.3%
Platelets	333,000/mm^3

7. Are these values normal? If not, what are the abnormalities?

8. K.B.'s physician notes that she is anemic, which most likely is the cause of her increasing fatigue. Why is K.B. anemic?

CASE STUDY PROGRESS

K.B. is sent for an HD treatment. Over the next 24 hours, K.B.'s nausea subsides, and she is able to eat normally. While you are helping her with her morning care, she confides in you that she doesn't understand her diet. "I just get blood drawn every week and meet with the dialysis dietitian every month—I just eat what she tells me to eat. It's so hard!"

9. Because K.B. is on HD and has DM, what are her special nutritional needs? Name at least four specific components of the diet recommended for K.B.

5 Genitourinary Disorders

10. Patients in renal failure have the potential to develop comorbid conditions. Identify five potential problems, determine how you would assess the problem, then delineate nursing interventions and patient education strategies for each.

CASE STUDY PROGRESS

The following day, K.B. is discharged feeling much better and with a good understanding of her dietary restrictions. Her iron stores have been evaluated and found to be low. Her physician has instructed her to resume her preadmission medications, with the addition of ferrous fumarate oral suspension 100 mg PO tid between meals with water, if tolerated (or with meals if GI distress occurs) and epoetin (Epogen) to be given three times a week intravenously with dialysis. She is also given a prescription for Nephrocaps vitamin supplements to be taken daily.

11. Explain the purpose of the new medications for K. B.

12. You spend some time with K.B. to explain the new medications. Which statement by K.B. reflects need for further teaching?
    a. "I won't need to take the iron supplements as long as I get the Epogen during dialysis."
    b. "The liquid iron will cause my bowel movements to turn black or dark green."
    c. "Hopefully I will feel less tired all the time when these medicines start building up my red blood cells."
    d. "I should dilute the liquid iron and drink it with a straw so that it won't stain my teeth."

13. K.B. asks, "Why do I need a prescription for vitamins? I can just take something on sale at the drugstore, right?" How do you respond?

14. The ferrous fumarate suspension comes in a bottle that is labeled 100 mg/5 mL. Indicate on the measuring cup how much medication will be used for each dose.

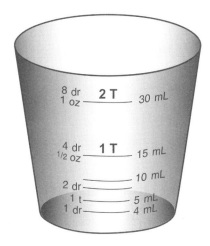

15. In monitoring K.B.'s response to the epoetin, what adverse effect would you expect?
   a. Arthralgia
   b. Tachycardia
   c. Drowsiness
   d. Diarrhea

17. Which vital sign will you monitor carefully while K.B. is on epoetin therapy? Explain your answer.

18. During the following weeks, which laboratory result is most important to monitor while K.B. is on the epoetin? Explain.

CASE STUDY OUTCOME

K.B. is discharged to home and goes to the local dialysis center three times a week. She also keeps appointments with the registered dietitian and reports that she is feeling much better.

Case Study **57**

Name _____ Class/Group _____ Date _____

Group Members _____

5 Genitourinary Disorders

▶ Scenario

A.B. is a 55-year-old man who was referred to the urology clinic by his primary care provider (PCP) because of an elevated prostate-specific antigen (PSA) level. He reports that he has been feeling well and has no specific complaints. He had a complete blood count (CBC), basic metabolic panel, urinalysis (UA), lipid profile, and screening PSA completed the week before when he was seen by his PCP. His CBC, lipid profile, UA, and blood chemistry findings are all within normal limits. His PSA is elevated at 11.9 ng/mL, and the prostate is slightly tender on examination.

1. A.B. wonders whether he has prostate cancer. What can you tell A.B. about his PSA level?

2. A.B. is scheduled for a transrectal ultrasound (TRUS) of the prostate. What is the purpose of this test?

3. Based on the PSA and TRUS results, A.B. is scheduled for a prostate biopsy. He wonders what he needs to do to prepare for this test. Explain a prostate biopsy procedure and how to prepare for the procedure.

CASE STUDY PROGRESS

A.B.'s prostate biopsy is positive for cancer, with a Gleason grade of 7. He has discussed his diagnosis with the urologist. He is now thinking about his treatment options and asks you to answer some questions. He was told about his Gleason grade but is not sure what this is.

4. What is a Gleason grade?

5. The urologist discusses possible treatment options with A.B. Identify three treatment options for prostate cancer.

CASE STUDY PROGRESS

After consulting with his urologist, A.B. has decided to have his prostate removed with the laparoscopic procedure. He is planning on having surgery in 2 weeks but is concerned about the possible consequences of surgery.

6. Identify the major immediate postoperative concerns for A.B.

7. What are the two main long-term consequences of prostatectomy?

8. The urologist you work for has asked you to give A.B. preoperative instructions. What should you tell him?

CASE STUDY PROGRESS

A.B. returns status post–laparoscopic radical prostatectomy (LRP). Initial postoperative orders are written.

9. Which orders are appropriate for A.B.? Select all that apply, and correct the inappropriate answers.
   a. Vital signs per hospital protocol
   b. Notify physician if urinary output is less than 30 mL/hr
   c. Up ad lib
   d. Change Foley catheter if clotting occurs
   e. Oxybutynin (Ditropan XL) 10 mg PO every morning
   f. Docusate (Colace) 100 mg PO qd
   g. Morphine 4 mg IV push q4h prn pain

10. Which of these assessment findings would be of most concern in the first 24 hours after surgery?
    a. A.B. complains of bladder spasms.
    b. A few blood clots are noted in the urine drainage bag.
    c. Bright red blood suddenly appears in the Foley catheter tubing.
    d. The urine is light pink in color.

11. Choose the type of catheter that you expect A.B. to have after surgery, and explain the rationale for it.

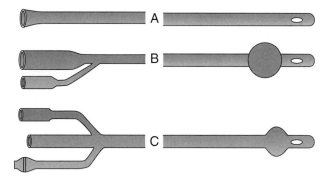

    a. Catheter A
    b. Catheter B
    c. Catheter C

5 Genitourinary Disorders

12. What would be ordered if clotting of the Foley catheter were to occur?

13. A.B. complains of bladder spasms and is given a dose of oxybutynin (Ditropan XL). The nurse will monitor for which adverse effects? Select all that apply.
    a. Dry mouth
    b. Watery eyes
    c. Dizziness
    d. Diarrhea
    e. Palpitations

CASE STUDY PROGRESS

A.B. does not require any additional therapy after surgery. At his 6-month follow-up visit, he reports he can get an erection but has difficulty maintaining an erection for sexual relations.

14. The physician discusses erectile aids with A.B. What options are possible? Name at least three types.

Case Study 58

Name _____ Class/Group _____ Date _____

Group Members _____

▶ Scenario

You are a registered nurse in the emergency department. It is a hot summer day and S.R., a 25-year-old woman, comes to the ED with severe left flank and abdominal pain and nausea and vomiting. S.R. looks very tired, her skin is warm to the touch, and she is perspiring. She paces about the room doubled over and is clutching her abdomen. S.R. tells you the pain started early this morning and has been pretty steady for the past 6 hours. She gives a history of working outside as a landscaper and takes little time for water breaks. Her past medical history includes three kidney stone attacks, all occurring during late summer. Examination findings are that her abdomen is soft and without tenderness, but her left flank is extremely tender to touch, palpation, and percussion. You place S.R. in one of the examination rooms and take the following vital signs: 188/98, 90, 20, 99° F (37.2° C). A voided urinalysis shows RBCs of 50 to 100 on voided specimen and WBCs of zero.

1. What could be the cause of the blood in her urine? How could you rule out some of these causes?

2. The physician orders an intravenous pyelogram (IVP). What questions do you need to ask S.R. before the test is conducted? What blood test results do you need to check before she has an IVP?

3. S.R. states she had an allergic reaction during her last IVP and was instructed, "Don't let anyone give you dye for any testing." The physician cancels the IVP. What alternative test will be conducted?

CASE STUDY PROGRESS

The noncontrast CT scan shows a left 2-mm ureteral vesicle junction stone.

4. What are the most common types of stones? Select all that apply.
   a. Calcium oxalate
   b. Calcium phosphate
   c. Struvite
   d. Uric acid
   e. Cystine

5. What is the most likely cause of S.R.'s stone?

6. What is a possible complication if S.R.'s stone is not removed?
   a. Nephrosclerosis
   b. Hydronephrosis
   c. Trabeculation
   d. Nephrotic syndrome

7. Identify two methods of treating a patient with a ureteral vesicle junction stone.

CASE STUDY PROGRESS

S.R. was discharged with instructions to strain all urine and return if she experienced pain unrelieved by the pain medication or increased nausea and vomiting.

8. What specific instructions will you give S.R. about straining her urine, fluid intake, medications, and activity?

CASE STUDY PROGRESS

S.R. returns to the ED in 6 hours with complaints of pain unrelieved by the pain medication and increased blood in her urine. She is being held in the ED until she can be transported to surgery.

9. What is the immediate plan of care for S.R.?

CASE STUDY PROGRESS

A 2-mm calculus was removed by basket extraction. Pathologic examination reported the stone to be calcium oxalate.

10. If S.R. continues to form calcium oxalate stones, what recommendations would the physician make for S.R.?

11. Because S.R.'s stone has been reported as calcium oxalate, she is referred to a registered dietitian for guidance on a diet that will prevent further development of stones. Which statements are true regarding recommendations for S.R.'s diet? Select all that apply.
    a. Decrease animal protein intake.
    b. Avoid eating organ meats, poultry, fish, gravies, red wine, and sardines.
    c. Avoid spinach, black tea, coffee, rhubarb, chocolate, beets, asparagus, and nuts.
    d. Decrease sodium intake.
    e. Drink at least 3 to 4 liters of water each day.

CASE STUDY OUTCOME

S.R. recovers from this most recent episode and continues to follow the protocol for fluid intake and dietary measures. One year later, she has yet to report a recurrence of stones.

Case Study **59**

Name _____ Class/Group _____ Date _____

Group Members _____

▶ Scenario

F.F., a 58-year-old man with type 2 diabetes mellitus, comes to the emergency department with severe right flank and abdominal pain and nausea and vomiting. The abdomen is soft and without tenderness. The right flank is extremely tender to the touch and to palpation. Vital signs are 142/80, 88, 20, 99° F (37.2° C). Urinalysis shows hematuria. An IV of 0.9% normal saline is started at 125 mL/hr. An IV pyelogram (IVP) confirms the diagnosis of a staghorn-type stone in the right renal pelvis. The right kidney looks enlarged. F.F. states that he did not sleep well last night and has not eaten much today. He is obviously fatigued. His laboratory results are listed in the chart. F.F. weighs 277 pounds.

Chart View

Admission Laboratory Test Results

Sodium	144 mEq/L
Potassium	4.0 mEq/L
Chloride	101 mEq/L
Carbon dioxide	26 mEq/L
BUN	30 mg/dL
Creatinine	3.6 mg/dL
Glucose	260 mg/dL
Uric acid	5.0 mg/dL
Calcium	9.0 mg/L
Phosphorus	3.2 mg/dL
Total protein	7.8 g/dL
Albumin	4.0 g/dL
Total bilirubin	0.3 mg/dL
Direct bilirubin	0.1 mg/dL
Cholesterol	200 mg/dL
ALP	61 units/L
LDH	Total 100 units/L
ALT	13 units/L
AST	38 units/L
Amylase	98 units/L

1. Review F.F.'s lab work, and note any value that might be of concern.

2. Analyze the relationship between creatinine and glomerular filtration rate (GFR) and prediction of kidney function.

3. F.F.'s pain is treated in the ED with IV morphine. It is late afternoon before he is admitted to your unit, and he is scheduled for lithotripsy in the morning. What specific priorities do you identify for F.F.?

4. What problems are possible as a result of the staghorn stone?

5. The physician has ordered gentamicin (Garamycin) 6 mg/kg/day IV piggyback in divided doses q8h. The pharmacist will calculate the dose of gentamicin for F.F., but you decide to double-check with your own calculations. How much will she receive per dose? After considering the results, are there any specific concerns?

5 Genitourinary Disorders

6. Use SBAR (*Situation, Background, Assessment, Recommendation*) to communicate your concerns about this dose of gentamicin to the physician.

7. The physician reduces the dose of gentamicin to 1 mg/kg q12h and orders daily creatinine and BUN levels, as well as trough gentamicin levels after day 2. You will monitor F.F. for what signs of gentamicin toxicity? Select all that apply.
   a. Tinnitus
   b. Headache
   c. Dizziness
   d. Hypotension
   e. Restlessness

CASE STUDY PROGRESS

Later, as you walk past F.F.'s bed, you notice him crawling off the end of the bed.

 8. What are you going to do?

CASE STUDY PROGRESS

You tell F.F. that radiology called, and you let him know what time the lithotripsy procedure is scheduled for on the next day. He looks at you, panicked, and says, "If that doesn't work, will they do surgery? I can't do that. I don't have any insurance. This is costing me so much already."

9. How will you respond?

5 Genitourinary Disorders

CASE STUDY OUTCOME

F.F. undergoes the lithotripsy procedure successfully and is discharged the next day. Before his discharge, F.F. met with the hospital social worker who assisted him with applying to the hospital's indigent fund and available insurance programs.

Case Study **60**

Name _____ Class/Group _____ Date _____

Group Members _____

▶ Scenario

N.H., an 89-year-old widow, recently experienced a left-sided cerebrovascular accident (CVA). She has right-sided weakness and expressive aphasia with minimal swallowing difficulty. N.H. has a past medical history of a minor left-sided CVA 2 ½ years ago, chronic atrial flutter, and hypertension. She has lived with her daughter's family in a rural town since her previous stroke. Since admission to an acute care facility 5 days ago, N.H. has gained some strength, has become oriented to person and place, and is anxious to begin her rehabilitation program. She is transferred for rehabilitation to your skilled nursing facility with the orders shown in the chart.

Chart View

Admission Orders

Hydrochlorothiazide (HydroDIURIL) 25 mg/day PO

Digoxin (Lanoxin) 0.125 mg/day PO

Warfarin (Coumadin) 5 mg/day PO

Acetaminophen (Tylenol) 325 mg q6h PO prn for pain

Zolpidem (Ambien) 5 mg PO at bedtime prn for sleep

Diet: mechanical soft, low sodium with ground meat

Foley catheter to gravity drainage, and then begin bladder training

Referrals for speech therapy, occupational therapy, and physical therapy to evaluate and treat swallowing, communication, and functional abilities

1. What laboratory orders would you anticipate as a result of this specific list of orders? With each response, describe your rationale.

CASE STUDY PROGRESS

A week later, at the interdisciplinary care conference, you report that bladder training is progressing and recommend removing the catheter if N.H.'s mobility and communication abilities have progressed sufficiently. The group and N.H. agree that she is ready for the Foley catheter to be removed.

2. Identify three problems that N.H. is at risk for developing after catheter removal, and describe specific interventions for each problem.

CASE STUDY PROGRESS

Two days after the Foley catheter is removed, you observe that N.H.'s urine is cloudy and concentrated and has a strong odor.

3. What are your immediate actions?

CASE STUDY PROGRESS

N.H. is started on sulfamethoxazole 800 mg/trimethoprim 160 mg (Bactrim DS) 1 tab PO bid × 10 days. However, 2 days later, N.H. is in the bathroom and she is very upset. She has just voided; there is blood on the toilet, and the water is bright red with blood. You help the nursing assistive personnel (NAP) clean N.H. and help her into bed.

4. Describe your assessment steps.

5. Identify at least two potential causes for N.H.'s hematuria.

6. Using SBAR, what information would you provide to the physician when you call?

CASE STUDY PROGRESS

N.H.'s physician changes her antibiotic to oral ciprofloxacin (Cipro) and holds the warfarin for 2 days. Two days later, N.H.'s urinary tract infection (UTI) is responding to antibiotics and she has had no further bleeding in the urine. You want to prepare her and her daughter for eventual discharge.

7. What specific issues must be considered in the teaching and discharge planning to prevent a recurrence of infection?

8. You discuss with N.H.'s daughter how certain foods and drinks may irritate the bladder and should be avoided. These foods include which of the following? Select all that apply.
   a. Caffeinated beverages
   b. Citrus juices
   c. Bananas
   d. Chocolate
   e. Spicy foods

9. You talk with N.H.'s daughter about her understanding of caregiving responsibilities for her mother. What kind of questions do you ask to assess whether she is capable of taking care of her mother since her mother's health has declined? List at least four.

CASE STUDY OUTCOME

N.H.'s right-sided weakness and expressive aphasia do not resolve. Her daughter takes N.H. home and, with the help of her sister, nieces, and a home health aide, they have adjusted well to living together.

5 Genitourinary Disorders

Neurologic Disorders

Case Study 61

Name _____ Class/Group _____ Date _____

Group Members _____

▶ Scenario

M.E. is a 66-year-old woman who has a 2-year history of progressive forgetfulness. After a neurologic evaluation, M.E. was diagnosed as having Alzheimer disease (AD). She is no longer able to care for herself, has become increasingly depressed and paranoid, and recently started a fire in the kitchen. Her husband and children have come to the Alzheimer unit at your extended care facility to seek information about AD and discuss the possibility of placement for M.E. You assure the family that you have experience dealing with the questions and concerns of most people in their situation.

1. How would you explain AD to the family?

2. M.E.'s husband asks, "How did she get Alzheimer's? We don't know anyone else who has it." How would you respond?

3. After asking the family to describe M.E.'s behavior, you determine that she is in stage 2 of Alzheimer's three stages. Describe common signs and symptoms for each stage of the disease.

4. M.E.'s daughter expresses some frustration at the number of tests M.E. had to undergo and the length of time it took someone to diagnose M.E.'s problem. What tests are likely to be performed, and how is AD diagnosed?

CASE STUDY PROGRESS

M.E.'s husband states, "How are you going to take care of her? She wanders around all night long. She cannot find her way to the bathroom in a house she has lived in for 43 years. She cannot be trusted to be alone anymore; she almost burnt the house down. We're all exhausted; there are three of us, and we can't keep up with her." You acknowledge how exhausted they must be from trying to keep her safe. You tell the family that Alzheimer units have been created to provide a structured, safe environment.

5. Describe specific nursing interventions to place in M.E.'s plan of care that are part of National Patient Safety Goals aimed at minimizing her risk of falling.

6. M.E.'s son asks why you can only access the unit through a door that has a keypad control. He wants to know if there are violent patients on the unit. How will you respond?

 7. Describe the Alzheimer-related nursing interventions related to each of the following problems: chronic confusion, inability to perform self-hygiene, disrupted sleep pattern, impaired verbal communication, and agitation.

8. M.E.'s son asks whether medications can help her AD. How would you respond?

9. What other medications might be prescribed for M.E. and why?

6 Neurologic Disorders

CASE STUDY PROGRESS

You try to comfort the family by telling them that the problems that they are experiencing are common. You explain that family support is a major focus of your program.

10. List four ways in which M.E.'s family might receive the support they need.

Case Study **62**

Name _____ Class/Group _____ Date _____

Group Members _____

▶ **Scenario**

C.B. is a single, self-supporting 48-year-old man. Three weeks ago, he saw his family physician because of symptoms of fatigue, myalgia, fever, and chills, which were accompanied by a hacking cough. He was diagnosed with viral influenza. Today he has complaints of weakness, numbness, and tingling of both lower extremities, which rapidly progressed into his upper body. He was brought to the emergency department after his brother recognized the seriousness of his condition. The attending physician immediately suspects Guillain-Barré syndrome (GBS).

1. Describe the cause of GBS.

2. What factors in C.B.'s medical history support a diagnosis of GBS?

3. What are the clinical manifestations of GBS?

4. How is GBS diagnosed, and what tests would you expect to be performed?

5. What is your immediate concern for C.B. and why?

6 Neurologic Disorders

6. What assessment findings would tell you this is occurring?

7. Which set of arterial blood gases would be consistent with the presence of this complication?
   a. pH 7.50, Pco_2 52 mm Hg
   b. pH 7.35, Pco_2 40 mm Hg
   c. pH 7.25, Pco_2 60 mm Hg
   d. pH 7.51, Pco_2 31 mm Hg

8. Which assessment finding, if present, would not be directly related to C.B. having GBS?
   a. Confusion
   b. Diaphoresis
   c. Facial flushing
   d. Diminished bowel sounds

CASE STUDY PROGRESS

Shortly after arrival, C.B. becomes completely paralyzed and requires endotracheal intubation and mechanical ventilation. He is transferred to the neurologic intensive care unit for further support.

9. What are the goals of medical management in GBS?

10. What are the overall goals of nursing care for C.B. at this time?

11. Which procedure would you expect the attending physician to order for C.B. and why?

12. You are concerned about the possibility of disuse syndrome related to C.B.'s paralysis. Describe an outcome of nursing care for C.B., and describe the independent nursing interventions you would implement to meet that outcome.

6 Neurologic Disorders

13. How would C.B.'s nutritional needs be met?

14. What evaluative parameters could you use to determine whether C.B.'s nutritional needs were being met?

15. What interventions can you implement to help decrease C.B.'s fear and anxiety? Select all that apply.
    a. Speak calmly to him when providing care.
    b. Administer continuous intravenous sedation.
    c. Limit visitors only to immediate family members.
    d. Continually reassure him that his needs are being met.
    e. Use a communication system that allows C.B. to let his needs be known.

16. C.B.'s brother asks how long C.B. will be paralyzed. How should you respond?

Case Study **63**

Name _____ Class/Group _____ Date _____

Group Members _____

▶ Scenario

L.C. is a 78-year-old man with a 3-year history of Parkinson disease (PD). He is a retired engineer, is married, and lives with his wife in a small farming community. He has four adult children who live close by. Since his last visit to the clinic 6 months ago, L.C. reports that his tremors are "about the same" as they were; however, further questioning reveals that he feels his gait is perhaps a little more unsteady, and his fatigue is slightly more noticeable. L.C. is also concerned about increased drooling. Among the medications L.C. takes are carbidopa-levodopa 25/100 mg (Sinemet) four times daily and amantadine (Symmetrel) 100 mg at breakfast and bedtime. On the previous visit the Sinemet was increased from three to four times daily. He reports that he has become very somnolent with this regimen and that his dyskinetic movements appear to be worse just after taking his carbidopa-levodopa (Sinemet).

1. What is PD?

2. What is parkinsonism?

3. What are the clinical manifestations of PD? Place a star next to the symptoms L.C. has mentioned.

6 Neurologic Disorders

4. L.C.'s wife asks you, "How do the doctors know he really has Parkinson disease? They never did a lot of tests on him." How is PD diagnosed?

5. L.C. asks, "Why don't they give me a dopamine pill? Wouldn't that just fix everything?" Why is oral dopamine not a replacement therapy?

6. Why is levodopa given in combination with carbidopa?

7. Why did L.C.'s dyskinetic movements appear to be worse just after taking his carbidopa-levodopa? What might be done about it?

8. Because L.C. takes Sinemet, what serious adverse effect should you assess for in him?
   a. Steven-Johnson syndrome
   b. Suicidal thoughts
   c. Spontaneous tendon rupture
   d. Permanent loss of hearing

9. L.C.'s wife asks, "They can do surgery for everything else. Why can't they do some kind of surgery to fix Parkinson's?" How would you describe the surgical treatments available for patients with PD?

CASE STUDY PROGRESS

After examining L.C., the physician decides not to hospitalize him but to decrease the dosage of the Sinemet. He tells L.C. and his wife that he feels that L.C. is likely experiencing some advancement in his disease and says that it is time for some changes in L.C.'s care. The physician looks at you and asks you to coordinate the "usual referrals."

10. What team members would likely be involved in L.C.'s care and how?

11. What factors do you need to take into consideration when assisting L.C. with these referrals?

12. L.C. is reporting an increase in drooling; you are concerned about the possibility of his ability to swallow. What further assessment could you perform to determine whether L.C. is at immediate risk for aspirating?

13. What are three nutrition interventions that should be implemented for L.C.?

14. Because L.C. is reporting that his gait is more unsteady, there is an increased risk for falls. Which suggestion could you offer to diminish this risk?
   a. Only use a wheelchair to get around.
   b. Stand as upright as possible and use a walker.
   c. Keep the feet close together while ambulating.
   d. Consciously think about walking over imaginary lines on the floor.

15. What are some suggestions you can make to L.C. to assist with managing fatigue?

16. You are giving instructions to L.C. and his wife about maintaining mobility safely. You determine that they understand the directions if they state that L.C. will:
   a. Use a step stool to obtain difficult-to-reach items.
   b. Schedule his PT appointments in the evening.
   c. When rising from a seat, rock back and forth to start moving.
   d. Sit on a large, soft sofa with supportive pillows.

17. As L.C.'s case manager, identify six things that you would need to assess to determine whether L.C. could be cared for in his home.

Case Study **64**

Name _____ Class/Group _____ Date _____

Group Members _____

▶ Scenario

N.T., a 79-year-old woman, arrives at the emergency room with expressive aphasia, left facial droop, left-sided hemiparesis, and mild dysphagia. Her husband states that when she awoke that morning at 0600, she stayed in bed, complaining of a mild headache over the right temple and feeling slightly weak. He went and got coffee, then thinking it was unusual for her to have those complaints, went back to check on her. He found she was having some trouble saying words and had developed a left-sided facial droop. When he helped her up from the bedside, he noticed weakness in her left hand and leg and brought her to the emergency department. Her past medical history includes paroxysmal atrial fibrillation (PAF), hypertension (HTN), and hyperlipidemia. A recent cardiac stress test had normal findings, and her blood pressure (BP) has been well controlled. N.T. is currently taking flecainide (Tambocor), hormone replacement therapy, amlodipine (Norvasc), aspirin, simvastatin (Zocor), and lisinopril (Zestril). The physician suspects N.T. has experienced an acute cerebrovascular accident (CVA).

1. What role do diagnostic tests play in evaluating N.T. for a suspected CVA?

2. Explain how knowing the type of CVA is an important factor in planning care.

3. Which factor in N.T.'s history is the most likely contributor to her having experienced a CVA?

CASE STUDY PROGRESS

After a noncontrast CT scan, she is diagnosed with a thrombolytic CVA. The physician writes the orders shown in the chart.

Chart View

Physician's Orders

IV 0.9% NaCl at 75 mL/hr
Activase (tPA) per protocol
Stat CBC, PT/INR, CPK isoenzymes
Neurologic assessment every hour
Obtain patient weight
Vital signs every hour
Oxygen at 2 L per nasal cannula (NC)
NPO until swallowing evaluation

4. Outline a plan of care for implementing these orders.

5. Which interventions can you delegate to the nursing assistive personnel (NAP)? Select all that apply.
    a. Obtaining N.T.'s weight
    b. Assisting N.T. in repositioning every 2 hours
    c. Initiating oxygen therapy by nasal cannula
    d. Performing N.T.'s neurologic checks every hour
    e. Obtaining a manual BP per protocol

6. What is the purpose of monitoring the CK isoenzyme levels?

7. Complete the National Institutes of Health Stroke Scale (NIHSS) scores for each of N.T.'s symptoms.

Symptom	Score
Alert	
Knows month and age	
Able to follow commands	
Extraocular movements (EOMs) intact	
No visual loss	
Partial left facial paralysis	
Left leg no movement	
Left arm no movement	
No ataxia	
Sensation intact	
Moderate aphasia	
Neglect of left side	
TOTAL SCORE	

8. Based on your scoring, what level of CVA did N.T. experience?

9. The instructions on the tPA vials read to reconstitute with 50 mL of sterile water to make a total of 50 mg/50 mL (1 mg/mL). The hospital protocol is to infuse 0.9 mg/kg over 60 minutes with 10% of the dose given as a bolus over 1 minute. N.T. weighs 143 pounds. What is the amount of the bolus dose, in both milligrams and milliliters, you will administer in the first minute? What is the amount of the remaining dose that you will need to administer?

10. Contraindications for beginning fibrinolytic therapy include which of the following? Select all that apply.
    a. Currently on Coumadin with an INR of 2.4
    b. Major surgery in the last 14 days
    c. Systolic BP of 150
    d. Platelet count of less than 100,000
    e. Blood glucose of less than 50 mg/dL
    f. History of myocardial infarction 1 year ago
    g. Improving neurologic status

11. What are your responsibilities during the administration of Activase (tPA)?

CASE STUDY PROGRESS

N.T. is admitted to the neurology unit. A second CT scan (18 hours later) reveals a small CVA in the right hemisphere. She is placed on flecainide (Tambocor), amlodipine (Norvasc), clopidogrel (Plavix), aspirin, simvastatin (Zocor), and lisinopril (Zestril).

12. If N.T.'s deficits are temporary, how long might it take before they completely reverse?

13. During the first 24 hours after receipt of Activase (tPA), the primary concern is controlling N.T.'s:
  a. Cardiac rhythm
  b. BP
  c. Glucose level
  d. Oxygen saturation

14. While assessing N.T., you note the following findings. Which one is unrelated to the CVA?
  a. Headache
  b. Lethargy
  c. Lumbar pain
  d. Blurred vision

15. Why was N.T. placed on clopidogrel (Plavix) post-CVA?

16. Because N.T. had a thrombolytic infusion, how many hours should you wait before beginning administration of any anticoagulant or antiplatelet medications?

17. Is there any benefit from continuing simvastatin (Zocor) after her CVA?

18. As you walk into the nurses' station, the charge nurse is coordinating the swallowing evaluation, including a modified barium swallow study and referral for a speech-language pathologist (SLP). Give the rationale for these orders.

6 Neurologic Disorders

Case Study 65

Name _____ Class/Group _____ Date _____

Group Members _____

▶ Scenario

T.H. is a 55-year-old man with an 8-month history of progressive muscle weakness. Initially, he tripped over things and seemed to drop everything. He lost interest in activities because he was always exhausted. He sought medical assistance when his speech became slurred and he started to drool. During the initial evaluation, the physician noted frequent, severe muscle cramps, muscle twitching, and inappropriate, uncontrollable periods of laughter. After undergoing a series of tests, T.H. was diagnosed with amyotrophic lateral sclerosis (ALS). He is upset and bewildered about a disease that he has "never even heard of." You are a home health nurse who is seeing T.H. for the first time.

1. How would you explain ALS to T.H.?

2. Who gets ALS?

3. How common is ALS?

4. T.H. has many questions. He asks you, "How long can I expect to live?" How should you respond?

5. T.H. asks, "Will I lose my mind?"

6. T.H. then asks, "Are there any treatments for this?"

7. T.H. thinks a moment, then says, "How is the doctor even sure this is what I have?" What is your response?

8. As part of this initial visit, you will begin to coordinate care with speech, occupational, respiratory, and physical therapists, as well as a dietitian and a psychologist. Describe the role that each of these professionals will play in T.H.'s treatment.

9. Which of the following actions will support communication among T.H.'s care providers? Select all that apply.
   a. Maintaining one central medical record
   b. Designating the physician as the team leader
   c. Having open communication among team members
   d. Holding periodic team conferences to communicate goals
   e. Inviting T.H. and his caregiver to participate in team conferences

10. You hold a family meeting to recruit adequate help for the caregiver—in this case, T.H.'s spouse. Why is this important?

11. What are some suggestions you can give T.H.'s spouse to help her reduce caregiver strain?

12. How would you assess if T.H.'s spouse were experiencing caregiver strain?
    a. Ask how well T.H. feels his spouse is caring for him.
    b. Assess the caregiving situation and health of T.H. and his spouse.
    c. Evaluate his spouse for any symptoms of anxiety and depression.
    d. Determine if his spouse is feeling overwhelmed by her responsibilities.

13. T.H. asks you, "How will the end probably come for me?" What should you tell him?

14. T.H. wants to know whether he "has to be put on a breathing machine." What factors will you take into consideration when deciding what to tell him?

15. Which legal document should T.H. formulate to describe his wishes regarding being placed on a "breathing machine"?
    a. Standard will
    b. Living will
    c. Health care power of attorney
    d. Living trust

Case Study 66

Name _____ Class/Group _____ Date _____

Group Members _____

▶ **Scenario**

J.B. is a 58-year-old retired postal worker who has been on your floor for several days receiving plasma-pheresis every other day for myasthenia gravis (MG). About a year ago, J.B. started experiencing difficulty chewing and swallowing, diplopia, and slurring of speech, at which time he was placed on pyridostigmine (Mestinon). Before this admission he had been relatively stable. His medical history includes hyperten-sion controlled with metoprolol (Lopressor) and glaucoma treated with timolol (ophthalmic preparation). Recently J.B. was diagnosed with a sinus infection and treated with ciprofloxacin (Cipro). On admission, J.B. was unable to bear any weight or take fluids through a straw. There have been periods of exacerbation and remission since admission.

Chart View

Vital Signs

Blood pressure	170/68 mm Hg
Heart rate	118 beats/min
Respiratory rate	32 breaths/min
Temperature	101.8° F (38.8° C)

1. You note that the nursing assistive personnel (NAP) has just entered these vital signs into J.B.'s record. What is your immediate concern and why?

2. What action do you need to take based on this concern?

3. What other assessment findings would support this complication being present?

4. What medical treatment do you anticipate for J.B.?

5. What is your nursing priority at this time?

6. Based on this priority, what nursing interventions do you need to perform?

 7. Which actions do you need to implement to administer edrophonium (Tensilon) safely? Select all that apply.
   a. Have intravenous (IV) atropine sulfate readily available.
   b. Monitor for changes in level of consciousness.
   c. Place J.B. on continuous cardiac monitoring.
   d. Initiate precautions to prevent excessive bleeding.
   e. Administer a prophylactic antiemetic before injection.

8. What is the difference between a cholinergic crisis and myasthenic crisis?

9. J.B.'s wife asks you, "What may have caused my husband to get worse, and why does he keep having these episodes?" What explanation should you give her?

CASE STUDY PROGRESS

J.B.'s condition improves after the administration of edrophonium (Tensilon). Two days later, after his condition has stabilized, you sit down to discuss discharge plans with J.B. and his wife.

10. J.B.'s wife tells you she does not have a lot of information about MG and she would like to know more about it. What should you tell her?

11. They ask you to explain what to expect in terms of symptoms as his illness progresses. What should you tell them?

12. J.B.'s wife asks, "How do they know that my husband has myasthenia gravis?" What should you tell her about how MG is diagnosed?

13. J.B.'s wife asks why he receives plasmapheresis for the treatments of MG. Which of the following best describes the purpose of this procedure?
    a. It replaces affected blood with unaffected blood.
    b. It decreases the production of antireceptor antibodies.
    c. It reduces inflammation by infusing immunoglobulins.
    d. It removes circulating abnormal antibodies from the blood.

14. J.B. wants to know when he will be able to go home. How will you respond?

15. J.B.'s wife asks you what information they will need before he goes home. Outline the points you need to teach J.B. and his wife.

6 Neurologic Disorders

16. You teach J.B. and his wife that the most effective means of preventing myasthenic and cholinergic crises is by:
    a. Doing all errands early in the day.
    b. Eating three large, well-balanced meals.
    c. Taking medications at the same time each day.
    d. Doing muscle-strengthening exercises twice a day.

17. How will you know that your teaching has been effective?

18. What community resources might J.B. and his wife find helpful?

Case Study 67

Name _____ Class/Group _____ Date _____

Group Members _____

6 Neurologic Disorders

▶ Scenario

D.V., a 32-year-old man, is being admitted to the medical floor from the neurology clinic with symptoms of multiple sclerosis (MS). D.V. has experienced increasing urinary frequency and urgency over the past 2 months. Because his female partner was treated for a sexually transmitted infection, D.V. underwent treatment, but the symptoms did not resolve. D.V. has also recently had two brief episodes of eye "fuzziness" associated with diplopia and flashes of brightness. He has noticed ascending numbness and weakness of the right arm with the inability to hold objects over the past few days. Now he reports rapidly progressing weakness in his legs along with blurred, patchy vision.

1. MS is associated with scattered, patchy demyelinization of the central nervous system (CNS). What does myelin do? What is demyelinization?

2. MS is characterized by remissions and exacerbations. What happens to the myelin during each of these phases?

3. Is D.V. too young to get MS? What is the etiology of MS?

4. Outline the subjective and objective assessment data associated with MS. Place a star next to the symptoms D.V. has.

5. How will the neurologist determine whether D.V. has MS?

6. The neurologist orders a magnetic resonance imaging (MRI) scan of the brain and spine. What role does this test play in diagnosing MS?

7. What is the goal of care in a patient with MS?

8. D.V. asks, "If this turns out to be MS, how will I be treated?" How would you respond?

 9. The neurologist orders 500 mg methylprednisolone (Solu-Medrol) IV daily. What do you need to do to administer this medication safely? Select all that apply.
   a. Reconstitute with 8 mL of benzyl alcohol
   b. Administer a total dose of 8 mL of reconstituted solution
   c. Use the solution within 60 minutes of reconstitution
   d. Begin the medication infusion before 0900 each day
   e. Deliver the dose over 30 minutes using IV pulse administration

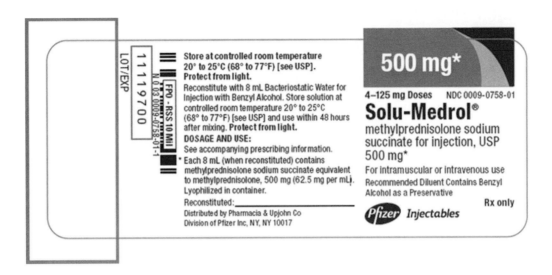

10. Because D.V. is experiencing urinary frequency and urgency, the neurologist orders oxybutynin (Ditropan) 30 mg orally each day. In addition to medication teaching, what will you teach him to do to assist in controlling urinary symptoms?

11. When planning D.V.'s care, what is the most appropriate goal for the clinical problem of activity intolerance related to muscle weakness?
    a. "D.V. will maintain muscle strength in his arms and legs."
    b. "D.V. can identify three factors that aggravate muscle weakness."
    c. "D.V. will participate in daily activities as desired without fatigue."
    d. "D.V. is free of trauma related to muscle weakness."

12. As part of your teaching plan, you want D.V. to be aware of situations or factors that are known to exacerbate symptoms. List four.

6 Neurologic Disorders

CASE STUDY PROGRESS

After testing is complete, D.V. is diagnosed with MS. He confides in you that he has been depressed since his parents' divorce and the onset of these symptoms. He tells you that he knows his girlfriend has been unfaithful, but he is afraid of being alone. He is afraid if he tells her about his MS diagnosis, she will leave him.

13. What are you going to do with this information?

14. You are concerned with D.V.'s psychological status, particularly the negative feelings he expresses regarding himself and the concerns he has voiced. Write a nursing outcome addressing this issue, and identify independent nursing actions you would implement.

15. In view of his personal history and current diagnosis, what two critical psychosocial issues require monitoring in his follow-up visits?

16. List several resources available in the community that D.V. might find helpful.

CASE STUDY OUTCOME

D.V. takes advantage of his time with a psychiatric nurse specialist, joins a local MS support group, and tells his girlfriend to move out. He later marries a woman from the support group.

Case Study 68

Name _____ Class/Group _____ Date _____

Group Members _____

▶ **Scenario**

J.G. is a 34-year-old woman who underwent an emergency cesarean delivery after a prolonged labor, during which she exhibited a sudden change in neurologic functioning and started seizing. Since that time she has experienced three tonic-clonic (grand mal) seizures. She was diagnosed with a basal ganglion hematoma with infarct and was started on phenytoin (Dilantin). Postdelivery, J.G. demonstrated dyskinesia, resulting in frequent falls during ambulation. Once the seizure disorder appeared to be under control, she was transferred to a rehabilitation facility for evaluation and 2 weeks of intensive physical therapy (PT). She is now home. She still has occasional falls but has had no seizures. She is receiving PT three times a week in her home. As case manager for J.G.'s health maintenance organization, you make a home visit with her and her family for evaluation of long-term follow-up care.

1. A seizure is not a disease in itself but a symptom of a disease. What is the term for chronically recurring seizures?

2. Does J.G. have epilepsy?

3. In addition to the brain injury, what are some other possible conditions that could be contributing to J.G.'s lowered seizure threshold?

4. What is the pathophysiology of a seizure?

5. J.G. had tonic-clonic, or grand mal, seizures. Describe this type of seizure.

6. They ask how phenytoin (Dilantin) works in preventing seizures. How would you respond?

7. What factors are considered when determining which seizure medication a patient should take?

8. J.G. tells you she is having trouble remembering to take her medication. Why does this concern you?

9. What are some strategies that you should review with J.G. and her husband to increase the likelihood of compliance?

10. You check the chart and note that J.G.'s last phenytoin (Dilantin) level was 12.7 mcg/mL. What action do you expect based on this level?
    a. J.G. at immediate risk for a seizure and she should go to the emergency department.
    b. Because this level is within normal limits, J.G. would continue therapy as prescribed.
    c. Because this level is on the border of therapeutic, notify the physician.
    d. This level is dangerously high, and an immediate reduction in dose is necessary.

11. J.G. asks, "Will my blood levels stay under control as long as I take my medicine?" How would you answer her question?

12. J.G.'s husband asks whether the Dilantin could harm his wife in any way. What general information would you review with them about Dilantin?

13. J.G. states that because she has not had a seizure since she was in the hospital, she questions how long she will have to continue taking the phenytoin (Dilantin). Which is your best response?
   a. "Your seizures are cured only as long as you take the medication."
   b. "This medication might need to be continued for the rest of your life."
   c. "This medication can be stopped after you are seizure free for 6 months."
   d. "This medication will have to be taken only when you are experiencing stress."

14. J.G.'s husband asks you what he should do if she has a seizure at home. What should you teach him?

15. Her husband states that he is afraid for J.G. to take care of the baby. What would you say to him?

6 Neurologic Disorders

16. What aspects of the home environment do you need to inspect and why?

 17. Describe safety measures you can teach J.G. that will minimize her risk of injury should she experience a seizure.

 18. You would determine further teaching is needed regarding modifying their home environment to reduce J.G.'s risk of falling if J.G. or her spouse states:
   a. "We will keep the stairway free of clutter and turn the light on as needed."
   b. "J.G. will need some new socks to wear so she is not going barefoot indoors."
   c. "We will put some nonskid strips in the shower in the master bath."
   d. "The decorative rugs are going to be put into storage."

6 Neurologic Disorders

Case Study **69**

Name _____ Class/Group _____ Date _____

Group Members _____

▶ Scenario

F.N. is a 57-year-old homemaker, happily married with grown children and two new grandchildren. F.N. made an appointment with her optometrist to explore progressive left eye visual loss over a 9-month period. Her eye examination findings were essentially normal, and the optometrist referred her to a neurologist. A magnetic resonance imaging (MRI) scan revealed a 2.5-cm primary brain mass, and she is now scheduled for a supratentorial craniotomy. Her past medical history is significant only for hypertension, for which she takes long-acting metoprolol (Toprol XL) 100 mg/day. Her past surgical history includes tonsillectomy and adenoidectomy as a child, cholecystectomy at age 35, and a total hysterectomy at age 42.

1. List six other general symptoms associated with many brain tumors to assess for in F.N.

2. F.N. and her family must be involved in the plan for treatment. Treatment can include surgery, radiation, chemotherapy, or any combination of these. F.N. also has the right to refuse treatment. Identify four other factors that the medical team, F.N., and her family would consider in devising a treatment plan.

3. F.N. is immediately placed on dexamethasone (Decadron) 40 mg intravenously twice daily. What is the expected goal of therapy with dexamethasone (Decadron)?

Chart View

Medication Administration Record

Phenytoin (Dilantin) 100 mg IV every 6 hours
Ondansetron (Zofran) 4 mg IV every 4 hours as needed for nausea
Morphine sulfate 2 mg IV every 1 hour as needed for pain
Mannitol 100 gram IV every 6 hours
Famotidine (Pepcid) 20 mg IV every 12 hours

4. Identify the expected outcome associated with each of the medications F.N. is receiving.

5. Describe common psychological responses to a diagnosis of a brain tumor.

6. F.N. draws up a living will and health care power of attorney after she hears the diagnosis. She also sits down with her family and makes her wishes known. Why is this important for F.N., in particular, and for everyone in general?

7. You enter F.N.'s room to take vital signs, and she says, "What if I come out of surgery and I'm different? Or what if I die? My grandbabies will never know me." You hear the concern in her voice and want to provide realistic reassurance about expected outcomes. Suggest several ways that F.N. can communicate with her loved ones in the event that her surgery is unsuccessful.

8. Describe your preoperative teaching for F. N. and her family.

CASE STUDY PROGRESS

After the craniotomy, F.N. is admitted to the intensive care unit (ICU) postoperatively. Her head dressing is dry and intact with a patent Hemovac. She has two peripheral intravenous (IV) lines, sequential compression devices (SCDs), oxygen at 4 L by nasal cannula, and a Foley catheter. She is neurologically intact with a Glasgow Coma Scale (GCS) score of 15.

9. What is the most serious complication that can occur after a craniotomy?

10. What assessment findings would indicate this complication may be occurring?

11. Outline the general nursing interventions you will need to implement to care for F.N. during the first 24 hours after surgery.

12. F.N. has ICP monitoring in place with an intraventricular catheter. Nursing interventions while the catheter is in place include which of the following? Select all that apply.
    a. Continuously monitoring the ICP waveforms
    b. Using aseptic technique when setting up the device
    c. Maintaining a cerebral perfusion pressure of 60 mm Hg
    d. Leveling the transducer even with the foramen of Monroe
    e. Administering prophylactic antibiotic therapy
    f. Notifying the physician if the ICP is greater than 30 mm Hg

13. Which of these care activities can be delegated to the nursing assistive personnel (NAP)? Select all that apply.
    a. Performing a capillary blood sugar measurement
    b. Positioning and turning F.N. every 2 hours
    c. Counseling F.N. on pain control measures as needed

6 Neurologic Disorders

d. Assessing F.N.'s status on the Glasgow Coma Scale
e. Emptying the Foley catheter collection bag
f. Monitoring F.N.'s serum potassium levels

Chart View

Laboratory Testing

Potassium	2.5 mmol/L
Sodium	138 mEq/L
Chloride	103 mEq/L
Glucose	202 mg/dL

14. Interpret F.N.'s laboratory values. State the rationale for any abnormalities and identify any treatment needed.

15. Is there any other assessment you need to obtain?

 16. You notify the neurosurgeon of the laboratory values and receive an order to infuse 40 mEq of IV potassium chloride (KCl). Which is the best option for administering the medication safely?
    a. Put the KCl in 250 mL 0.9% saline and infuse over 4 hours as a secondary infusion.
    b. Add the KCl to 1000 mL 0.9% saline and infuse over 12 hours as a primary IV solution.
    c. Dilute the KCl in a syringe with 100 mL 0.9% saline and infuse through a pump as a secondary infusion.
    d. Prepare four separate IV piggybacks, each containing 10 mEq KCl in 100 mL 0.9% saline, and infuse each over 1 hour.

17. After your prompt recognition of a critical laboratory value you need to document what happened. Write an example of a documentation entry describing this event.

CASE STUDY OUTCOME

F.N.'s condition stabilizes and the remainder of her hospital stay is uneventful. She did sustain mild neurologic damage as a result of the surgery and was discharged to a rehabilitation facility where she eventually recovered most of her lost function. F.N. continues to enjoy an active life and is involved in helping others face similar experiences.

6 Neurologic Disorders

Case Study **70**

Name _____ Class/Group _____ Date _____

Group Members _____

6 Neurologic Disorders

▶ Scenario

T.W. is a 22-year-old man who fell 50 feet from a chairlift while skiing and landed on hard-packed snow. He is now at the emergency department (ED) with a suspected T5-T6 fracture with paraplegia.

Chart View

Physician's Orders

Insert Foley catheter
ECG monitoring
Immobilize the cervical spine
Oxygen at 4 L per nasal cannula
Initiate two large bore IVs
Neurologic assessment every hour
Apply warming blankets as needed

1. Describe a plan for implementing these physician's orders.

2. What are the nursing priorities at this time?

3. Which assessment would you complete first?
   a. Assessing ability to move the extremities
   b. Determining pupil response to light
   c. Auscultating breath sounds
   d. Testing the peripheral reflexes

4. What other interventions would likely be done by the ED nurse?

5. Awareness of the prehospital management of a spinal cord injury (SCI) is critical to T.W.'s ultimate neurologic outcome. What actions will the nurse take to ensure this goal is met?

 6. The physician orders the following for T.W.: Intravenous (IV) methylprednisolone (Solu-Medrol), bolus of 30 mg/kg over 15 minutes, followed by a maintenance infusion of 5.4 mg/kg body weight per hour. T.W. weighs 176 pounds. How many milligrams of methylprednisolone (Solu-Medrol) will T.W. receive with the bolus? How many milligrams per hour will T.W. receive with the maintenance infusion? What effect will this medication have on T.W.?

CASE STUDY PROGRESS

Although T.W.'s injury is at a level where independent respiratory function is expected, he experiences low oxygen saturation levels and is placed on a mechanical ventilator. The physician states that this is because of spinal shock.

7. How would you explain spinal shock to T.W.'s family and why T.W. requires mechanical ventilation at this time?

8. List three critical potential infections that T.W. will be monitored for throughout his hospitalization.

6 Neurologic Disorders

CASE STUDY PROGRESS

The diagnosis of the fracture is confirmed and T.W. is transferred from the ED to the surgical intensive care unit (SICU). T.W. is taken to surgery 48 hours after the accident for spinal stabilization. He spends 2 additional days in SICU and 5 days in the neurology unit and now is in the rehabilitation unit. He continues to have paralysis of his lower extremities. Shortly after the transfer, T.W. turns on his call light and asks for medication for headache. As you walk into the room, you immediately note that T.W.'s face is flushed and he is profusely sweating.

9. What complication do you suspect T.W. is experiencing and why?

10. What further assessment data do you need to collect?

11. What could happen if autonomic dysreflexia (AD) is left untreated?

12. What interventions do you need to perform for T.W.?

13. After your prompt intervention, T.W.'s AD resolves and you need to document what happened. Write an example of a documentation entry describing this event.

14. Part of rehabilitation care includes teaching T.W. how to manage his continuous urinary drainage system (UDS). What would this teaching include?

15. T.W. is taking vitamin C 2 g orally four times daily. What is the purpose of this and what other nursing actions should accompany vitamin C therapy?

16. What outcome parameters would you use to determine whether your efforts to promote urinary excretion have been effective?

17. T.W. needs to be taught bowel-training techniques. What will this teaching include?

18. T.W. asks whether he will ever be able to have sex again. What do you tell him, and what are some possible referrals?

19. Realizing T.W. has special dietary needs, you request a consultation with the registered dietitian. Describe an optimal diet for T.W.

20. While you are assisting T.W. with his morning hygienic care, he states, "Why would anyone want to live like this? No woman will ever want me. I just wish you would have let me die." How should you initially respond?
    a. "You wish you would have died?"
    b. "Tell me why you are talking like this."
    c. "Let's finish your bath and then we can talk."
    d. "I know this is hard now, but things will work out."

21. Consider a hierarchy of rehabilitation needs for patients such as T.W. Number the following options from highest (1) to lowest (8) priority as they apply to T.W.
    a. Community integration
    b. Gainful employment
    c. Accomplishment of self-care and activities of daily living (ADLs)
    d. Self-actualization
    e. Stabilization of the physiologic systems and early psychological support
    f. Adjustment to living at home
    g. Participating in physical therapy, occupational therapy, using assistive devices; bowel and bladder training
    h. Independence

Case Study 71

Name _____   Class/Group _____   Date _____

Group Members _____

▶ Scenario

Y.W. is a 23-year-old male student from Thailand studying electrical engineering at the university. He was ejected from a moving vehicle, which was traveling at 70 mph. His injuries included a severe closed head injury with an occipital hematoma, bilateral wrist fractures, and a right pneumothorax. During his neurologic intensive care unit (NICU) stay, Y.W. was intubated and placed on mechanical ventilation, had a feeding tube inserted and was placed on tube feedings, had a Foley catheter placed, and had a central venous catheter (CVC) inserted for medication administration.

1. Differentiate between primary and secondary head injury.

2. Why is increased intracranial pressure (ICP) clinically important?

3. Identify at least six signs and symptoms of increased ICP.

4. This is how Y.W. responded to painful stimuli when he was initially admitted. What is this response called and what does it signify?

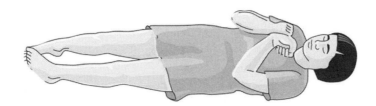

5. After the CVC was inserted, Y.W. had a stat portable chest x-ray (CXR) examination. Why?

6. List eight independent nursing measures and the rationale for the use of each that nurses implement to decrease or control increased ICP in closed head injury.

7. What outcome criteria would determine whether the independent nursing measures for Y.W. were effective?

8. Y.W.'s medication list includes ranitidine (Zantac elixir) 150 mg per percutaneous endoscopic gastrostomy (PEG) tube bid, phenytoin (Dilantin) 100 mg per PEG tube every 8 hours, propofol (Diprivan) 10 mcg/kg/min continuous intravenous (IV) infusion, and acetaminophen (Tylenol) 650 mg per PEG tube every 6 hours as needed for temperature greater than 101.0° F. Indicate the reason Y.W. received each medication.

9. Y.W. weighs 158 pounds. The pharmacy-supplied infusion bottle reads "propofol (Diprivan) 500 mg/50 mL." At how many milliliters per hour would you set the infusion pump? (Round to the nearest hundredth.)

10. The pharmacy supplies phenytoin (Dilantin) 125 mg/5 mL. How many milliliters would you administer to correctly fulfill the order of 100 mg per dose?

11. Which actions would you perform to safely administer Y.W.'s medications through the PEG tube? Select all that apply.
    a. Position Y.W. in a side-lying position with the head of bed flat.
    b. Temporarily stop the feeding while administering the medications.
    c. Flush the PEG tube with water after medication administration.
    d. Hold the tube feeding for 2 hours after administering the medication.
    e. Place the medications into the feeding bag with his tube feed formula.
    f. Aspirate for gastric residual before administering the medications.

6 Neurologic Disorders

CASE STUDY PROGRESS

Y.W. spent 2 months in acute care and is now on the rehabilitation unit. He follows commands but tends to get agitated with too much stimulation. He is receiving supplemental tube feedings and has periodic incontinence of his bowel and bladder. Y.W. has a supportive group of fellow university friends, several of them are also from Thailand.

12. Outline a general rehabilitation plan for Y.W.

13. Are you surprised by Y.W.'s periodic agitated behavior? Explain.

14. When Y.W. is agitated, which of the following interventions would be most helpful?
    a. Placing him in a solitary, quiet room
    b. Asking him to share his feelings verbally
    c. Ignoring his behavior until he is more calm
    d. Medicating him with an as-needed sedative

15. What dietary instructions are important for Y.W. that will assist him in regaining bowel control?

16. Y.W.'s mother has just arrived in the United States and speaks no English. What measures can be taken to facilitate communication between medical personnel and the mother?

17. Y.W.'s mother will need a place to stay while in the United States. What can you do to facilitate the initial contact with the Thai community?

18. What special discharge planning considerations are present for Y.W.?

Case Study 72

Name _____ Class/Group _____ Date _____

Group Members _____

▶ Scenario

K.B. is a 21-year-old man with a past medical history (PMH) of seizure disorder controlled with carbamazepine (Tegretol). He was accidentally struck in the head by a pitched baseball while batting in a baseball game. He was unconscious for about 5 seconds, then awakened and was alert and responsive. After a few hours, K.B. returned home with complaints of a "splitting" headache, drowsiness, slight confusion, and some nausea. K.B. was taken to the local hospital emergency department (ED), where a computed tomography (CT) scan revealed a left subdural hematoma. He was been transferred to your medical center 70 miles away, which has a neurosurgeon on call, and is being admitted from the ED to the medical unit.

1. The ED nurse gives you the previous information during a phoned report. What other information do you need to prepare for K.B.?

2. Because you have not taken care of a patient with a head injury recently, you look up *subdural hematoma* before K.B. arrives. What do you find?

3. Draw a shaded oval in the area where a subdural hematoma occurs.

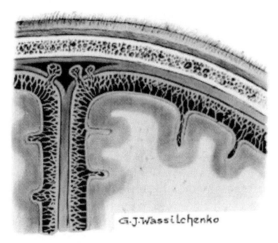

4. What are common signs and symptoms of an acute subdural hematoma?

5. Other than death, what is the most serious complication that can occur with a subdural hematoma?

6. What assessment would you need to perform to determine if this complication is occurring?

7. The neurosurgeon orders a stat serum carbamazepine (Tegretol) level. Why?

8. The decision was made in K.B.'s case not to do a craniotomy. When would a neurosurgeon decide to treat medically versus perform surgery?

9. The resident writes an order for D5W to infuse intravenously at 125 mL/hr. Does this order concern you? If so, why?

10. How would you instruct the nursing assistive personnel (NAP) to position K.B. in bed and why?

11. You are concerned about managing K.B.'s pain. Write a pain-related outcome for K.B.

12. Describe five interventions that could assist in managing K.B.'s pain.

13. What other interventions would be appropriate to implement while caring for K.B. that would assist in reducing intracranial pressure (ICP)?

14. How would you support his family?

CASE STUDY PROGRESS

You go in to assess K.B. and find that he is complaining of a headache. His heart rate is 120 and his blood pressure (BP) is 90/60. His urine output for the past hour was 685 mL with a specific gravity of 1.002.

15. What do you immediately suspect is occurring and why?

16. Using SBAR, what information would you provide to the neurosurgeon when you call?

17. What do you anticipate your care of K.B. will include over the next several hours?

18. The neurosurgeon orders vasopressin (Pitressin) continuous IV infusion: 0.0005 unit/kg/hr initially, then double dose q30min to reach the desired effect, not to exceed 0.01 unit/kg/hr. Which findings would best indicate the desired effect has been achieved? Select all that apply.
    a. BP of 100/60
    b. Glucose 90 mEq/L
    c. Heart rate 100 beats/min
    d. Serum sodium 135 mEq/L
    e. Urine specific gravity of 1.12

6 Neurologic Disorders

Case Study 73

Name _____ Class/Group _____ Date _____

Group Members _____

6 Neurologic Disorders

▶ Scenario

C.J. is a 48-year-old concert pianist. Before her performance this evening, she told a friend that she was experiencing what she called "the worst headache I've ever had" and that she had taken two extra-strength acetaminophen (Tylenol ES), but they "didn't touch my headache." During her performance, she stopped playing, reached up, grasped her head, and then fell unconscious. When the paramedics arrived, she was intubated and an intravenous (IV) line was started with normal saline.

On arrival at the emergency department, she has a Glasgow Coma Scale (GCS) score of 3. Her husband reports a history of hypertension and states she recently quit taking her medication because it made her feel tired. She is trying to quit smoking; she has cut down to a half pack of cigarettes per day, she drinks alcohol only socially on weekends, and she has a remote history of cocaine use. He says that she has complained of worsening, intermittent headaches for the past few weeks.

1. Describe C.J.'s neurologic presentation that equates with a GCS score of 3.

2. The physician immediately suspects a subarachnoid hemorrhage (SAH). Why?

CASE STUDY PROGRESS

After a noncontrast computed tomography (CT) scan is done, C.J. is diagnosed with a massive grade V SAH. She is transported to the intensive care unit (ICU) for close monitoring. She is ventilator dependent, is unresponsive to verbal or painful stimuli, and has no physical movement. Her husband, mother, and children are at her bedside; several relatives and friends are in the waiting area.

3. What is an SAH?

4. What are common causes of an SAH?

5. What are C.J.'s risk factors for SAH?

6. Describe a patient with a grade V SAH.

7. What are common complications of SAH you would anticipate?

8. What is the likely goal of treatment for C.J.?

9. Treatment of a SAH can include surgery, embolization, medications, and watchful waiting. What factors are considered in determining treatment?

Chart View

Physician's Orders

Nimodipine (Nimotop) 60 mg every 4 hours IV
0.9% normal saline at 100 mL/hr
Nicardipine (Cardene IV) IV, titrate to maintain systolic blood pressure (SBP) less than 150
Acetaminophen (Tylenol) 650 mg q6h for temperature greater than 101.0° F (38.3° C)
Insulin aspart (Novolog) subcut per sliding scale every 6 hours

10. Identify the expected outcome associated with each treatment C.J. is receiving.

11. Outline the general nursing interventions F.N. would receive during the next 24 hours.

12. Describe how you would support C.J.'s family during this time.

CASE STUDY PROGRESS

After C.J. has been in the ICU for 12 hours, the physician decides to begin testing C.J. to determine whether she is clinically brain dead.

13. What is brain death?

14. What are the criteria for declaring a patient clinically brain dead?

15. It is determined that C.J.'s condition meets the criteria and she is declared legally brain dead. She had previously indicated her willingness to be an organ donor, and her husband agrees to honor her wishes. C.J.'s husband asks you to explain the donation process. How will you explain it to him?

6 Neurologic Disorders

16. While you are waiting for the transplant team to arrive, you are working to maintain C.J.'s hemodynamic stability. Which of the following parameters would indicate your efforts are successful?
    a. Urine output of 30 mL/hr
    b. Cardiac index greater than 2.4 L/min
    c. Mean arterial BP is greater than 50 mm Hg
    d. Left ventricular ejection fraction greater than 30%

Case Study **74**

Name _____ Class/Group _____ Date _____

Group Members _____

6 Neurologic Disorders

▶ **Scenario**

D.H., a 54-year-old resort owner, has had multiple chronic medical problems, including type 2 diabetes mellitus (DM) for 25 years, which has progressed to his having been insulin dependent for the past 10 years; a kidney transplant 5 years ago with no signs of rejection at last biopsy; hypertension; and peptic ulcer disease. His medications include insulin, immunosuppressive agents, and two antihypertensive drugs. Three days ago he visited his local physician with complaints of left ear, mastoid, and sinus pain. He was diagnosed with sinusitis and *Candida albicans* infection (thrush); cephalexin (Keflex) and nystatin were prescribed. Later in the afternoon he developed nausea, hematemesis, and weakness and was taken to the emergency department. He was admitted and started on intravenous (IV) antibiotics, but his condition worsened throughout the night; his dyspnea increased and he developed difficulty speaking. He was flown the next morning to your tertiary referral center and was intubated en route. On arrival, D.H. had decreased level of consciousness with periods of total unresponsiveness, weakness, and cranial nerve deficits. His admitting diagnosis is meningitis. He has since developed aspiration pneumonia and atrial fibrillation. D.H. has continued fever and leukocytosis despite aggressive antibiotic therapy.

1. Why was D.H. at particular risk for infection?

2. Describe bacterial meningitis.

3. Describe how meningitis is diagnosed.

4. What is the probable route of entry of bacteria into D.H.'s brain?

5. When D.H. was admitted, the nurse charted that he could not extend his legs without complaining of extreme pain. This sign would be charted as a positive:
   a. Kernig sign
   b. Trousseau sign
   c. Babinski sign
   d. Brudzinski sign

6. How do you think D.H. developed aspiration pneumonia?

7. What transmission-based precautions need to be instituted for D.H.? Select all that apply.
   a. Placing D.H. in a private room
   b. Wearing a gown for all patient contacts
   c. Wearing gloves during contact with oral secretions
   d. Wearing a respirator each time on entering the room
   e. Placing D.H. in a room with negative airflow pressure
   f. Wearing a surgical mask each time on entering the room

8. What factors influenced the physician's decision to transport D.H. from a smaller hospital to a tertiary care center?

9. Describe how you evaluate D.H. for cranial nerve deficits.

Chart View

Medication Administration Record

Neutral protamine Hagedorn (NPH) insulin subcut 20 units bid
Insulin aspart (NovoLog) subcut per sliding scale ac/hs
Digoxin 0.125 mg IVP daily
Sucralfate (Carafate) 1 g PO q6h
Azathioprine (Imuran) 100 mg daily IV piggyback (IVPB) in 150 mL D5W
Imipenem–cilastatin sodium (Primaxin) 1 g IVPB q8h in 100 mL 0.9% NaCl
Metronidazole (Flagyl) 500 mg IVPB q6h in 75 mL 0.9% NaCl
Methylprednisolone (Solu-Medrol) 125 mg IVP q8h in 75 mL 0.9% NaCl

10. Indicate the expected outcome for D.H. that is associated with each of the medications he is receiving.

6 Neurologic Disorders

11. The order for the imipenem–cilastatin sodium (Primaxin) reads to infuse 1 g in 100 mL 0.9% NaCl q8h over 30 minutes. You have IV tubing that supplies 15 gtt/mL. At how many drops per minute will you regulate the infusion?

12. When evaluating D.H.'s expected fluid intake over the next 24 hours, how many total milliliters should he receive from the administration of IVPBs?

13. The nursing assistive personnel (NAP) reports to you that D.H. has a glucose result of 450 mg/dL. Identify two factors that could contribute to D.H.'s elevated glucose level.

14. What should you do regarding the elevated glucose level, and why?

As D.H.'s primary nurse, you are responsible for his nursing care plan. In addition to his risk for increased intracranial pressure, you determine you are concerned about managing pain and avoiding seizure-related injury. You decide to address each of these areas in his plan of care.

15. You plan to administer prescribed as-needed analgesics. What are three other strategies that will facilitate the expected outcome of managing his acute pain?

 16. Which of the following interventions to decrease the risk of seizure-related injury can you delegate to the nursing assistive personnel (NAP)? Select all that apply.
a. Keeping D.H.'s bed in low position
b. Reorienting D.H. as needed to the environment
c. Setting up oxygen and suction equipment at the bedside
d. Ensuring that D.H.'s call light is within easy reach at all times
e. Teaching D.H. why he should not get up without assistance if he is dizzy

17. D.H.'s family is staying at a nearby motel. His adult son brings his mother to the hospital. Mrs. H. says she just wants to stay with her husband around the clock. She states, "I took care of him for 35 years now, and I'm not going to abandon him now when he needs me the most." Recognizing that these are stressful times for all involved, how will you respond?

Unfortunately, D.H.'s infection destroys his cadaver kidney. He develops multiple system organ failure and dies 7 weeks later.

Case Study 75

Name _____ Class/Group _____ Date _____

Group Members _____

▶ Scenario

S.B. is a 22-year-old man who lost control of an all-terrain utility vehicle and struck a tree. He was not restrained and his face hit the windshield on impact. When paramedics arrived, S.B. was responsive but confused, had significant facial swelling, and complained of pain in his right wrist and left forearm. The paramedics initiated cervical spine precautions, started oxygen at 15 L/min via a non-rebreather mask, and started a 16-gauge intravenous (IV) line with 0.9% normal saline. His vital signs (VS) were 120/75, 125, 36, and Spo$_2$ 94%. On arrival at the local emergency department (ED) 15 minutes later, his VS are 110/62, 110 regular, 28 to 32 and shallow, and Spo$_2$ 99%. An additional 16-gauge IV is inserted, and samples are drawn for the following laboratory tests: complete blood count (CBC), type and crossmatch, complete metabolic panel, prothrombin time/partial thromboplastin time (PT/PTT) and international normalized ratio (INR), and alcohol level. The trauma physician completes a head-to-toe assessment; the findings are shown in the chart.

Chart View

Physician Note

Obeys commands, responds to voice, but not oriented to time or place. Generalized facial edema with full-thickness 2-cm cheek laceration. Blood behind left tympanic membrane, edema with slight discoloration over left mastoid process. Clear drainage coming from the left naris. Mid- to upper-chest contusions without crepitus, breath sounds clear. Abdomen slightly firm but not tender. Catheterized for 500 mL clear yellow urine; negative for blood, glucose, ketones. Positive deformity of right wrist and diffuse tenderness of left lower forearm.

1. What is the significance of the slight discoloration over the left mastoid process, blood behind the left tympanic membrane, and drainage from the nose?

2. What are the typical signs and symptoms of a basilar skull fracture (BSF)? Place a star next to those S.B. has.

3. What physical condition does this picture depict, and why is it a significant finding in a patient with a BSF?

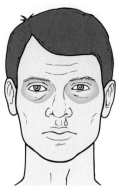

4. S.B.'s skull x-ray study is negative for BSF. How significant is this finding?

5. What is the most reliable diagnostic indicator for BSF?

6. Identify three serious complications associated with BSF.

7. How would you test S.B. for evidence of cerebrospinal fluid (CSF) leakage?

8. What are the symptoms of a posterior fossa fracture (fracture of temporal petrous bone), and how does it compare with a BSF?

9. The medical student gets a nasogastric tube and begins preparation to insert one into S.B. Why do you stop the student?

10. What implications do S.B.'s injuries have in relation to discharge planning?

CASE STUDY PROGRESS

CT scan confirms a basilar skull and left maxillary (Le Fort) fractures. Both arms are placed in splints because of right and left radial fractures. Because of his multiple injuries, he is admitted to the surgical unit.

11. What is the treatment strategy for a BSF with a limited CSF leak?

12. Which neurologic interventions could you delegate to the nursing assistive personnel (NAP)? Select all that apply.
    a. Reminding S.B. not to cough or sneeze
    b. Assessing his pupillary response to light
    c. Noting S.B.'s intake and output with each incidence
    d. Assisting S.B. to sit in the bed with the head elevated
    e. Evaluating S.B.'s response to his as-needed pain medications
    f. Instructing S.B. on the importance of deep breathing every hour

Chart View

Vital Signs

Blood pressure	170/68 mm Hg
Heart rate	118 beats/min
Respiratory rate	32 breaths/min
Temperature	101.8° F (38.8° C)
Oxygen saturation	93%

13. You note that the NAP has entered these vital signs into S.B.'s record. What are your immediate concerns and why?

14. What action do you need to take based on this concern?

15. What are your nursing priorities at this time?

16. Describe four nursing interventions you will perform over the next few hours based on these priorities.

17. Identify three expected outcomes for S.B. as a result of your interventions.

CASE STUDY PROGRESS

After S.B. stabilizes from this the brief episode of increased intracranial pressure (ICP), he stays in the hospital for 72 hours, during which time his condition remains relatively stable. Before discharge, bilateral short arm casts are applied. Arrangements have been made for him to go to his family home for recuperation.

18. As you are evaluating discharge teaching for S.B., you would understand that further teaching would be required if he stated:
    a. "I will try to avoid blowing my nose for the next 2 weeks."
    b. "If I start vomiting, I will return to the hospital immediately."
    c. "If I do not move my bowels each day, I will take a Dulcolax."
    d. "Because a headache is expected, I can take aspirin for the pain."

6 Neurologic Disorders

Endocrine Disorders

Case Study 76

Name _____ Class/Group _____ Date _____

Group Members _____

▶ **Scenario**

Y.L., a 34-year-old Southern Asian woman, comes to the clinic with complaints of chronic fatigue, increased thirst, constant hunger, and frequent urination. She denies any pain, burning, or low-back pain on urination. She tells you she has a vaginal yeast infection that she has treated numerous times with over-the-counter medication. She works full time as a clerk in a loan company and states she has difficulty reading numbers and reports, resulting in her making frequent mistakes. She says, "By the time I get home and make supper for my family, then put my child to bed, I am too tired to exercise." She reports her feet hurt; they often "burn or feel like there are pins in them." She has a history of gestational diabetes and reports that after her delivery she went back to her traditional eating pattern, which is high in carbohydrates.

In reviewing Y.L.'s chart, you note she last saw the provider 6 years ago after the delivery of her last child. She has gained considerable weight; her current weight is 173 pounds. Today her blood pressure (BP) is 152/97 mm Hg, and a random plasma glucose level is 291 mg/dL. The provider suspects that Y.L. has developed type 2 diabetes mellitus (DM) and orders the laboratory studies shown in the chart.

Chart View

Laboratory Test Results	
Fasting glucose	184 mg/dL
Hemoglobin A_{1c} (HbA$_{1c}$)	8.8%
Total cholesterol	256 mg/dL
Triglycerides	346 mg/dL
Low-density lipoprotein (LDL)	155 mg/dL
High-density lipoprotein (HDL)	32 mg/dL
Urinalysis (UA)	+glucose, −ketones

1. Interpret Y.L.'s laboratory results.

2. Identify the three methods used to diagnose DM.

3. Describe the functions of insulin.

4. Describe the major pathophysiologic difference between type 1 and type 2 DM.

5. Name six risk factors for type 2 DM. Place a star or asterisk next to those that Y.L. exhibits.

CASE STUDY PROGRESS

Y.L. is diagnosed with type 2 DM. The provider starts her on metformin (Glucophage) 500 mg and glipizide (Glucotrol) 5 mg orally each day at breakfast and atorvastatin (Lipitor) 20 mg orally at bedtime. She is referred to the dietitian for instructions on starting a 1200-calorie diet using an exchange system to facilitate weight loss and lower blood glucose, cholesterol, and triglyceride levels. You are to provide education regarding pharmacotherapy and exercise.

6. How can you incorporate Y.W.'s cultural preferences as you develop her education plan?

7. What is the rationale for starting Y.L. on metformin (Glucophage) and glipizide (Glucotrol)?

8. Outline the teaching you need to provide to Y.L. regarding oral hypoglycemic therapy.

9. What benefits should Y.L. receive from encouragement to exercise?

7 Endocrine Disorders

CASE STUDY PROGRESS

Y.L. comments, "I've heard many people with diabetes lose their toes or even their feet." You take this opportunity to teach her about neuropathy and foot care.

10. Which of the symptoms that Y.L. reported today led you to believe she has some form of neuropathy?

11. What other findings in Y.L.'s history place her at increased risk for developing neuropathy?

12. What would you teach Y.L. about neuropathy?

13. Because Y.L. has symptoms of neuropathy, placing her at risk for foot complications, you realize you need to instruct her on proper foot care. Outline what you will include when teaching her about proper diabetic foot care.

14. What monitoring will Y.L. need regarding nephropathy and retinopathy?

Case Study **77**

Name _____ Class/Group _____ Date _____

Group Members _____

7 Endocrine Disorders

▶ **Scenario**

You graduated 3 months ago and are working with a home care agency. One patient in your caseload is J.S., a 60-year-old man with chronic obstructive pulmonary disease (COPD) related to cigarette smoking. He has been on home oxygen, 2 L oxygen by nasal cannula, for several years. Approximately 10 months ago, he started on chronic oral steroid therapy. His current medications include an ipratropium/albuterol (Combivent) inhaler, beclomethasone (Beclovent) inhaler, dexamethasone (Decadron), digoxin (Lanoxin), and furosemide (Lasix).

1. On the way to J.S.'s home, you make a mental note to check him for signs and symptoms of Cushing syndrome. Why?

2. Differentiate between Cushing syndrome and Cushing disease.

3. Your assessment includes the following findings. Determine whether the findings are attributable to J.S.'s COPD or possible Cushing syndrome. Place an *L* beside the symptoms consistent with COPD and a *C* next to those consistent with Cushing syndrome.
   _____ 1. Barrel chest
   _____ 2. Full-looking face (moon face)
   _____ 3. BP 180/94 mm Hg
   _____ 4. Pursed-lip breathing, especially when patient is stressed
   _____ 5. Striae over trunk and thighs
   _____ 6. Bruising on both arms
   _____ 7. Acne
   _____ 8. Diminished breath sounds throughout lungs
   _____ 9. Truncal obesity with thin extremities
   _____10. Supraclavicular and posterior upper back fat

4. You inform the physician of J.S.'s assessment. The physician believes J.S. has developed Cushing syndrome and decides to change his prescription from dexamethasone (Decadron) daily to prednisone (Deltasone) given on alternate days. Explain the rationale for this change.

5. Identify possible consequences of suddenly stopping dexamethasone (Decadron) therapy.

6. You advise J.S. to take the prednisone (Deltasone) at breakfast. Why?

7. Cushing syndrome can affect memory. Patients can easily forget what medications have been taken, especially when there are several different medications and some are taken on alternating days. List at least three ways you can help J.S. remember to take his medications as prescribed.

8. J.S. states that his appetite has increased but he is losing weight. He reports trying to eat, but he gets short of breath and cannot eat any more. How would you address this problem?

9. You ask him questions related to the presence gastric discomfort, vision, and joint pain. Why?

10. Differentiate between the glucocorticoid and mineralocorticoid effects of prednisone (Deltasone).

11. How would your assessment change if J.S. were taking a glucocorticoid that had significant mineralocorticoid activity?

12. Review J.S.'s list of medications. Based on what you know about the side effects of loop diuretics and steroids, discuss the potential problem of administering these in combination with digoxin.

13. You need to assess J.S. for signs and symptoms of an infection. Why?

14. What signs and symptoms of infection do you assess for in J.S.? Select all that apply.
    a. Pain
    b. Fever
    c. Loss of function
    d. Palpitations
    e. Unusual drainage
    f. Localized edema

15. Realizing J.S. is susceptible to infection, you review with him ways to reduce the risk of infection. Identify four major points to include.

16. In addition to measures to reduce the risk of infection, what other information would you want to stress to J.S. at your visit? Select all that apply.
    a. Drink at least 4000 mL of fluids daily.
    b. Increase intake of foods high in sodium.
    c. Weigh yourself first thing in the morning.
    d. Take vitamin and electrolyte supplements as prescribed.
    e. Notify the physician if your pulse is lower than 60 beats/min.
    f. Call the doctor if your weight increases more than 2-3 pounds in 1 day.
    g. Take the furosemide (Lasix) first thing in the morning and again at bedtime.

Case Study 78

Name _____ Class/Group _____ Date _____

Group Members _____

7 Endocrine Disorders

▶ Scenario

You are working in a community outpatient clinic where you perform the intake assessment on R.M., a 38-year-old woman who is attending graduate school and is very sedentary. Her chief complaint is overwhelming fatigue that is not relieved by rest. She is so exhausted that she has difficulty walking to classes and trouble concentrating when studying. She reports a recent weight gain of 15 pounds over 2 months without clear changes in her dietary habits. Her face looks puffy, she has experienced excessive hair loss, and her skin is dry and pale. She complains of generalized body aches and pains with frequent muscle cramps and constipation. You notice she is dressed inappropriately warmly for the weather.

Chart View

Vital Signs (VS)	
Blood pressure (BP)	142/84 mm Hg
Heart rate	52 beats/min
Respiratory rate	12 breaths/min
Temperature	96.8° F (36° C)

1. Compare her VS with those of a healthy person her same age.

2. List eight general questions you might ask R.M. to assist in determining what is going on.

3. You know that potential causes for some of R.M.'s symptoms include depression, hypothyroidism, anemia, cardiac disease, fluid and electrolyte imbalance, and allergies. As part of your screening, describe how you would begin to investigate if any of these conditions explain R.M.'s symptoms.

4. What diagnostic tests are the most appropriate for R.M., and why?

Chart View

Laboratory Test Results

Thyroid-stimulating hormone (TSH)	20.9 mU/L (2-10 mU/L)
Thyrotropin-releasing hormone (TRH)	18.8 ng/dL (2-10 ng/dL)
T_3	24 mU/L (70-205 ng/dL)
Free T_4	0.2 ng/dL (0.8-2.4 ng/dL)

5. Interpret R.M.'s laboratory results.

6. The practitioner affirms a diagnosis of hypothyroidism. With this diagnosis, what other signs and symptoms would you want to assess for in R.M.?

7. The practitioner prescribes levothyroxine (Synthroid) 1.7 mcg/kg body weight per day. At this time, R.M. weighs 130 pounds. What should be her daily dose of levothyroxine in milligrams? How would her prescription read?

8. What general teaching issues will you address with R.M. concerning hypothyroidism?

9. What teaching needs will you review with R.M. with regard to her medication?

10. What should you teach R.M. regarding prevention of myxedema coma?

11. Which statements indicate R.M. understands your teaching regarding hypothyroidism and using Synthroid? Select all that apply.
    a. "It may take several weeks before I feel better."
    b. "The best time to take my medicine is with breakfast."
    c. "If my heart rate is over 100, I will hold my medication until it is back below 100."
    d. "I will be able to discontinue my medication after the symptoms are under control."
    e. "I will come in when you need me to so my blood levels can be checked to make sure the medicine is working."

7 Endocrine Disorders

12. Before R.M. leaves the clinic, she asks how she will know whether the medication is "doing its job." Outline simple expected outcomes for R.M.

13. A few weeks later, R.M. calls the clinic stating she cannot remember whether she took her thyroid medication. What additional data should you obtain, and how would you advise her?

CASE STUDY OUTCOME

R.M. comes in 2 months later for a follow-up visit. You cannot believe she is the same person. She looks and walks as if she were 10 years younger. Her skin appears more radiant, and her hair looks much healthier. "You can't believe how different I'm feeling," she says. "I didn't know how bad off I was; I'm starting to live again."

Case Study **79**

Name _____ Class/Group _____ Date _____

Group Members _____

7 Endocrine Disorders

▶ Scenario

K.B. is a 65-year-old man admitted to the hospital after a 5-day episode of "the flu" with complaints of dyspnea on exertion, palpitations, chest pain, insomnia, and fatigue. K.B. was diagnosed with Graves' disease 6 months ago and placed on methimazole (Tapazole) 15 mg/day. His other past medical history includes heart failure and hypertension requiring antihypertensive medications; however, he states that he has not been taking these medications on a regular basis. Vital signs (VS) are: 150/90, 124 irregular, 20, 100.2° F (37.9° C). Admission assessment findings are: height 5 ft, 8 in; weight 132 lb; appears anxious and restless; loud heart sounds; 1+ pitting edema noted in bilateral lower extremities; diminished breath sounds with fine crackles in the posterior bases. K.B. begins to cry when he tells you he recently lost his wife; you notice someone has punched several more holes in his belt so he could tighten it.

Chart View

Laboratory Test Results

Hemoglobin (Hgb)	11.8 g/dL
Hematocrit (Hct)	36%
Erythrocyte sedimentation rate (ESR)	48 mm/hr
Sodium	141 mmol/L
Potassium	4.7 mmol/L
Chloride	101 mmol/L
Blood urea nitrogen (BUN)	33 mg/dL
Creatinine	1.9 mg/dL
Free thyroxine (T_4)	14.0 ng/dL
Triiodothyronine (T_3)	230 ng/dL

1. Which of K.B.'s assessment findings represent manifestations of hypermetabolism?

2. Interpret K.B.'s laboratory results.

3. You go to assess K.B. What additional data do you need to obtain because he has Graves' disease?

Chart View

Physician's Orders

Propranolol (Inderal) 20 mg PO q6h
Dexamethasone (Decadron) 10 mg IV q6h
Verapamil (Calan SR) 120 mg/day PO
Furosemide (Lasix) 80 mg IV push now, then 40 mg/day IVP
Diet as tolerated
STAT ECG and echocardiogram
Up ad lib
IV of D5W at 125 mL/hr
Daily weights with intake and output (I&O)

4. The physician writes these admission orders. Which will you question, and why?

5. Describe four priority problems related to K.B.'s nursing care.

CASE STUDY PROGRESS

Later on your shift, you note that K.B. is extremely restless and disoriented to person, place, and time. VS are 174/82, 180 and irregular, 32 and labored, 104° F (40° C). His electrocardiogram (ECG) shows atrial fibrillation.

6. What is likely happening with K.B.? State your rationale.

7. What will you do first?

8. You need to call the physician regarding K.B.'s status. Using SBAR, what will you report to the physician?

CASE STUDY PROGRESS

The physician evaluates K.B. and determines he is in thyroid crisis. The physician's orders are shown in the chart.

Chart View

Physician's Orders

Oxygen at 2 L per nasal cannula
STAT arterial blood gases, brain natriuretic peptide (BNP), and cardiac enzymes
Digoxin (Lanoxin) 0.25 mg IV push now, then 0.125 mg IVP q8h × 2 doses
Diltiazem (Cardizem) bolus dose of 0.25 mg/kg IV; after 15 minutes, give a second dose of 0.35 mg/kg IV for heart rate greater than 140
Increase methimazole (Tapazole) to 15 mg PO q6h
Lugol's solution 10 drops PO tid: start 1 hour after first methimazole dose
Hydrocortisone (HydroCort) 50 mg IVP q6h
Absolute bed rest
Acetaminophen (Tylenol) 650 mg PO q6h prn for temp over 100° F (37.8° C)

9. Describe how you would care for K.B. in the next hour.

10. The label on the vial of diltiazem (Cardizem) states that there are 5 mg/mL. How many total milliliters will you administer for the first dose? How many for the second (if needed)?

 11. Describe how to safely administer Lugol's solution.

12. What is your primary nursing goal at this time?

13. Describe six interventions you will perform over the next few hours for K.B. based on this priority.

14. Why was K.B. at risk for developing thyroid storm?

15. Identify three outcomes that you expect for K.B. as a result of your interventions.

CASE STUDY PROGRESS

After several hours of treatment, K.B.'s condition stabilizes. The physician discusses two treatment options with K.B. and his family: radioactive iodine (RAI) therapy, also known as I-131, and subtotal thyroidectomy.

16. K.B. is fearful of radiation treatment and asks you for your opinion. How would you respond?

17. K.B. decides to receive RAI. During pretreatment instructions, the family asks whether he will be radioactive and what precautions they should take. Outline important guidelines for instructing K.B. and his family regarding home precautions.

18. In the midst of all this, you remain concerned over K.B.'s bereavement after the loss of his wife. How would you address this issue?

19. K.B. does have some exophthalmos and is experiencing periodic photophobia and dry eyes. What should you include in teaching him how to manage these problems? Select all that apply.
    a. Wear sunglasses at all times when outside.
    b. Report any changes in vision to the physician.
    c. Use artificial tears to provide moisture as needed.
    d. Tape the eyes closed at night with nonallergenic tape.
    e. Apply warm compresses to the eyes if they are irritated.

7 Endocrine Disorders

20. Which statement indicates K.B. understands the discharge instructions?
   a. "I will take this medication on a full stomach."
   b. "If I get a sore throat, ice chips should help me feel better."
   c. "I should see an improvement in my symptoms by tomorrow."
   d. "I will follow the precautions for 2 weeks to keep my family safe."

CASE STUDY OUTCOME

Six months later, K.B.'s heart rate, blood pressure, and thyroid hormone levels are within normal limits. He has gained 14 pounds and has started walking in the mornings without any dyspnea. He says he has started to do woodworking and has been doing some volunteer work at the senior center.

7 Endocrine Disorders

Case Study **80**

Name _____ Class/Group _____ Date _____

Group Members _____

▶ Scenario

You are working on the surgical floor and will be receiving a patient from the postanesthesia care unit. The nurse calls and gives the following report: C.P. is a 55-year-old woman who underwent a subtotal thyroidectomy for papillary carcinoma. Estimated blood loss was 25 mL. Vital signs (VS) are 130/82, 80 to 90, 20, and Sao_2 94% on room air. She is receiving a peripheral intravenous (IV) infusion of D5.45NS at 100 mL/hr. She has received a total of 3 mg morphine sulfate IV push, and she remains awake, but drowsy, and fully oriented. C.P.'s past medical history includes a total abdominal hysterectomy for fibroids and low-level radiation treatments to the neck 30 years ago for eczema. Both parents are living; her father had a myocardial infarction at 70 years of age; her mother has hypothyroidism but never had thyroid tumors.

1. What specific preparations will you make before C.P. arrives?

2. You receive C.P. from the recovery room. How will you focus your initial assessment, and why?

3. During your initial assessment, you document negative Chvostek and Trousseau signs. Describe data that would support this conclusion.

4. Identify the major risk factor that might have contributed to the development of thyroid adenoma in C.P.

5. Identify interventions to use to reduce the risk of postoperative swelling.

6. List four complications that C.P. is at risk for postoperatively. Describe actions you should include in C.P.'s plan of care related to each complication.

7. Which assessment findings would indicate C.P. has laryngeal nerve damage? Select all that apply.
   a. Stridor
   b. Hoarseness
   c. Breathy voice
   d. Circumoral numbness
   e. Difficulty swallowing

8. After surgery, C.P.'s thyroid hormone levels are elevated. The physician orders propranolol (Inderal) 80 mg ER orally twice daily for "surgically induced thyrotoxicosis." Is this reaction expected after thyroid surgery, or did something go wrong during surgery? Explain.

CASE STUDY PROGRESS

Eighteen hours after surgery, C.P. calls you into her room complaining of numbness around her mouth, tingling at the tips of her fingers, and jitteriness. She appears restless but denies any pain at the operative site. She is able to swallow and speak without difficulty.

9. What is your immediate concern and why?

10. What actions do you need to take based on this concern?

11. The physician orders you to give C.P. 1 gram of calcium gluconate intravenously over 15 minutes now, and then initiate an infusion of 2 grams of calcium gluconate in 500 mL D5W over 12 hours. After the bolus is complete, at what rate will you set the IV pump?

12. What precautions do you need to take while administering the calcium gluconate infusion?

CASE STUDY PROGRESS

Six hours after initiation of the calcium gluconate infusion, C.P. is no longer complaining of numbness around her mouth or tingling in her fingertips and toes. Chvostek and Trousseau signs remain negative.

Chart View

Laboratory Test Results

Serum calcium	7.4 mg/dL
Ionized calcium	3.4 mg/dL
Parathyroid hormone (PTH)	<3.0 pg/mL

13. Has C.P.'s status improved or not? Defend your response.

7 Endocrine Disorders

CASE STUDY PROGRESS

C.P. is started on oral calcium gluconate. Her calcium levels stabilize within 24 hours and she recovers without further complications. Two days postoperatively, you are preparing her for discharge.

14. As part of your discharge instructions, what would you teach C.P.? Select all that apply.
    a. Keep her head raised while sleeping for 3 -4 days
    b. The importance of keeping follow-up medical appointments
    c. Not to return to work until her thyroid hormone level is normal
    d. Cover her incision with clothing or sunscreen when she is in the sun
    e. Proper care of the incision and signs of infection to report to the physician
    f. To avoid foods containing iodine because they increase her risk of recurrent cancer

Case Study **81**

Name _____ Class/Group _____ Date _____

Group Members _____

7 Endocrine Disorders

▶ Scenario

You work in the diabetes mellitus (DM) center at a large teaching hospital. The first patient you meet is K.W., a 25-year-old Hispanic woman, who was just released from the hospital 2 days ago after being diagnosed with type I DM.

Nine days ago K.W. went to see the physician after a 1-month history of frequent urination, thirst, severe fatigue, blurred vision, and some burning and tingling in her feet. She attributed those symptoms to working long hours at the computer. Her random glucose level was 410 mg/dL. The next day her laboratory values were as follows: fasting glucose 335 mg/dL, hemoglobin A_{1c} (HbA_{1c}) 8.8%, cholesterol 310 mg/dL, triglycerides 300 mg/dL, high-density lipoprotein (HDL) 25 mg/dL, low-density lipoprotein (LDL) 160 mg/dL, ratio 12.4, and creatinine 0.9 mg/dL. Her body mass index is 37.6. Her blood pressure (BP) is 160/96 mm Hg. She was admitted to the hospital for control of her glucose levels and the initiation of insulin therapy with carbohydrate (CHO) counting. After discharge, K.W. has been referred to you for comprehensive education. You are to cover four basic areas: pharmacotherapy, glucose monitoring, medical nutrition therapy (MNT), and exercise.

1. K.W. was started on sliding scale lispro (Humalog) four times daily and glargine (Lantus) insulin 30 units at bedtime. What is the most significant difference between these two insulin therapies?

2. K.W. says she knows people who "only take 2 shots" because they are on NPH and regular insulin and wants to know why she can't do that. Explain the advantages of using the glargine (Lantus) and lispro (Humalog) insulin regimen.

3. Identify important content to be included under pharmacologic therapy.

4. What specific points would you include regarding managing insulin therapy? Select all that apply.
   a. Store unused insulin in the freezer.
   b. The insulin can be used if it is yellow but not expired.
   c. Administer the lispro (Humalog) within 15 minutes of eating.
   d. Ideally, the glargine (Lantus) should be administered at bedtime.
   e. Always administer the injections in the same, easy-to-reach location.
   f. The current vial of lispro (Humalog) can be kept at room temperature for 1 month.
   g. Two injections will be needed to administer lispro (Humalog) and glargine (Lantus).

5. Identify important content to review regarding glucose monitoring.

6. K.W. states her diet is mostly fast foods, and the foods cooked at home are high in starch and fat. She says because of her work schedule, mealtimes often vary from day to day. What is CHO (carbohydrate) counting, and why would this method work well for K.W.?

7. Identify important points to be covered in a basic nutrition plan with CHO counting.

8. K.W. states that she currently does not exercise at all. What benefits will K.W. receive from participating in an exercise program?

9. What do you need to teach K.W. regarding safe exercise?

10. K.W. states she and her husband were planning to have another child in a year to two. She wants to know if her DM will affect a pregnancy. Pregnancy in persons with DM is a complex issue. What basic information can you share with K.W. today without overwhelming her?

11. What evaluative parameters could you use to determine whether your teaching with K.W. was effective?

7 Endocrine Disorders

CASE STUDY PROGRESS

K.W. calls the clinic several days later complaining of having "the flu." She says that she has been nauseated and vomited once during the night. She says she has had two loose stools. On questioning, she states that she does have a few chills and might have a low-grade fever but does not have a thermometer to check her temperature. She states she did not check her glucose level this morning or take her insulin because she has "not eaten."

12. Describe the instructions that you need to give K.W. regarding the management of her illness and DM.

13. Describe how you will document the phone call with K.W.

Immunologic Disorders

Case Study 82

Name _____ Class/Group _____ Date _____

Group Members _____

▶ **Scenario**

You are a nurse at a university health clinic. Twenty-year-old T.Q. comes in and informs you he is a new student and he has an immunodeficiency problem. He gives you a letter from his attending physician, hands you a vial of gamma globulin, and asks you to give him his "shot." The letter from T.Q.'s physician states T.Q. was diagnosed with primary immunodeficiency disease (PIDD) at age 2. He has an adequate number of B cells, but they fail to mature properly and become plasma cells or immunoglobulin. T.Q. states he has a history of chronic respiratory and gastrointestinal infections. He is maintained on 0.66 mL/kg of gamma globulin (GamaSTAN) given intramuscularly every 3 weeks and has tolerated this well. He has no known drug allergies (NKDA). His vital signs are stable.

1. Can you honor T.Q.'s prescription? Why or why not? How could you provide him with his injection?

2. While the provider is verifying the information, you place T.Q. in a treatment room and obtain his permission to perform a history and physical assessment so the clinic has baseline information. What essential components do you need to include and why?

3. You note on T.Q.'s health record that he has not received an MMR (measles, mumps, rubella) vaccine. Why?

4. The provider receives confirmation from T.Q.'s physician that T.Q. has a PIDD and orders the gamma globulin (GamaSTAN). Differentiate between primary and secondary immunodeficiency.

5. Explain why T.Q. is at greater risk for developing infections than his classmates.

6. What role does gamma globulin play in managing PIDD?

7. What questions would you ask T.Q. that would assure you the medication itself is safe to administer?

8. Your assessment of T.Q. is unremarkable. After you administer the gamma globulin, you assess T.Q.'s knowledge and give specific precaution instructions. What will you assess and what precautions will you review?

9. Write a sample SOAP note documenting T.Q.'s visit to the clinic.

CASE STUDY PROGRESS

Several weeks later, on T.Q.'s return visit for an injection, he complains of a stuffy nose.

10. What is your immediate concern?

11. What assessment do you need to perform to evaluate his stuffy nose?

12. If T.Q. were developing a sinus infection, what manifestations would you likely see when examining him?

13. T.Q. denies any cough, headache, sore throat, fatigue, or muscle ache. T.Q.'s nares do not appear swollen or red, although he does have some clear mucous drainage. External auditory canals and tympanic membranes clear. There is no adenopathy or sinus tenderness, and his lung sounds are clear to auscultation. Oral cavity and pharynx normal; there is no inflammation, swelling, exudate, or lesions. Vital signs are 110/60, 76, 18, 98.4° F (36.9° C). Should you give the medication or ask him to return when he is no longer having nasal stuffiness? Why or why not?

14. What do you need to teach T.Q. before he leaves the clinic?

15. Write a sample SOAP note documenting T.Q.'s visit to the clinic.

8 Immunologic Disorders

Case Study 83

Name _____ Class/Group _____ Date _____

Group Members _____

▶ **Scenario**

You are working in a community health clinic and you have just taken C.Q., a 38-year-old woman, into the consultation room. C.Q. has been divorced for 5 years, has two daughters (ages 14 and 16), and works full time as a legal secretary. She is here for her yearly routine physical examination C.Q. states she is in a serious relationship, is contemplating marriage, and just wants to make certain she is "okay." No abnormalities were noted during C.Q.'s physical examination. Blood was drawn for routine blood chemistries and hematology studies; since she has never been tested, C.Q. agrees to a human immunodeficiency virus (HIV) test. The physician requests you perform a rapid HIV test, which is an antibody test. Within 20 minutes, the results are available and are positive.

1. Does a positive rapid HIV test mean that C.Q. definitely has HIV? If it is negative, does it mean she definitely does not have HIV?

2. What counseling do you need to provide to C.Q.?

CASE STUDY PROGRESS

C.Q. returns to the clinic two days later. The physician informs you that C.Q.'s Western blot test results confirm that she is HIV positive; he requests that you be present when he talks to her. Before leaving C.Q.'s room, the physician requests that you give C.Q. verbal and written information about local HIV support groups and help C.Q. call a friend to accompany her home this evening. She looks at you through her tears and states, "I can't believe it. J. is the only man I've had sex with since my divorce. He told me I had nothing to worry about. I can't believe he would do this to me."

3. C.Q.'s statement is based on three assumptions: (1) J. is HIV positive; (2) he intentionally withheld the information from her; and (3) he intentionally transmitted the HIV to her through unprotected sex. Based on your knowledge of HIV infection, how would you counsel C.Q.?

4. In addition to offering alternative explanations and exploring options, what is your most important role at this time?

5. C.Q. asks you whether she has AIDS. What do you tell her?

6. Why is it a good idea for C.Q. to have someone she trusts transport her home this evening?

7. C.Q. gives you the name and phone number of a relative she wants you to call. You remain with her until she leaves with her relative. Has C.Q.'s right to privacy been violated? Explain why or why not.

CASE STUDY PROGRESS

C.Q. returns to the clinic 4 days later to discuss her diagnosis.

8. What are your goals for C.Q. at this time?

9. What additional laboratory tests would you anticipate for C.Q. and why?

8 Immunologic Disorders

10. C.Q. asks whether there is any treatment available. How would you respond?

11. C.Q. asks why she has to take so many drugs instead of a "big dose" of one drug. What would you tell her?

12. The physician starts C.Q. on a regimen of Truvada (tenofovir and emtricitabine) and efavirenz (Sustiva). What general information will you give C.Q. about ART therapy?

13. What other issues will you discuss with C.Q. at this visit?

14. C.Q. asks if she has to tell J. of her HIV status. Does she have a legal responsibility to inform him?

15. What reporting obligations does the clinic have?

16. Before C.Q. leaves the clinic, you recognize the need for further teaching when she says:
    a. "Joining a support group can help me deal with my HIV diagnosis."
    b. "I will not use any other medications without checking with my health care provider."
    c. "If my viral load becomes undetectable, I will not have to worry about transmitting HIV to someone else."
    d. "If my skin turns yellow, I have unusual muscle pain or feel dizzy or weak, I will call the provider immediately."

CASE STUDY PROGRESS

Two weeks later, C.Q. visits the office and asks to speak to you in private. She thanks you for talking to her the day she received the news of her diagnosis. She tells you that J. confessed to her that he has hemophilia and tested positive for HIV after having been infected through contaminated recombinant factor VIII products. He was afraid to tell her about his diagnosis because she might leave him. C.Q. tells you that she is angry with J. They are going through counseling and the wedding is "off" at the moment.

8 Immunologic Disorders

Case Study 84

Name _____ Class/Group _____ Date _____

Group Members _____

▶ Scenario

K.D. is a 56-year-old gay professional man who has been human immunodeficiency virus (HIV) infected for 6 years. He had been on antiretroviral therapy (ART) with Combivir (zidovudine and lamivudine) and nelfinavir (Viracept). He stopped taking his medications 6 months ago because of depression. The appearance of purplish spots on his neck and arms persuaded him to make an appointment with his physician. At the physician's office, K.D. stated he had been feeling fatigued for several months and was experiencing occasional night sweats. He also related he had been working long hours, skipping meals, and was stressed over a project at work. Other than the purplish spots, the remainder of K.D.'s physical examination findings were within normal limits. The doctor took three skin biopsy specimens and ordered a chest x-ray examination, a complete blood count (CBC), lymphocyte studies including CD4 T-cell count, an ultrasensitive viral load, a cytomegalovirus (CMV) assay, and a tuberculin test.

Over the next week, K.D. developed a nonproductive cough and increasing dyspnea. Last night, he developed a fever of 102° F and was acutely short of breath, so his roommate brought him to the emergency department. He was admitted to the medical unit with probable *Pneumocystis jiroveci* pneumonia (PJP), which was confirmed with bronchoalveolar lavage examination under light microscopy. K.D.'s admission white blood cell count (WBC) and lymphocyte studies demonstrate an increased pattern of immunodeficiency compared with earlier studies. K.D. is on nasal oxygen, intravenous (IV) fluids, and IV trimethoprim-sulfamethoxazole (Bactrim). His current vital signs (VS) are 138/86, 100, 30, 100.8° F (38.2° C) and Spo_2 92%.

1. What is PJP?

2. The skin biopsies return a diagnosis of Kaposi sarcoma (KS). What is KS?

3. What is the significance of K.D.'s developing KS and PJP?

4. K.D. has been seropositive for several years, yet he has been asymptomatic for acquired immunodeficiency syndrome (AIDS). What factors might have influenced K.D.'s development of PJP and KS?

5. Identify four problems you must manage at this time regarding K.D.

 6. What type of isolation precautions do you need to use when caring for K.D.?
   a. Droplet
   b. Contact
   c. Standard
   d. Airborne

7. What immediate complication is K.D. at risk for experiencing?

8. To detect this complication, what will be the focus of your ongoing assessment?

9. What major antibiotic side effects do you need to monitor for in K.D.?

10. What aspects of K.D.'s care can you delegate to the licensed practical nurse (LPN)? Select all that apply.
    a. Providing instructions about a high-calorie, high-protein diet
    b Repositioning K.D. and having him deep breathe every 2 hours
    c. Developing a plan of care to improve K.D.'s oxygenation status
    d. Reinforcing teaching with K.D. about good hand washing techniques
    e. Administering first dose of IV trimethoprim-sulfamethoxazole (Bactrim)
    f. Monitoring K.D.'s pulse oximetry readings and reporting values under 95%

8 Immunologic Disorders

11. K.D. has 20 KS lesions on his neck, upper chest, and both upper arms, all of which are closed and painless. How will you care for the KS lesions?
    a. Keep each lesion covered with a clear, transparent dressing
    b. Place sterile, saline-soaked gauze over each lesion twice daily
    c. Keep the lesions dry, cleaning the affected areas gently as needed
    d. Apply topical antibiotic ointment twice daily to the affected areas

12. Because of compromised immune function, K.D. is at risk for developing other opportunistic infections. List at least five.

13. Describe the assessment you need to perform to determine if these problems are present.

14. What interventions can you use to assist K.D. in managing his depression?

15. Recognizing that K.D. has multiple posthospital needs, you begin discharge planning. What type of assessment do you need to complete as part of K.D.'s discharge planning?

16. What other health care team members may you involve in K.D.'s discharge planning?

8 Immunologic Disorders

CASE STUDY PROGRESS

K.D. is responding well to treatment for PJP and plans are being made for discharge. His ART regimen is restarted and he will soon begin radiation treatments for the KS. He will receive follow-up care at the outpatient clinic.

17. K.D. is kept on trimethoprim/sulfamethoxazole (Bactrim) two tablets once daily. He asks why he has to keep taking the drug "since the pneumonia is gone." How would you respond?

18. What ongoing laboratory monitoring will K.D. need?

19. K.D. was taught about disease transmission and safer sex and encouraged to maintain moderate exercise, rest, and dietary habits when he was first diagnosed as HIV positive. Give at least four additional topics that should be discussed with K.D. before he goes home.

Case Study 85

Name _____ Class/Group _____ Date _____

Group Members _____

8 Immunologic Disorders

▶ Scenario

J.P., a 56-year-old man, developed a severe viral infection with fatigue, fever, and myalgia. Although he recovered from the acute episode, J.P. never quite regained his normal activity level. Six months later, J.P. continued to find it difficult to work a 10-hour day as a brick mason, so he returned to his physician. Diagnostic studies revealed heart failure related to postviral cardiomyopathy. After medical management with metoprolol (Toprol XL) and furosemide (Lasix), his condition stabilized and he returned to work.

After several months, J.P.'s condition began to deteriorate and his work attendance became erratic. Sixteen months later he is being admitted complaining of dyspnea with minimal exertion, fatigue, orthopnea, chest pain, anorexia, and feelings of abdominal fullness. He has 2+ peripheral edema and is diaphoretic. Further studies reveal that J.P. has cardiac dilation, moderate to gross ventricular hypertrophy, and a systolic ejection fraction of 17%, consistent with severe congestive cardiomyopathy. Because J.P.'s only other health problem is mild hypertension, a heart transplant evaluation is recommended. J.P. and his wife discuss his prognosis, and he agrees to an evaluation for possible heart transplantation.

1. If J.P. is accepted for cardiac transplantation, what data will be collected in addition to his past medical history, current diagnostic findings, and cardiac evaluation?

2. What criteria does J.P. meet that will make him eligible for cardiac transplantation?

3. Identify five contraindications for cardiac transplant.

4. What compatibility tests are performed to determine eligibility for transplantation and to ensure as close a match as possible?

5. J.P. is accepted for cardiac transplant and placed on the waiting list. He asks you where his new heart will come from. How would you respond?

6. What fears or concerns might J.P. experience during this waiting period?

CASE STUDY PROGRESS

Seven weeks later J. P. receives a donor heart. His surgery and recovery are uncomplicated. He is sent home on immunosuppressive therapy using cyclosporine (Sandimmune), mycophenolate mofetil (Cellcept), and steroids and is referred to cardiac rehabilitation.

7. What is the rationale for immunosuppression after the transplant?

8. J.P. is at increased risk for contracting an infection because of the immunosuppressive therapy. Describe four strategies for preventing infections that you would include in his discharge teaching plan.

CASE STUDY PROGRESS

Twenty-four days after surgery, J.P. is readmitted to the coronary care unit (CCU) after a cardiac biopsy demonstrates moderate acute rejection.

9. What is the cause of acute rejection? How does it differ from chronic rejection?

10. Why did J.P. have a cardiac biopsy?

11. Which of J.P.'s assessment findings would suggest he is experiencing transplant rejection? Select all that apply.
    a. Angina at rest
    b. Temperature 99.4° F (37.4° C)
    c. Not urinating as much as usual
    d. Presence of 1+ peripheral edema
    e. Complaints of increasing dyspnea
    f. Intermittent nighttime diaphoresis

12. J.P. requires aggressive immunosuppressive therapy. What drugs will be used? How do these alter the rejection process?

8 Immunologic Disorders

13. The tacrolimus (Prograf) dose is 0.03 mg/kg/day IV as a continuous infusion. J.P. currently weighs 187 pounds. The pharmacy sends 5 mg of tacrolimus (Prograf) in 100 mL of 0.9% sodium chloride injection. How many total milligrams per day will J.P. receive? At how many milliliters per hour would you set the infusion pump? (Round to the hundredth.)

CASE STUDY PROGRESS

J.P. responds positively to therapy and is released home after 6 days. J.P. is admitted to the hospital 7 months later with complaints of dyspnea, low-grade fever, and ankle swelling. Both J.P. and his wife are anxious and fearful.

14. Explain what might be happening to J.P. physiologically.

15. Compare the treatment for this episode of graft rejection with the treatment from his earlier episode of rejection.

16. J.P.'s prognosis will depend on what factors?

17. How would you best provide J.P. psychological support at this time?

8 Immunologic Disorders

Case Study 86

Name _____ Class/Group _____ Date _____

Group Members _____

8 Immunologic Disorders

▶ Scenario

W.V. is a 57-year-old man who lives with his wife and two teenage sons. W.V. developed chronic kidney disease 20 years ago after using a drug for migraine headaches that was later shown to cause severe nephrotoxicity. W.V. underwent hemodialysis for 5 years before receiving a cadaveric transplant, or cadaver kidney. He recovered without complications, and his serum laboratory values returned to normal. He was placed on triple immunosuppression therapy, including prednisone (Deltasone), cyclosporine (Imuran), and tacrolimus (Prograf), and was discharged to home.

1. What histocompatibility studies are generally performed before renal transplant, and why are they important?

2. By what criteria was W.V. considered a good candidate for renal transplantation?

3. Identify at least four ways in which W.V. might experience difficulty adjusting after organ transplant.

4. If W.V.'s kidney is producing sufficient urine and he is feeling well, why is ongoing laboratory monitoring necessary?

5. Why must W.V. be concerned about infection?

6. Which statement would indicate W.V. needs more teaching regarding posttransplant care and immunosuppressant therapy?
   a. "I should wash my hands frequently."
   b. "I will need to have regular laboratory testing."
   c. "I will call the doctor if I urinate less frequently."
   d. "It will be nice to go to all of my grandkid's activities now."

CASE STUDY PROGRESS

Today, W.V. reports to his physician for a 12-week follow-up. W.V. has gained 5 pounds since his last appointment 2 weeks ago.

Chart View

Vital Signs

Blood pressure (BP)	148/82 mm Hg
Pulse rate	88 beats/min
Respiratory rate	24 breaths/min
Temperature	99.2° F (37.3° C)

Laboratory Test Results

Sodium	148 mmol/L
Potassium	4.0 mmol/L
Glucose	198 mg/dL
Calcium	10.1 mg/dL
Creatinine	2.2 mg/dL
Blood urea nitrogen (BUN)	42 mg/dL

7. What is the possible significance of W.V.'s BP?

8. Interpret W.V.'s laboratory results.

9. What other signs and symptoms would be present if W.V. was experiencing acute rejection?

10. What are the collaborative care options to save the kidney if rejection is present?

11. The physician decides to add mycophenolate (CellCept) 1 gram orally twice daily to W.V.'s immunosuppressive regimen. How does mycophenolate protect W.V.'s kidney from rejection?

12. What do you need to teach W.V. regarding therapy with mycophenolate?

13. Glipizide (Glucotrol), a sulfonylurea, is prescribed for W.V.'s hyperglycemia. W.V. asks if this means he is now a diabetic. How would you answer him?

14. How can you best support W.V. and his family during this time?

8 Immunologic Disorders

CASE STUDY OUTCOME

W.V. does not experience any further episodes of acute rejection and within 6 months is able to be on lower doses of immunosuppressive therapy. With the lower level of immunosuppression, his elevated glucose resolves and he does not develop diabetes. His kidney continues to function well, and he says that despite a few challenges that come with being a posttransplant patient, "I feel better than I have in years."

8 Immunologic Disorders

Case Study **87**

Name _____ Class/Group _____ Date _____

Group Members _____

▶ **Scenario**

D.W. is a 25-year-old married woman with three children under 5 years old. She came to her physician 7 months ago with vague complaints of intermittent fatigue, joint pain, low-grade fever, and unintentional weight loss. Her physician noted small, patchy areas of vitiligo and a scaly rash across her nose, cheeks, back, and chest at that time. Laboratory studies revealed that D.W. had a positive antinuclear antibody (ANA) titer, positive anti-dsDNA test, positive anti-Sm test, elevated C-reactive protein (CRP) and erythrocyte sedimentation rate (ESR), and decreased C3 and C4 serum complement. Joint x-ray films demonstrated joint swelling without joint erosion. D.W. was diagnosed with systemic lupus erythematosus (SLE). Her initial treatment consisted of hydroxychloroquine (Plaquenil) 400 mg and prednisone (Deltasone) 20 mg orally per day, bed rest, and ice packs. D.W. responded well and the steroid was tapered and discontinued. She was told she could report for follow-up every 6 months unless her symptoms became acute. D.W. resumed her job in environmental services at a large geriatric facility.

1. What is the significance of each of D.W.'s laboratory findings?

2. Given that most tests are nonspecific, how is SLE diagnosed?

3. What priority problems would be addressed in D.W.'s care plan at that time of diagnosis?

8 Immunologic Disorders

CASE STUDY PROGRESS

Twenty-eight months after diagnosis, D.W. seeks out her physician with complaints of puffy hands and feet and increased fatigue. D.W. reports that she has been working longer hours because of the absence of two of her fellow workers.

Chart View

Laboratory Test Results

Sodium	129 mmol/L
Potassium	4.2 mmol/L
Chloride	119 mmol/L
Total CO_2	21 mmol/L
Blood urea nitrogen (BUN)	34 mg/dL
Creatinine	2.6 mg/dL
Glucose	123 mg/dL
Urinalysis	2+ protein

4. Which laboratory findings concern you, and why?

5. The goal of therapy in lupus nephritis is to normalize or prevent the loss of renal function. To attain this goal, what additions to D.W.'s care can you anticipate?

 6. The physician orders cyclophosphamide (Cytoxan) 100 mg/m^2/day orally in two divided doses. D.W. weighs 140 pounds and is 5 feet, 4 inches tall. How much will she receive with each dose?

7. What key points should you include in a teaching plan for D.W. regarding cyclophosphamide therapy?

CASE STUDY PROGRESS

D.W. is seen in the immunology clinic twice monthly during the next 3 months. Although her condition does not worsen, her BUN and creatinine remain elevated. While at work one afternoon, D.W. begins to feel dizzy and develops a severe headache. She reports to her supervisor, who has her lie down. When D.W. starts to become disoriented, her supervisor calls 911, and D.W. is taken to the hospital. D.W. is admitted for probable lupus cerebritis related to acute exacerbation of her disease.

8. What other findings indicative of central nervous system involvement should you assess for in D.W.?

 9. What protective measures need to be instituted at this time?

10. In caring for D.W., which care activities can be delegated to the UAP? Select all that apply.
    a. Monitoring D.W.'s BUN and creatinine levels
    b. Counseling D.W. on seizure safety precautions
    c. Assisting D.W. with personal hygiene measures
    d. Assessing D.W.'s neurologic status every 2 hours
    e. Measuring D.W.'s blood pressure (BP) every 2 hours
    f. Emptying the urine collection device and measuring the output

CASE STUDY PROGRESS

The physician orders pulse therapy with methylprednisolone (Solu-Medrol) 125 mg IV every 6 hours and plasmapheresis once daily.

11. What major complications associated with immunosuppression therapy will D.W. have to be monitored for?

8 Immunologic Disorders

12. D.W. asks about what plasmapheresis does and why it might help her feel better. Describe how you would respond.

Chart View

Vital Signs

BP	80/43 mm Hg
Pulse rate	118 beats/min
Respiratory rate	18 breaths/min
Temperature	97.2 ° F (36.2 ° C)

13. D.W. returns to the floor after the plasmapheresis. The UAP reports to you D.W.'s vital signs. Based solely on her vital signs, what could be happening with D.W. and why?

14. You go to assess D.W. What do you need to include in your assessment?

15. D.W. is complaining of dizziness and is slightly diaphoretic but denies any headache, nausea, or paresthesia. What do you immediately suspect is occurring and why?

16. You need to call the physician regarding D.W.'s status. Using SBAR, what would you report to the physician?

17. What do you anticipate your care of D.W. will include over the next 2 to 3 hours?

18. What outcome criteria would support that D.W.'s condition is stabilizing?

19. You note that D.W.'s husband is visiting her. You enter the room to ask whether they have any questions. D.W.'s husband states, "I have tried to tell her that she cannot go back to work. Sure, we need the money, but the kids and I need her more. I'm afraid that this lupus has weakened her whole body and it will kill her if she goes back to work. Is that right?" How should you respond to his concerns?

Oncologic and Hematologic Disorders

Case Study 88

▶ **Scenario**

You are a home health nurse seeing for the first time P.C., a 64-year-old divorcee diagnosed with small cell lung cancer approximately 1 year ago. She was treated with radiation and chemotherapy; however, her oncologist recently informed her that her cancer is no longer treatable because it has spread to her bones and liver. Now the focus of her treatment will change from curative to symptom relief. She is confused and somewhat bewildered. She vaguely remembers the term *palliative treatment* from the discussion of her situation with her oncologist but does not know what it means.

1. How would you describe palliative treatment?

2. Describe the assessment you need to perform at this time.

3. Palliative care is delivered by an interprofessional team. What role will each of the following professionals play in P.C.'s care?

CASE STUDY PROGRESS

P.C. confides that she has not formally written down her wishes concerning what types of treatments she would or would not want. You advise her to complete an advance directive, a living will, and a medical durable power of attorney or surrogate decision maker form.

4. How would you describe the purpose of these documents to her?

5. What health care decisions are considered in these documents?

6. How are advance directives and living wills formalized?

7. P.C. states that she is confused and has mixed feelings about her health care wishes right now. She asks, "If I fill out these forms, can I change my mind down the road?" How should you answer this question?

8. As P.C. becomes more frail and incoherent, how will these documents guide her treatment?

You inform P.C. that one of your roles will be to help with the symptom control as her illness progresses. You begin with pain control because it has a powerful effect on quality of life.

9. What interventions will you use to help her be as pain free as possible?

10. Because her advancing lung cancer will likely result in respiratory distress, which interventions should you include in her plan of care? Select all that apply.
    a. Perform a respiratory assessment at each visit.
    b. Administer low-dose morphine sulfate if vital signs are adequate.
    c. Maintain room at a warm temperature and have blankets available.
    d. Have her space activities and rest as needed in a position of comfort.
    e. If oxygen saturation falls below 90% on room air, begin oxygen at 2 L.

11. Why is P.C. at risk for impaired skin integrity?

12. Realizing that loss of appetite frequently accompanies the dying process, describe how you can maintain P.C.'s oral nutrition and hydration.

13. Toward the end of your visit, P.C. looks at you and says, "You know, I just really thought I had more time." The most appropriate response is:
    a. "Dying is a natural process; we will help you through it."
    b. "Your feelings are understandable; most people aren't ready to die."

9 Oncologic/Hematologic

    c. "Tell me more about what you mean when you say, 'I thought I had more time.'"
    d. "No one ever really knows when it is their time, even if they don't have cancer."

14. You are concerned with P.C.'s psychological status, particularly because she is expressing feelings of grief. Write a nursing outcome addressing this issue, and identify independent nursing actions that you would implement to provide her emotional support.

CASE STUDY OUTCOME

P.C. discusses her wishes with her family and completes the documents describing what she would like her plan of care to be over the remainder of her life span. She dies peacefully 7 weeks later in her home, supported by her family and friends, on her terms.

Case Study 89

Name _____ Class/Group _____ Date _____

Group Members _____

9 Oncologic/Hematologic

▶ **Scenario**

G.C. is a 78-year-old widow who relies on her late husband's Social Security income for all of her expenses. Over the past few years, G.C. has eaten less and less meat because of her financial situation and the trouble of preparing a meal "just for me." She struggles financially to buy medicines for the treatment of hypertension and arthritis. She goes to the outpatient clinic complaining that over the past 2 to 3 months she has felt increasingly tired, despite sleeping well at night. Her vital signs (VS) are 136/76, 16, 80. She denies any dyspnea or palpitations. The nurse practitioner orders blood work. G.C.'s chemistry panel findings are all within normal limits and a stool guaiac test result is negative. Her other results are shown in the chart.

Chart View

Laboratory Test Results

White blood cell (WBC) count	$7600/mm^3$
Hematocrit (Hct)	27.3%
Hemoglobin (Hgb)	8.3 mg/dL
Platelets	$151,000/mm^3$

Red Blood Cell (RBC) Indices

Mean corpuscular volume (MCV)	$65 \, mm^3$
Mean corpuscular hemoglobin (MCH)	31.6 pg
MCH concentration (MCHC)	35.1%
Red cell distribution width (RDW)	15.6%
Iron (Fe)	30 mcg/dL
Total iron-binding capacity (TIBC)	422 mcg/dL
Ferritin	8 mg/dL
Vitamin B_{12}	414 pg/mL
Folate	188 ng/mL

1. Which laboratory values are normal and which are abnormal?

2. Explain the significance of each abnormal result.

3. Based on these results and her history, what condition does G.C. have?

4. What individuals are at risk for this condition?

5. What other signs and symptoms of this condition do you assess for in G.C.?

6. Which question would best help you determine the impact of fatigue on her activities of daily living?
   a. "Are you upset about feeling more tired?"
   d. "Do you sleep more now than you used to?"
   b. "How far can you walk until you get short of breathe?"
   c. "Have you been able to do what you would like to do?"

7. Discuss the treatment options for her condition.

8. The physician starts G.C. on ferrous sulfate (Feosol) 325 mg orally once per day. What teaching needs to be done regarding this medication?

9. As you are evaluating your teaching about ferrous sulfate, you determine that additional instruction is needed if G.C. says:
   a. "My stools will likely turn a tarry, black color soon."
   b. "I can take the iron and my calcium supplements at the same time."
   c. "I will increase my fluid and fiber intake as long as I am on the iron."
   d. "Taking the tablets when I eat my meals will help my stomach not be upset."

10. Discuss some ideas that might help her with her meal planning.

11. You teach G.C. about foods she should include in her diet. You determine that she understands your teaching if she states she will increase her intake of which of the following foods?
    a. Whole-wheat pastas and skim milk
    b. Lean cuts of poultry, pork, and fish
    c. Beans and dark green, leafy vegetables
    d. Cooked cereals, such as oats, and bananas

12. What evaluative parameters could you use to determine whether G.C.'s condition is improving?

9 Oncologic/Hematologic

13. Using SOAP, write a sample documentation entry for this encounter.

Case Study 90

Name _____   Class/Group _____   Date _____

Group Members _____

▶ Scenario

You are a nurse working as a preoperative evaluation nurse. J.B., a well-known 62-year-old homeless alco-holic, is sent to you before a left radical neck dissection with total laryngectomy and placement of a permanent tracheostomy to treat stage III hypopharyngeal cancer. He has a long history of tobacco use, poor diet, and no dental care. Over the past several months, he has experienced increasing shortness of breath, hoarseness, and odynophagia. A piriform sinus mass was found on bronchoscopy. The large mass extends and is fixed to the left true vocal cord. His chest x-ray film is normal with the exception of changes related to chronic tobacco use. Past medical history includes reactive airway disease and hypertension. On examination, you find one palpable left-sided cervical node, which is firm and fixed.

1. Identify J.B.'s risk factors for cancer.

2. Name the warning signals listed on the American Cancer Society's list of warning signs of cancer. Place a star by those J.B. has.

3. Describe the surgical intervention J.B. will undergo.

9 Oncologic/Hematologic

4. J.B. has several important postoperative needs. Identify two serious complications for which he is most at risk.

5. What type of follow-up therapy is J.B. likely to undergo after his initial wound heals?

6. You note placement of a percutaneous endoscopic gastrostomy (PEG) feeding tube is also on the operative procedure list. Why is J.B. having a PEG tube placed?

7. Which of the following points would you include his preoperative teaching plan?
   a. "The head of your bed will be kept up at all times."
   b. "You will not be able to eat or drink for 7 to 14 days."
   c. "We will be encouraging you to whisper frequently after surgery."
   d. "You will have to avoid all coughing until the sutures are removed."

8. J.B. asks you, "How will I talk after the surgery?" Which of the following is the best response?
   a. "Unfortunately, you will not be able to communicate orally ever again."
   b. "You will be able to speak again after the tracheostomy tube is removed."
   c. "If you work hard at speech therapy, you may regain some of your normal voice."
   d. "You won't be able to speak. There are some alternative devices you can learn to use."

9. J.B. asks how he will be able to let the nurses know what he needs if he cannot talk. How will you respond?

10. J.B. has several factors that make discharge planning especially problematic. Describe two specific discharge problems and list possible solutions.

CASE STUDY PROGRESS

J.B. undergoes surgery. His postoperative course is complicated by pneumonia and poor wound healing. After being hospitalized for 6 weeks, he is discharged to a long-term care facility for care while recuperating for external radiation therapy. He is scheduled to receive 2000 cGy to the head and neck three times weekly for the next 8 weeks.

11. As J.B.'s nurse, which adverse effects of external radiation therapy would most concern you?

12. Outline independent nursing actions that will assist J.B. in managing mucositis and xerostomia.

9 Oncologic/Hematologic

13. What instructions will you provide the UAP caring for J.B. regarding skin care? Select all that apply.
    a. "Assist J.B. with selecting loose-fitting shirts."
    b. "After his shower, apply lotion to the irradiated area."
    c. "Dry the area with patting motions using a soft cloth."
    d. "Make sure you thoroughly rinse away all of the soap."
    e. "Remove the ink marked on his neck with a washcloth."
    f. "He can have an ice pack applied to the red areas for 15 minutes."

 14. What interventions would you place in a plan of care to reduce J.B.'s risk of infection?

15. How can the nurse assist J.B. in combating fatigue during his treatment?

CASE STUDY OUTCOME

Despite radiation therapy, J.B.'s disease progresses and he develops metastases to his lung and brain. He chooses to remain in the long-term care facility, and he dies from pneumonia 5 months later.

Case Study **91**

Name _____ Class/Group _____ Date _____

Group Members _____

▶ **Scenario**

R.T. is a 64-year-old man who went to his primary care provider's office for a yearly examination. He initially reported having no new health problems; however, on further questioning, he admitted to having developed some fatigue, abdominal bloating, and intermittent constipation. His physical examination findings were normal except for stool positive for occult blood. He had a complete blood count (CBC) with differential, basic metabolic panel (BMP), and carcinoembryonic antigen (CEA) testing and was referred to a gastroenterologist for a colonoscopy. Colonoscopy revealed a 5-cm mass in the sigmoid colon, which was diagnosed as adenocarcinoma of the colon. A distant metastatic workup is negative, and R.T. is being scheduled for a laparoscopic sigmoidectomy with anastomosis.

1. What is a risk factor?

2. Identify six risk factors for colon cancer.

3. Outline the American Cancer Society's current evidence-based screening procedures for colon cancer.

4. What are the warning signs of colon cancer? Place a star next to those that R.T. has.

9 Oncologic/Hematologic

5. What is CEA? How does it relate to the diagnosis of colon cancer?

6. Shade in the area of the colon that will be removed during R.T.'s surgery.

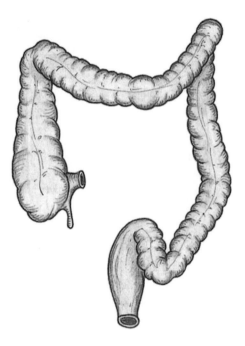

7. The preoperative chart includes detailed instructions for R.T. for a bowel preparation regimen with polyethylene glycol and a prescription for neomycin (Mycifradin). What is the purpose of the neomycin?

8. What are some suggestions you can make to help R.T. successfully complete the bowel preparation?

9. Describe the rest of your preoperative teaching for R.T. and his family.

CASE STUDY PROGRESS

R.T.'s surgical course is uneventful and he is discharged after 5 days. Based on the final pathology report, his cancer is designated stage IIIB. The cancer had spread to the muscle layer of the colon wall with nine lymph nodes being positive. Four weeks after surgery, R.T. is scheduled to begin 6 months of adjuvant chemotherapy.

10. Describe three chemotherapy regimens used to treat stage IIIB colon cancer. Underline the two drugs common to all three regimens.

11. The purpose of the leucovorin (folinic acid) is to:
    a. Rescue healthy cells from the toxic effects of methotrexate
    b. Improve R.T.'s nutritional status by supplementing vitamin intake
    c. Reduce the incidence of renal failure associated with methotrexate
    d. Help the methotrexate be more effective by inhibiting cancer cell mitosis

12. Discuss the major toxicities and side effects associated with 5-fluorouracil (5-FU) and leucovorin (folinic acid).

13. When prioritizing R.T.'s plan of care, which of these effects is the most serious?

14. When R.T.'s white blood cell (WBC) count begins to drop, which is the **most** important means to teach him to protect himself from infection?
    a. Brushing and flossing his teeth after meals and before bed
    b. Having someone else clean the litterbox of all household pets
    c. Staying away from people who are visibly sick or have a cold
    d. Washing his hands frequently, especially after using the restroom and before eating

15. Develop a teaching plan for R.T. focusing on the common effects of diarrhea, alopecia, and nausea and vomiting.

9 Oncologic/Hematologic

16. R.T. demonstrates he understands the adverse effects of methotrexate when he states:
   a. "I should take ibuprofen if I have a mild headache or joint pain."
   b. "If I develop a bad rash, there is no need to worry. This is normal."
   c. "Coffee and black tea are good choices to help me maintain my fluid intake."
   d. "If I have any chills or unusual pain, I need to let my doctor know immediately."

9 Oncologic/Hematologic

Case Study **92**

Name _____ Class/Group _____ Date _____

Group Members _____

▶ **Scenario**

M.D. is a 50-year-old woman whose routine mammogram showed a 2.3-×4.5-cm lobulated mass at the 3 o'clock position in her left breast. M.D. underwent a stereotactic needle biopsy and was diagnosed with infiltrating ductal carcinoma, estrogen receptor positive. The staging workup was negative for distant metastasis. Her final staging was stage IIB. She had a modified radical mastectomy with lymph node dissection. The sentinel lymph node and 4 of 16 lymph nodes were positive for tumor cells. An implanted port was placed during surgery.

1. Describe the biopsy technique used to diagnose M.D.'s cancer.

2. Discuss the implications of a positive sentinel node.

3. According to the TNM staging system, what would her classification be?

4. Is she a candidate for tamoxifen (Nolvadex) therapy? Explain your rationale.

5. Surgical intervention is the primary treatment for breast cancer. Describe the surgical procedure that M.D. had.

9 Oncologic/Hematologic

429

6. Describe M.D.'s risk for lymphedema.

7. What actions will you teach M.D. to reduce her risk of developing lymphedema?

CASE STUDY PROGRESS

Eight weeks after surgery, M.D. is now beginning a prescribed a chemotherapy regimen of six cycles of CAF (cyclophosphamide [Cytoxan], fluorouracil [5-FU], and doxorubicin [Adriamycin]).

8. M.D. asks you why she has to have chemotherapy with so many drugs if the surgeon removed all of the cancer. How would you respond?

9. Compare the drug actions of cyclophosphamide (Cytoxan), 5-FU, and doxorubicin (Adriamycin).

10. Describe any side effects and special considerations associated with the use of CAF.

11. M.D. is ordered doxorubicin at 75 mg/m². Her height is 5 feet, 7 inches, and her weight is 155 pounds. Calculate the dose she will receive.

12. M.D. is prescribed filgrastim (Neupogen) as part of her treatment regimen. You teach her filgrastim is used is to do which of the following?
   a. Improve the number and function of neutrophils
   b. Help CAF be more effective in treating her cancer
   c. Replace abnormal cells in the bone marrow with normal cells
   d. Decrease the level of fatigue she will experience during treatment

13. You have finished teaching M.D. regarding the effects of CAF. You know that she understands instructions regarding cyclophosphamide (Cytoxan) when she states:
   a. "This medication should be taken with food."
   b. "I will drink 2000 to 3000 mL of fluids each day."
   c. "Taking this drug at nighttime will reduce nausea."
   d. "I will increase my intake of foods with potassium."

14. However, after reviewing with her how to manage alopecia, you determine further teaching is required after she states:
   a. "I should go buy a wig now, before I start losing my hair."
   b. "Wearing a scarf or hat when outside will help to protect me."
   c. "My hair should begin to return 2 months or so after treatment ends."
   d. "I can prevent hair loss if I wash every other day with a gentle shampoo."

15. What information would you want to review with M.D. regarding the signs and symptoms of infection and when to seek treatment?

9 Oncologic/Hematologic

CASE STUDY PROGRESS

M.D. has now completed three cycles of CAF, with her last treatment being approximately 12 days ago. She comes to the emergency department with a 2-day history of fever, chills, and shortness of breath. On arrival, she is disoriented and agitated. Vital signs are 86/43, 119, 28, 103.6°F (39.8°C), Spo$_2$ 85% on room air. The chest x-ray examination demonstrates diffuse infiltrates in the left lower lung. Her basic metabolic panel (BMP) is within normal limits, with the exception of blood urea nitrogen (BUN) 28 mg/dL, creatinine 1.6 mg/dL, and lactic acid 2.4 mg/dL.

Chart View

Complete Blood Count

White blood cells (WBCs)	1200/mm^3
Neutrophils	34%
Segmented ("polys")	30%
Bands	4%
Lymphocytes	60%
Monocytes	3%
Eosinophils and basophils	2%
Hematocrit (Hct)	24.9%
Hemoglobin (Hgb)	8.7 g/dL
Platelets	85,000/mm^3

16. Interpret M.D.'s laboratory results and explain the rationale for abnormal results.

17. Calculate M.D.'s absolute neutrophil count (ANC) and describe its significance.

18. What is the single most important nursing intervention for a patient with an ANC below 500/mm^3?

19. What treatment do you anticipate for M.D.?

20. The physician orders a 500-mL normal saline bolus now, with orders to infuse over 2 hours. You decide to use M.D.'s implanted port for intravenous (IV) access. After you access the port and connect the fluid, the infusion pump alarms that the line is occluded. What will you do?

CASE STUDY OUTCOME

M.D. is transferred to the intensive care unit (ICU), where she soon requires endotracheal intubation. She spends 3 days in the ICU receiving IV antibiotics and respiratory support. After she is extubated, she returns to the oncology unit, where she remains for a few more days before being discharged to home.

9 Oncologic/Hematologic

Case Study 93

Name _____ Class/Group _____ Date _____

Group Members _____

▶ **Scenario**

C.P. is a 71-year-old married farmer with a past medical history of hernia surgery in 1986 and prostate surgery in 2005 for benign prostatic hyperplasia. C.P. has smoked for 40 years; for the past 3 years, he has smoked two to three packs per day. Two weeks ago, C.P. visited the local rural health clinic with complaints of a progressive cough and chest congestion. Despite a week of antibiotic therapy, C.P.'s condition continued to worsen; he experienced progressive dyspnea and productive cough, and he began to have night sweats. C.P. refused to be admitted to the hospital because "there's no one to look after the cows," but he agreed to go for a chest x-ray (CXR) study. The radiologist reads C.P.'s CXR film as "left hilar lung mass, probable lung cancer." C.P. is scheduled for a diagnostic fiberoptic bronchoscopy with endobronchial lung biopsy as an outpatient this morning to confirm the diagnosis.

1. What information does a fiberoptic bronchoscopy with endobronchial lung biopsy provide?

2. As the nurse who works with the pulmonologist, it is your responsibility to prepare C.P. for the fiberoptic bronchoscopy procedure. What will you include in your teaching plan?

3. What is your responsibility during and immediately after the bronchoscopy?

4. C.P. tolerates the procedure well. He returns to the office 4 days later to learn the results of his test. The pulmonologist tells C.P. and his wife that he has poorly differentiated oat cell lung cancer and explains that it is a very fast-growing cancer with a poor prognosis. This kind of lung cancer is directly related to C.P.'s history of smoking. What is your role at this time?

9 Oncologic/Hematologic

5. What does poorly differentiated mean?

CASE STUDY PROGRESS

C.P. undergoes a metastatic workup and is found to have disease in a number of lymph nodes, his liver, and sternum. The physician tells C.P. and his wife that surgery is not an option and schedules C.P. to begin combination chemotherapy.

6. Using simple terms, how would you explain combination chemotherapy and how it works to C.P. and his wife?

7. C.P. says he doesn't know if he should undergo chemotherapy if he "isn't going to live anyway." What are the goals of administering chemotherapy to patients such as C.P.?

8. C.P.'s wife tells you she's heard that chemotherapy makes you really sick. Again, using simple terms, how would you explain chemotherapy side effects?

9. C.P. agrees to chemotherapy and is scheduled to receive cisplatin (Platinol) 60 mg in 100 mL normal saline (NS) IV over 1 to 2 hours daily, and etoposide (VePesid) 200 mg in 250 mL NS IV over 1 to 2 hours daily, both during the first 3 days of each month. What is the nadir for each drug, and what implications does the nadir have for C.P.?

10. Based on your knowledge of the most common side effects of cisplatin (Platinol) and etoposide (VePesid), list at least seven interventions that should be incorporated into C.P.'s care plan to assist him with managing these effects.

11. C.P. plans to continue to work the farm as long as possible and says his brother-in-law has promised to help him. C.P. needs to have a working understanding of how to balance his treatment with his work. You sit down with C.P. to plan a daily work, activity, and rest schedule to accommodate his treatments and side effects. List at least three points you would emphasize.

CASE STUDY PROGRESS

A month later, when C.P. returns for his second round of chemotherapy, he complains of shortness of breath, chest tightness, and palpitations. He looks exhausted. An electrocardiogram (ECG) reveals new-onset atrial fibrillation, and a CXR film suggests a large left lower lobe pleural effusion. C.P. is admitted to the hospital for supportive care. The pulmonologist performs a thoracentesis and drains 985 mL of fluid, immediately relieving some of C.P.'s dyspnea and chest discomfort.

Chart View

Laboratory Test Values

WBCs	2500 /mm^3
RBCs	4.9 million/mm^3
Hemoglobin (Hgb)	12.7 g/dL
Hematocrit (Hct)	37.6%
Platelets	152,000 /mm^3
Sodium	131 mmol/L
Potassium	4.2 mmol/L
Chloride	90 mmol/L

12. What do these laboratory values indicate?

13. You assess C.P. 2 hours after the thoracentesis. Which information is important to report to the physician?
    a. C.P. complains of occasional chest pain when taking deep breaths.
    b. C.P. has a small amount of serosanguineous drainage on the dressing.
    c. C.P. has a blood pressure of 90/50 mm Hg and some increase in dyspnea.
    d. C.P. states that he has some burning and stinging at the thoracentesis site.

14. C.P. tells you he doesn't want to live like this and that he would like to stop chemotherapy, but his physician wants him to continue with aggressive therapy. Discuss what role you can play in helping him.

15. How do you feel about this in relation to his condition?

CASE STUDY OUTCOME

C.P. refuses the second round of chemotherapy and is discharged to home. He receives no further treatment and dies 3 weeks later with his wife at his side.

Case Study **94**

Name _____ Class/Group _____ Date _____

Group Members _____

9 Oncologic/Hematologic

▶ Scenario

H.J. is a 46-year-old man diagnosed with non-Hodgkin lymphoma (NHL) 4 months ago. He just finished receiving his third of six chemotherapy courses 5 days ago. Earlier today, he was seen at his medical oncologist's office with complaints of malaise, muscle weakness, and palpitations. He had splenomegaly on examination. A computed tomography (CT) scan of the abdomen showed metastatic disease in the liver and spleen. He is admitted to the hospital with progressive disease.

Chart View

Basic Metabolic Panel (BMP)

Na	136 mmol/L
K	6.1 mmol/L
Cl	97 mmol/L
CO_2	28 mmol/L
Glucose	98 mg/dL
Blood urea nitrogen (BUN)	54 mg/dL
Creatinine	2.7 mg/dL
Ca	6.3 units/L
Total protein	5.4 g/dL
Albumin	2.8 g/dL
Phosphorus	4.5 mg/dL
Uric acid	23.7 mg/dL
Total bilirubin	0.8 mg/dL
Alkaline phosphatase	172 units/L
Aspartate transaminase (AST)	254 units/L
Alanine transaminase (ALT)	74 units/L
Lactate dehydrogenase (LDH)	214 IU/L

Complete Blood Count (CBC)

White blood cells (WBCs)	1500/mm³
Neutrophils	66%
Lymphocytes	16%
Monocytes	15%
Eosinophils	5%
Hemoglobin (Hgb)	8.3 g/dL
Hematocrit (Hct)	23.6%
Platelets	21,000/mm³

1. Interpret H.J.'s admitting BMP panel.

2. Based on these values, which common oncologic emergency is H.J. experiencing and why?

3. Which of his laboratory results confirm this diagnosis?

4. What assessment findings related to this diagnosis would you anticipate in H.J.?

5. Based on his laboratory values, identify two additional problems for which H.J. is at risk.

Chart View

Medication Record

IV 0.9% saline at 150 mL/hr
100 mEq sodium bicarbonate in the first liter of IV fluid
Allopurinol (Aloprim) 500 mg orally twice daily
Furosemide (Lasix) 40 mg IV now then every 6 hours
Sodium polystyrene (Kayexalate) 15 g orally every 6 hours
Aluminum hydroxide (Amphojel) two caps orally with meals

CASE STUDY PROGRESS

The physician confirms a diagnosis of acute tumor lysis syndrome (TLS) and writes a number of orders for H.J.

6. What is the expected outcome associated with each medication H.J. is receiving?

9 Oncologic/Hematologic

7. After administration of the sodium polystyrene (Kayexalate), it is important for you to monitor H.J.'s:
   a. Level of consciousness
   b. Urine output
   c. Bowel sounds
   d. Peripheral pulses

8. What major complication of TLS is H.J. at risk for and why?

9. Identify three signs and symptoms of this complication you will assess for in H.J.

10. List four independent nursing interventions that you would include in H.J.'s plan of care and the rationale for each.

 11. The best way to prevent infection in a patient such as H.J. is:
   a. Placing him in reverse isolation
   b. Administering prophylactic antibiotics
   c. Practicing good handwashing by all who are in contact with him
   d. Limiting his intake of fresh fruits and vegetables

CASE STUDY PROGRESS

Twenty-four hours after admission, H.J.'s laboratory tests are repeated.

9 Oncologic/Hematologic

Chart View

Basic Metabolic Panel

Na	138 mmol/L
K	4.8 mmol/L
Cl	109 mmol/L
CO_2	26 mmol/L
Glucose	148 mg/dL
BUN	34 mg/dL
Creatinine	2.4 mg/dL
Ca	7.3 units/L
Total protein	5.4 g/dL
Albumin	2.8 g/dL
Phosphorus	3.8 mg/dL
Uric acid less than	0.5 mg/dL
Total bilirubin	1.0 mg/dL
Alkaline phosphatase	96 units/L
AST	49 units/L
ALT	48 units/L
LDH	224 IU/L

12. Interpret H.J.'s laboratory results. Is his condition improving?

CASE STUDY PROGRESS

Because H.J.'s condition has stabilized, the oncologist orders another round of chemotherapy.

13. Because the TLS is just resolving, what interventions would you include in your plan of care?

14. What precautions should you take when administering H.J.'s chemotherapy to reduce the risk of injury? Select all that apply.
   a. Independently verify the completeness of the drug order and infusion rate.
   b. Dispose of any equipment that contained the drug in special biohazard containers.
   c. Scrub any skin that comes into contact with the drug for 5 minutes with a surgical brush.
   d. Wear goggles, powder-free gloves, and a disposable, fluid-resistant, long-sleeved gown.
   e. If using a peripheral site, place a disposable drape under the arm where the drug will be infused.
   f. Use a Luer-Lok connector to attach the drug tubing to the main IV line, using the IV port closest to H.J.

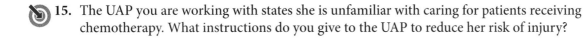

 15. The UAP you are working with states she is unfamiliar with caring for patients receiving chemotherapy. What instructions do you give to the UAP to reduce her risk of injury?

9 Oncologic/Hematologic

CASE STUDY OUTCOME

H.J. does not experience any acute kidney injury. He is discharged to home 3 days later after finishing this round of chemotherapy. He will be following up with the medical oncologist in 1 week.

Case Study 95

Name _____ Class/Group _____ Date _____

Group Members _____

▶ Scenario

R.M. is a 58-year-old woman with stage III ovarian carcinoma. Her initial treatment is an exploratory lapa-rotomy with a total abdominal hysterectomy, an ileocecal resection and anastomosis, omentectomy, and peritoneal biopsies. The postoperative CA-125 level is 69 units/mL. Family history analysis reveals a strong positive occurrence of breast and ovarian cancer in R.M.'s family. Her mother died of breast cancer at the age of 56, and a maternal aunt died of ovarian cancer at the age of 59. The oncologist suggests testing for the presence of the *BRCA1* and *BRCA2* genes and, if the results are positive, testing of R.M.'s two daughters and son.

1. Describe the meaning of this test.

2. Discuss the pros and cons of genetic testing for cancer.

3. In reviewing R.M.'s family history, which of the following would be considered significant? Select all that apply.
    a. Aunt who died from ovarian cancer at age 59
    b. Mother who died from breast cancer at age 56
    c. Sister was diagnosed with cervical cancer at age 50
    d. Grandmother who died from gastric cancer at age 84
    e. Aunt was diagnosed with endometrial cancer at age 65

9 Oncologic/Hematologic

4. R.M. tests positive for the *BRCA2* gene. What implications does this have for her children?

5. Why is ovarian cancer usually stage III or stage IV when initially diagnosed?

CASE STUDY PROGRESS

R.M. begins a chemotherapy regimen of paclitaxel (Taxol) and cisplatin (Platinol). After receiving the fourth course, she presents with shortness of breath, complaints of nausea, and early satiety with a recent weight loss of 10 pounds. Her abdomen is distended, and her Spo_2 is 86% on room air. Her current CA-125 level is 328 units/mL. You are admitting her directly from the oncologist's office to the medical floor.

6. Explain the significance of R.M.'s CA-125 level.

7. Knowing the chemotherapeutic agents R.M. has received, what laboratory tests will you expect the oncologist to order?

8. You perform R.M.'s admission assessment. Which finding must be reported to the oncologist immediately?
   a. Dark, amber-colored urine
   b. A temperature of 101°.8 F (38.8° C)
   c. Bleeding gums and mouth ulcerations
   d. Numbness in her lower legs bilaterally

9. R.M.'s chest x-ray film reveals bilateral pleural effusions. How do these relate to her underlying disease? How might they be treated?

CASE STUDY PROGRESS

After performing a thoracentesis, the oncologist orders a magnetic resonance imaging (MRI) scan of the chest, abdomen, and pelvis, which reveals a mass in the left lower quadrant and a malignant bowel obstruction. He immediately schedules R.M. for a tumor debulking and possible placement of an ostomy.

10. Scheduling R.M. for a debulking procedure implies which of the following?
    a. After this surgery, R.M. will be cured of her cancer.
    b. R.M. has advanced disease and the prognosis is poor.
    c. Chemotherapy will no longer be given after she recovers from surgery.
    d. R.M. will now need to have radiation therapy in addition to chemotherapy.

11. R.M. is undergoing a palliative surgical intervention. How will you explain this to R.M. and her family?

12. What additional risks does surgery pose for R.M.?

13. Describe four appropriate topics to be included in her preoperative teaching.

14. Later in your shift, you find R.M.'s daughter sitting in a chair at the end of the hall crying quietly. You pull up a chair and sit. She tells you, "I had always thought mom was going to fight this. It is really just kind of hitting me that she is actually dying. You just think after surgery and all the chemo everything is going to be fine." What is your best response?
    a. "Let's talk about what is going on with your mother's illness."
    b. "Don't worry about her dying now. Focus on getting her through this surgery."
    c. "Your mother is receiving the best care available. Let's talk about her surgery."
    d. "You are being rather pessimistic. You just need to maintain hope for your mother."

9 Oncologic/Hematologic

15. How can you support R.M. and her family at this time?

CASE STUDY OUTCOME

R.M. undergoes the debulking procedure. Because of the presence of multiple small tumors that were not detected on preoperative scanning, the oncologist elects not to place an ostomy. R.M. never fully recovers from surgery and does not resume chemotherapy. She experiences recurrent bowel obstructions and passes away in hospice care 7 weeks later.

9 Oncologic/Hematologic

Case Study **96**

Name _____ Class/Group _____ Date _____

Group Members _____

9 Oncologic/Hematologic

▶ **Scenario**

V.M. is a 29-year-old African American married man who has sickle cell disease (SCD) marked by frequent episodes of severe pain. His anemia has been managed with multiple transfusions. Six months ago he started showing signs of chronic renal failure. His regular medications are pentoxifylline (Trental), oxycodone-acetaminophen (Percocet), hydroxyurea (Droxia), and folic acid. In the hematology clinic this morning, V.M.'s hemoglobin measured 6.7 g/dL. He received 2 units of packed red blood cells (PRBCs) over 3 hours and then went home. He developed dyspnea and shortness of breath approximately 1 hour later, and his wife called 911. The emergency medical system crew initiated oxygen at 8 L per nasal cannula and transported V.M. to the emergency department (ED).

1. What is SCD?

2. True or False: Only African Americans get SCD. Explain your response.

3. Which statement is true about the inheritance pattern of SCD?
   a. If V.M.'s wife has sickle cell trait, each child will either have SCD or be a carrier.
   b. If V.M.'s wife does not have sickle cell trait, each child has a 50% risk of having SCD.
   c. If V.M.'s wife has sickle cell trait, each child will can either having SCD or be normal.
   d. If V.M. has children, each child will automatically have SCD regardless of his wife's status.

4. V.M.'s hemoglobin measured 6.7 g/dL. Why is anemia common in patients with SCD?

5. Why is it difficult to crossmatch blood to transfuse V.M.?

6. What role does hydroxyurea (Droxia) play in managing V.M.'s SCD?

CASE STUDY PROGRESS

When V.M. arrives at the ED, you perform a quick assessment and note a grade III systolic murmur and crackles in V.M.'s bases bilaterally. Vital signs (VS) are 176/102, 94, 28, 97.8° F (36.6° C), and Spo_2 78%. Peripheral pulses are equal and 4+. Acting according to the standing orders for your institution, you start an intravenous (IV) line, obtain arterial blood gases (ABGs), and draw blood for complete blood count (CBC) with differential and basal metabolic panel.

7. The physician asks him whether he is in pain and whether he needs pain medication. V.M. answers no to both questions. Why did the physician ask these two questions?

8. V.M.'s ABGs on 8 L O_2 by simple face mask show Pao_2 74 mm Hg. Is V.M. being adequately oxygenated?

9. Your assessment findings are consistent with fluid overload. What five findings led you to that conclusion?

10. Your institution uses electronic charting. Based on the assessment described, which of the following systems would you mark as "abnormal" as you document your findings? For abnormal findings, provide a brief narrative note.
    X Abnormal

☐ Neurologic
☐ Respiratory
☐ Cardiovascular
☐ Gastrointestinal (GI)
☐ Genitourinary (GU)
☐ Musculoskeletal
☐ Skin
☐ Psychosocial
☐ Pain

9 Oncologic/Hematologic

Chart View

Laboratory Test Values

Sodium	137 mmol/L
Potassium	4.9 mmol/L
Chloride	110 mmol/L
CO_2	16 mmol/L
BUN	27 mg/dL
Creatinine	2.7 mg/dL
White blood cells (WBC)	4300/mm³
Hemoglobin	7.8 g/dL
Hematocrit	20.9%
Platelets	208,000/mm³

11. Interpret V.M.'s laboratory results.

12. V.M. complains of being short of breath. Do you believe the low hemoglobin level is responsible for his complaints?

13. What action will you expect the physician to take next and why?

CASE STUDY PROGRESS

The physician prescribes furosemide (Lasix) 40 mg IV push (IVP) now, methylprednisolone (Solu-Medrol) 75 mg IVP now, and ceftriaxone (Rocephin) 1 g IV piggyback after the furosemide (Lasix).

14. Indicate the expected outcome for V.M. that is associated with each of the medications he is receiving.

15. The methylprednisolone (Solu-Medrol) 75 mg IV is supplied as a 125 mg/2 mL solution. Shade in the dose to be administered on the syringe.

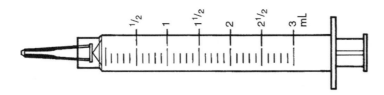

16. Identify three outcomes that you expect for V.M. as a result of your interventions.

CASE STUDY PROGRESS

V.M. voids 1900 mL within 2 hours of the furosemide (Lasix) administration. As V.M.'s dyspnea is relieved, he shakes the physician's hand and thanks him for asking about the presence of pain and the need for pain medication. V.M. states, "One of my biggest fears is that I'll come in here in crisis and the doctor won't treat my pain aggressively enough. I don't want to be labeled as a drug seeker or an emergency room abuser."

17. Why would V.M. be concerned about obtaining adequate pain control in the ED?

18. What issues will you address with V.M. before discharge?

Case Study 97

Name _____ Class/Group _____ Date _____

Group Members _____

▶ **Scenario**

C.O. is a 43-year-old woman who noted a nonpruritic nodular rash on her neck and chest approximately 6 weeks ago. The rash became generalized, spreading to her head, abdomen, and arms and was accompanied by polyarticular joint pain and back pain. About 2 weeks ago, she experienced three episodes of epistaxis in 1 day. Over the past week, her gums became swollen and tender and she was severely fatigued. Because of the progression of symptoms, she sought medical attention. Lab work was performed, and C.O. was directly admitted to the hematology/ oncology unit under the care of a hematologist for diagnostic evaluation. Her chest x-ray examination showed normal lung expansion and heart size, without lymphadenopathy. Skin biopsy showed cutaneous leukemic infiltrates, and bone marrow biopsy showed moderately hypercellular marrow and collections of monoblasts. Her lumbar puncture specimen was free of blast cells. The final diagnosis was acute myeloblastic leukemia.

C.O. is to begin remission induction therapy with cytarabine (Ara-C) 100 mg/m²/day as a continuous infusion for 7 days and idarubicin (Idamycin) 12 mg/m²/day intravenous (IV) push for 3 days. She is scheduled in angiography for placement of a triple-lumen subclavian Hickman catheter before beginning her therapy.

Chart View

Laboratory Test Results

Complete Blood Count (CBC)

White blood cells (WBCs)	39,000/mm³
Monocytes	64%
Lymphocytes	15%
Neutrophils	4%
Blasts	17%
Hemoglobin (Hgb)	10.4 g/dL
Hematocrit (Hct)	28.7%
Platelets	49,000/mm³

1. Interpret C.O.'s CBC results. What does the presence of blasts in the differential mean?

2. What was the purpose of the bone marrow biopsy?

 3. Considering all the admission data, what potential problem will the nurse be alert for when C.O. returns to the unit after insertion of the catheter?

4. What assessments regarding the central catheter are essential for the nurse to perform?

5. What unique adverse effects are associated with cytarabine and idarubicin?

6. Identify five nursing interventions related to these side effects to include in C.O.'s plan of care.

9 Oncologic/Hematologic

CASE STUDY PROGRESS

On the fifth day of continuous infusion of cytarabine, the UAP reports C.O.'s vital signs to you.

Chart View

Vital Signs

Blood pressure (BP)	110/54 mm Hg
Heart rate	115 beats/min
Respiratory rate	26 breaths/min
Temperature	101.6° F (38.7° C)

7. What additional assessments should you make at this time?

CASE STUDY PROGRESS

Your assessment findings are unremarkable and you notify the intern on duty of C.O.'s vital signs. After evaluating C.O., the orders shown in the chart are written.

Chart View

Physician's Orders

Blood cultures now × 2 sites
Acetaminophen (Tylenol) suppository 650 mg q4-6 h prn
Imipenem/cilastatin sodium (Primaxin) 500 mg intravenous piggyback (IVPB) q8h
Notify physician for temp over 100.0° F (37.8° C)

8. Do these orders seem appropriate for this patient? Explain.

9. What will your next action be?

Chart View

Laboratory Test Values

WBCs	1200/mm^3
Monocytes	25%
Lymphocytes	65%
Neutrophils	5%
Blasts	5%
Bands	0%
Hgb	6.8 g/dL
Hct	21.3%
Platelets	17,000/mm^3

10. These are C.O.'s laboratory findings on the last day of the continuous chemotherapy. What does this count indicate about her immune system?

11. Calculate C.O.'s absolute neutrophil count (ANC) and describe its significance.

9 Oncologic/Hematologic

12. Considering the previous data, what blood products will most likely be given to C.O.?

On day 14 after completion of her therapy, a bone marrow biopsy shows C.O. is in complete remission. With continued blood product support and antibiotic coverage, her marrow recovers and she is discharged from the hospital. HLA (human lymphocyte antigen) typing has been performed on all siblings. Her oldest brother is a perfect HLA match and has agreed to donate bone marrow or stem cells. C.O. is to be readmitted to the bone marrow transplant unit within the next few weeks.

13. What does "complete remission" mean for C.O., and what impact did it have on the decision to perform a bone marrow transplant?

14. What type of bone marrow transplant will she have? Briefly describe the transplant process.

15. Identify four priority problems C.O. will face in undergoing a bone marrow transplant. Put a star next to the most important priority, then develop interventions and an expected outcome for each problem.

Problem List	Interventions	Expected Outcomes

Problem List	Interventions	Expected Outcomes

9 Oncologic/Hematologic

16. After the transplant, C.O. will be at risk for graft-versus-host disease. Describe graft-versus-host disease.

Case Study 98

Name _____ Class/Group _____ Date _____

Group Members _____

▶ **Scenario**

You are working in the emergency department (ED) of a community hospital when the ambulance arrives with A.N., a 28-year-old woman who was involved in a house fire. She was sleeping when the fire started and managed to make her way out of the house through thick smoke. The emergency medical system crew initiated humidified oxygen at 15 L/min per non-rebreather mask and started a 16-gauge IV with lactated Ringer's solution. On arrival in the ED, her vital signs are 100/66, 125, 34, Spo$_2$ 93%. She appears anxious and in pain.

1. Describe the interventions needed to care for A.N. on her arrival in the ED.

2. As you perform your initial assessment, you note burns on A.N.'s right anterior leg, left anterior and posterior leg, and anterior torso. Shade the affected areas, and then, using the rule of nines, calculate the extent of A.N.'s burn injury.

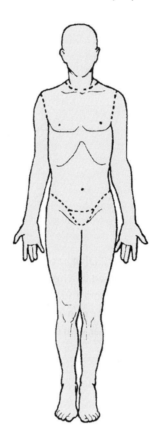

3. You suspect that A.N. has sustained deep partial-thickness burns. Which best describes this type of burn?
   a. The skin is blackened; the charred skin is numb.
   b. The wounds are red, blanch, and have accompanying edema.
   b. The skin is mixed red to waxy white, moist, has blisters and is painful.
   c. The wounds have severe edema, pain may or may not be present, and the color varies.

4. Because you are concerned about possible smoke inhalation, what will you monitor for in A.N.?

Laboratory Test Values

Hgb	20 g/dL
Hct	51%
K	4.9 mEq/dL
Na	133 mEq/dL
Cl	100 mEq/dL
Glu	159 mg/dL
BUN	28 mg/dL
Cre	1.0 mg/dL

5. Interpret A.N.'s laboratory results.

6. A.N. is undergoing burn fluid resuscitation using the standard Baxter (Parkland) formula. She was admitted at 0400. She weighs 154 pounds. Calculate her fluid requirements, specify the fluids used in the Baxter (Parkland) formula, specify how much will be given, and indicate what time intervals will be used.

10 Multiple Disorders

7. A.N. is in severe pain. What is the drug of choice for pain relief after burn injury, and how should it be given?

A.N. does not exhibit any signs of smoke inhalation injury and is admitted to the medical unit for further treatment. As her nurse, you are concerned about meeting her needs for infection prevention, skin integrity, nutrition, fluids, and psychologic support.

8. Because of her significant burn injury, A.N. is at high risk for infection. What measures will you institute to prevent this?

9. A.N.'s burns are being treated by the open method with topical application of silver sulfadiazine (Silvadene). In caring for A.N., which interventions will you perform? Select all that apply.
   a. Shave all hair within the wound beds
   b. Maintain the room temperature at 85° F (29.4° C)
   c. Use clean technique when changing A.N.'s dressings
   d. Monitor the CBC and WBC with differential frequently
   e. Do not allow her to bathe for the initial 72 hours after injury
   f. Apply a ¹⁄₁₆-inch film of medication, covering entire burn

10. A.N. has one area of circumferential burns on her right lower leg. What complication is she in danger of developing? How will you monitor for it?

11. What interventions will facilitate maintaining A.N.'s peripheral tissue perfusion?

12. A.N. is ordered a special burn diet. She has always gained weight easily and is concerned about the size of the portions. What diet-related teaching will you provide?

13. Describe interventions you can use to assist in meeting A.N.'s nutrition goals.

14. Tissues under and around A.N.'s burns are severely swollen. She looks at you with tears in her eyes and asks, "Will they stay this way?" What is your answer?

15. A.N. is concerned about visible scars. What will you tell her to calm her fears?

10 Multiple Disorders

Chart View

Vital Signs

Blood pressure	90/50 mm Hg
Heart rate	130 beats/min
Respiratory rate	24 breaths/min
Temperature	99.0° F (37.2° C)

CASE STUDY PROGRESS

Eighteen hours after the injury, the UAP reports these vital signs for A.N. and states that the urine output for the past hour was 20 mL.

16. What do you suspect is occurring, and why does this concern you?

17. What treatment do you anticipate?

Chart View

Laboratory Test Values

Hgb	24 g/dL
Hct	59%
K	5.3 mEq/dL
Na	128 mEq/dL
Cl	92 mEq/dL
Glu	122 mg/dL
BUN	38 mg/dL
Cre	1.9 mg/dL

18. The physician increases A.N.'s IV rate and orders a new set of lab work. Compare A.N.'s current laboratory results with those from admission.

19. By the end of your shift, which of the following assessment findings would best indicate that A.N. is responding to therapy?
    a. Respiratory rate 22; blood pressure 120/74
    b. Heart rate 110; urine output 20 mL/hr for past 4 hours
    c. Blood pressure 120/70; urine output 25 mL/hr for past 4 hours
    d. Blood pressure 104/64; urine output 40 mL/hr for past 4 hours

10 Multiple Disorders

Case Study **99**

Name _____ Class/Group _____ Date _____

Group Members _____

▶ **Scenario**

You are directly admitting a 30-year-old woman, J.L., to your telemetry unit with the diagnosis of status post–cardiac transplantation and fever of unknown origin. She was healthy until the birth of her only child at 27 years of age. She developed idiopathic cardiomyopathy after childbirth and underwent cardiac transplantation 10 months ago. All of her endomyocardial biopsies have been negative for signs of rejection; her last one was 3 weeks ago. She is currently maintained on a regimen of baby aspirin, multivitamins, tacrolimus (Prograf), nifedipine (Procardia), and metolazone (Zaroxolyn). The UAP reports her vital signs (VS) as 130/78, 104, 20, 101.7° F (38.7° C).

1. Admitting has assigned J.L. to a semiprivate room. Her roommate is on day 4 of IV antibiotic treatment for pneumonia and now has a near normal white blood cell (WBC) count. Is this assignment appropriate?

2. Fever is a sign of two major complications of organ transplantation. What are they?

3. Why is J.L. receiving tacrolimus (Prograf)? How will this influence your assessment?

4. Compare and contrast the signs and symptoms of organ rejection and sepsis that you need to assess for in J.L.

CASE STUDY PROGRESS

While you are performing your admission assessment, J.L. tells you she urinates frequently because of "that Zaroxolyn." She mentions, though, she has experienced burning with urination for the past 2 days. You decide to collect a urine specimen for laboratory analysis in addition to ordered blood cultures, complete blood count (CBC), and basic metabolic panel (BMP).

10 Multiple Disorders

5. What are possible causes of the burning and what type of urine specimen should you obtain?

Chart View

Urinalysis (UA)

pH	7.8
Color and appearance	Yellow, cloudy
WBCs	12
RBCs	≤2
Glucose	Negative
Ketones	Negative
Nitrates	Positive
Bacteria	≥100,000 colonies

6. Interpret J.L.'s UA results.

CASE STUDY PROGRESS

J.L.'s BUN and creatinine are within normal limits, and the CBC shows WBCs 11,000/mm³. Pending blood and urine culture results, the physician believes a urinary tract infection is the reason for J.L.'s symptoms and orders IV levofloxacin (Levaquin) 500 mg every 24 hours.

7. What are your primary nursing concerns for J.L. at this time?

8. Considering J.L.'s urinary infection and her immunosuppressed status, what other interventions should you implement when caring for J.L.?

9. Identify three expected outcomes for J.L. as a result of your interventions.

CASE STUDY PROGRESS

Thirty-six hours later, preliminary results of J.L.'s blood and urine cultures are available. The blood cultures show no growth.

Chart View

Urine Culture and Sensitivity (C&S)

Staphylococcus aureus	≥100,000 colonies
Amoxicillin	R
Ceftriaxone	R
Ciprofloxacin	R
Clindamycin	R
Doxycycline	S
Levofloxacin	R
Trimethoprim-sulfa	R
Vancomycin	S

10. Interpret J.L.'s urine C&S results.

11. What action do you need to take?

12. Describe the transmission-based precautions you need to institute for J.L.

10 Multiple Disorders

CASE STUDY PROGRESS

The physician changes J.L. to IV vancomycin (Vancocin) 500 mg every 8 hours and sends her to interventional radiology for placement of a peripherally inserted central catheter (PICC). Her first dose of vancomycin arrives from the pharmacy just as J.L. returns to the floor.

13. What other information do you need to know before you begin the vancomycin?

14. What interventions do you need to implement to safely administer vancomycin? Select all that apply.
  a. Hold the infusion if J.L. complains of tinnitus
  b. Obtain a trough level 6 hours after each infusion
  c. Monitor urine output, BUN, and creatinine levels
  d. Anticipate replacing the PICC line every 48 hours
  e. Administer each infusion over a minimum of 1 hour
  f. Assess for the onset of hypertension during the infusion

CASE STUDY PROGRESS

After 7 days, J.L. shows a positive response to antibiotic therapy, and she is preparing for discharge. She will continue her prehospital drug regimen, with the addition of 3 weeks of sulfamethoxazole 800 mg/trimethoprim 160 mg (Bactrim DS) PO twice daily.

15. While you are reviewing her discharge instructions, J.L. tells you that her husband's parents gave her son a pet cat. She jokingly says, "They gave him the play and me the work! My husband is going to have to help. I'm not up to looking after a cat, too." What job does her husband need to do, and why?

16. Because of her remark, you decide to reinforce teaching regarding things J.L. can do to protect herself from infection. List five points you will include.

17. What information would you want to review with J.L. regarding the signs and symptoms of infection and when to seek treatment?

18. Which of the following statements indicates that J.P. understands your discharge teaching?
a. "I will drink a minimum of eight glasses of fluid per day."
b. "I should wait 2 hours after taking this medicine before I eat."
c. "I will notify the health care provider if my hands and feet become numb."
d. "This drug may make me dizzy so I should not do an activity that requires alertness."

10 Multiple Disorders

Case Study **100**

Name _____ Class/Group _____ Date _____

Group Members _____

10 Multiple Disorders

▶ Scenario

You are working evenings on an orthopedic floor. One of your patients, J.O., is a 25-year-old man who was a new admission on day shift. He was involved in a motor vehicle accident during a high-speed police chase on the previous night. His admitting diagnosis is status post (S/P) open reduction internal fixation (ORIF) of the right femur, multiple rib fractures, sternal bruises, and multiple abrasions. He speaks some English but is more comfortable with his native language. He is under arrest for narcotics trafficking, so one wrist is shackled to the bed and a guard is stationed inside his room continuously. He says a drug dealer told him he is "coming to get him." Hospital security is aware of the situation.

Your initial assessment reveals stable vital signs (VS) of 116/78, 84, 16, 98.6° F. His only complaint is pain, for which he has a patient-controlled analgesia (PCA) pump. Lungs are clear to auscultation. His abdomen is soft and nontender. He has a nasogastric tube connected to intermittent low wall suction. He is receiving IV D5LR through the proximal port of a left subclavian triple-lumen catheter at 75 mL/hr; the remaining two ports are locked. The right femur is connected to 10 pounds of skeletal traction. The dressing is dry and intact over the incision site.

1. J.O. has not had a cigarette since the accident. He is irate because the day nurse would not let him smoke. Do you think J.O. would be a good candidate for a nicotine patch? State your rationale.

2. J.O. has an antiembolism stocking ordered for his left leg. What is the rationale for putting a stocking only on this leg?

 3. What other measures would be instituted as part of thromboembolism prevention?

4. J.O. has a Foley catheter inserted to drain his urine. What would you assess for in relation to the Foley catheter?

 5. In view of the threat made on J.O.'s life and his vulnerable situation, what precautions should the nursing unit take to protect him?

CASE STUDY PROGRESS

The nurse in the emergency department phones to tell you that J.O.'s immunization status could not be determined when he arrived, so no tetanus immunization was given. When you ask J.O. the date of his last tetanus shot, you find out that he was born and raised in Colombia and immigrated to the United States 5 years ago. He does not know whether he has ever had a tetanus shot. You inform the physician, and he orders diphtheria/tetanus toxoid 0.5 mL IM and tetanus immune globulin (HyperTET) 250 units deep IM.

6. Why is J.O. getting two injections?

7. When you give J.O. the tetanus injections, you find J.O. in the position shown in the illustration. Are any of these findings of concern to you? If so, how would you fix it?

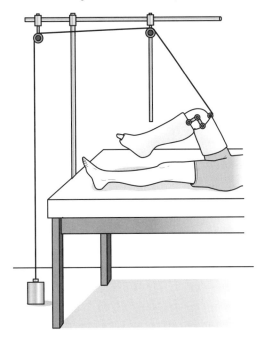

8. While assessing the leg distal to the fractured femur, you note that his toes are slightly cool to the touch. Why would this concern you?

9. What assessment do you need to complete?

10. J.O.'s assessment is negative for any further signs and symptoms of an evolving complication. What do you think your best course of action is?

10 Multiple Disorders

CASE STUDY PROGRESS

At 2100, J.O.'s guard summons you to his room. J.O. is pale, slightly confused, and complaining of chest pain and dyspnea. Vital signs are 90/60, 120, 28, 100.0° F (37.8° C), and Spo$_2$ of 84%. His pulse is weak and thready and there are petechiae on his chest.

11. What do you immediately expect is occurring and why?

12. Explain the pathophysiology of this complication and the reason J.O. is at risk for experiencing this complication.

13. List the priority actions you should take next and the rationale for each.

Chart View

Arterial Blood Gases (ABGs) on 2 L Nasal Cannula

pH	7.32
$Paco_2$	53 mm Hg
HCO_3	22 mmol/L
Pao_2	84 mm Hg

14. Interpret J.O.'s ABG results.

CASE STUDY PROGRESS

The physician comes and examines J.O. He writes the following orders, then leaves, stating he will be back in 1 hour to check on J.O.

Chart View

Physician's Orders

Bed rest
Oxygen (O_2) to maintain Spo_2 of 90%
Increase IV D5LR to 125 mL/hr
ECG monitoring
Repeat ABGs in 1 hour
CBC with differential and serum lipase now
STAT chest x-ray (CXR)
Methylprednisolone (Solu-Medrol) 12 mg IV push now
Furosemide (Lasix) 60 mg IV push now
Digoxin 0.25 mg IVP now

15. Describe a plan for implementing these orders in order of priority.

16. What is the expected outcome associated with each medication ordered for J.O.?

Chart View

ABGs on 10 L Face Mask

pH	7.29
$Paco_2$	56 mm Hg
HCO_3	22 mmol/L
Pao_2	74 mm Hg

17. J.O. is placed on oxygen at 10 L via face mask. ABGs are redrawn after 1 hour. Interpret the results.

18. What intervention do you anticipate based on your interpretation of these values?

CASE STUDY PROGRESS

The physician returns to reexamine J.O. Because J.O.'s status is deteriorating despite the application of oxygen and the administration of the IV medications, the physician writes to transfer J.O. to the ICU for ventilator support.

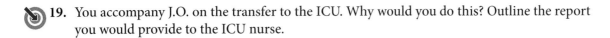 19. You accompany J.O. on the transfer to the ICU. Why would you do this? Outline the report you would provide to the ICU nurse.

CASE STUDY OUTCOME

J.O. recovers for several weeks in the hospital before being sent to jail to await trial. Shortly before his trial date, he is found stabbed to death in his cell. Although there is an investigation, the murder weapon is never found, and no one is ever charged in his death.

Case Study **101**

Name _____ Class/Group _____ Date _____

Group Members _____

10 Multiple Disorders

▶ Scenario

You are working on a telemetry unit and have just received a transfer from the ICU. The 50-year-old male patient, T.A., is postoperative day 2 after a repair of an abdominal aortic aneurysm (AAA) measuring 8 cm in diameter. He is an attorney with an active practice. Before surgery, he routinely took medication for gastritis and has a 10-year history of type 2 diabetes mellitus requiring insulin for the past 6 months to control glucose levels. Despite this, T.A. considered himself healthy before diagnosis of the aneurysm. The ICU nurse tells you during the report that since surgery, T.A. has experienced some weakness of his lower extremities and decreasing urinary output.

1. T.A. has questions about his surgery. He asks you, "I was fine before surgery. I'd still be fine now if I hadn't been operated on, wouldn't I?" Based on your knowledge of AAA, what will your response be?

2. Why are you concerned about the weakness in T.A.'s legs?

3. You are performing your initial assessment of T.A.'s legs. What should you include?

 4. In addition to ongoing assessment, describe specific nursing interventions to place in T.A.'s plan of care that are part of patient safety initiatives aimed at minimizing his risk of developing a deep vein thrombosis (DVT).

5. Four hours after his admission to your floor, you note that T.A. has had a total urinary output of 75 mL of dark amber urine. Why are you concerned?

6. You examine the urinary catheter and tubing for obstructions, and find none. What other assessments do you need to gather?

CASE STUDY PROGRESS

You notify the physician of the decrease in urine output. The physician orders a STAT electrolyte panel and asks you to call him with the results.

Chart View

Laboratory Test Results

Potassium	5.8 mEq/L
Sodium	132 mEq/L
Glucose	224 mEq/L
BUN	66 mg/dL
Creatinine	3.4 mg/dL

7. Interpret T.A.'s laboratory results.

CASE STUDY PROGRESS

The physician determines that T.A. is in the beginning phases of acute kidney injury. T.A. is sent to radiology for placement of a dialysis catheter. On T.A.'s return, the physician updates T.A.'s medical orders.

8. Indicate the expected outcome for T.A. that is associated with each of the medications he is receiving.

Chart View

Medication Administration Record

Lantus (insulin glargine) 30 units subcut daily
NovoLog (insulin aspart) subcut per sliding scale ac/hs
Imipenem–cilastatin sodium (Primaxin) 1 g IV piggyback (IVPB) q8h
Dopamine IV infusion at 2 mcg/kg/hr
Furosemide (Lasix) 20 mg IV push q8h
Sevelamer hydrochloride (Renagel) 800 mg PO with meals
Sodium polystyrene sulfonate (Kayexalate) 1 g PO bid

 9. The dialysis catheter is inserted into T.A.'s left subclavian vein. You are preparing to administer the IV antibiotic and find that his only other IV access, a peripheral line, is the site of the dopamine infusion. What are your options?

10. T.A. is placed on a fluid restriction and a renal diet. T.A. asks how much he is going to be able to drink. What is your reply?

11. Briefly describe a renal diet. What referral may be needed and why?

12. What are some interventions you can use to help T.A. be more comfortable while on a fluid restriction?

13. As you plan your care of T.A. for the remainder of the shift, identify which aspects of his care you can delegate to the UAP? Select all that apply.
    a. Measure vital signs every 2 hours
    b. Assist him with oral hygiene as needed
    c. Assess T.A.'s glucose level before dinner
    d. Monitor T.A.'s lung sounds every 4 hours
    e. Obtain and record an accurate daily weight
    f. Evaluate T.A.'s I/O trends for the past 48 hours

14. You note that T.A.'s blood glucose levels have ranged from 62 to 387 mg/dL over the past 3 days. He comments, "That's funny, you're giving me almost twice the amount of insulin that I give myself at home. I don't understand why it's not working." How should you respond?

15. Explain the relationship between his blood glucose readings and wound healing.

CASE STUDY PROGRESS

The next morning, T.A. goes for his first dialysis treatment. Shortly after his return, T.A. complains of headache and severe nausea. He is restless and slightly confused, and he has an elevated blood pressure.

16. What is the significance of these findings?

17. You page the physician. What will you do while waiting for the physician to return your call?

18. While waiting for the physician, T.A. begins to vomit severely. During the episode, he complains of something "not feeling right" in his abdomen. What is your immediate concern and why?

19. You remove his abdominal dressing and immediately see a few loops of intestine. You have another staff member page the physician. What care will you render before the physician's arrival?

CASE STUDY OUTCOME

After the repair of the evisceration, T.A. returns to the ICU. During the remainder of his hospitalization, he experiences delayed wound healing and difficulties with maintaining fluid and electrolyte balance between his dialysis treatments. His kidneys eventually regain function, and he spends two more weeks on the rehabilitation unit before being discharged with home health assistance for wound care.

10 Multiple Disorders

Case Study **102**

Name _____ Class/Group _____ Date _____

Group Members _____

▶ Scenario

You are a nurse working in the medical intensive care unit (ICU) and take the following report from the emergency department (ED) nurse: "We have a patient for you: R.L. is an 81-year-old frail woman who has been in a nursing home. Her primary admitting diagnoses are sepsis, pneumonia, and dehydration, and she has a known stage III right hip pressure ulcer. Past medical history includes remote cerebrovascular accident with residual right-sided weakness and paresthesia, remote myocardial infarction, and peripheral vascular disease. She is a full code. Her vital signs are 98/62, 88 and regular, 38 and labored, 100.4° F (38° C). Lab work is pending; she has oxygen at 4 L per nasal cannula and an IV of D5.45 at 100 mL/hr. We just inserted a Foley catheter. The infectious disease doctor has been notified, and respiratory therapy is with the patient—they are just leaving the ED and should arrive shortly."

1. What major factors increase risk for developing a pressure-induced ulcer?

2. Each health care setting should have a policy that outlines how to assess patients for their risk of developing a pressure ulcer. What should be included in that assessment?

3. As part of R.L.'s admission assessment, you conduct a skin assessment. What areas of R.L.'s body will you pay particular attention to?

4. What are the advantages of using a validated risk assessment tool to document her skin condition on admission?

CASE STUDY PROGRESS

During your assessment, you note that she has very dry, thin, almost transparent skin. She has limited mobility from her stroke and is currently bedridden. There are several areas of ecchymosis on her upper extremities. She is alert and oriented to person only. You review the transfer summary from the long-term care facility and note she has a history of urinary and fecal incontinence.

5. Evaluate R.L. with the Norton risk assessment scale.

	Physical Condition		Mental Condition		Activity		Mobility		Incontinence		
Date	Good	4	Alert	4	Ambulant	4	Full	4	Not	4	Total Score
	Fair	3	Apathetic	3	Walk/help	3	Slightly Limited	3	Occasional	3	
	Poor	2	Confused	2	Chairbound	2			Usually/urine	2	
	Very bad	1	Stupor	1	Bed rest	1	Very limited	2	Urinary and fecal	1	
							Immobile	1			

 6. Given R.L.'s Norton score, describe specific measures you would implement to prevent further skin breakdown.

7. Knowing that R.L. is frail, has right-sided weakness, and has a pressure ulcer, what consultations or referrals would you initiate?

CASE STUDY PROGRESS

As you are completing R.L.'s assessment, the wound nurse specialist comes in. She knows R.L. from a prior admission; as soon as she received the request for a wound care consultation, she ordered a specialty mattress. She states that an air overlay should be delivered to your unit before your shift ends.

8. Why is a specialty bed or mattress used for immobile or compromised patients?

9. Why do patients placed on specialty beds remain at risk for skin breakdown?

10. What essential points should all staff know about the specialty bed?

11. Why do the heels have the greatest incidence of breakdown, even when the patient is on the most advanced specialty bed?

12. What intervention can you initiate to protect R.L.'s heels?

13. Compare and contrast friction and shear.

14. What interventions are needed to reduce the possibility of shear?

15. What risk factor does using a draw sheet prevent or minimize?

16. In caring for R.L., it is important for you to instruct the UAP to do which of the following? Select all that apply.
    a. Assess R.L.'s skin status every shift
    b. Develop an every-2-hour turn schedule
    c. Use the appropriate sheets on the airflow bed
    d. Keep R.L.'s head of bed below a 30-degree angle
    e. Assist with hygiene measures when R.L. is incontinent
    f. Empty and measure output in the urine collection device

CASE STUDY PROGRESS

The wound nurse needs to evaluate the preexisting pressure ulcer. She gently removes the old dressing, using the push-pull method and adhesive remover wipes. After taking off the outside dressing, often called a *secondary dressing,* she pulls out the primary dressing and states that R.L. has a tunneled wound that was "packed too hard."

17. What problems can be created by packing a wound too full?

18. The nurse systematically assesses the ulcer and confirms the presence of a stage III wound with moderate drainage. There is no tissue necrosis or debris. What does it mean to "stage a pressure ulcer"?

19. What would you expect a stage III pressure ulcer to look like?

20. What is a tunneling wound? What risk factors are associated with tunneling?

CASE STUDY PROGRESS

After the wound nurse obtains a set of wound cultures, you watch as she packs the wound with gauze. The wound nurse charts the findings and makes formal recommendations for management of the wound to the primary care provider.

10 Multiple Disorders

21. Describe the technique for packing a tunneled wound.

22. What wound documentation is necessary at this time?

23. What factors influence the selection of wound dressing?

24. What do you feel would be the best option for dressing R.L.'s wound? State your rationale.

10 Multiple Disorders

Emergency Situations

11

Case Study **103**

Name _____ Class/Group _____ Date _____

Group Members _____

 Scenario

You are on duty in the emergency department (ED) when a "code blue" is called. As the code nurse, you grab the crash cart and run to the code, which is in the employee lounge of the operating room. On the couch, you find a nurse, Z.H., unconscious, dusky, and barely breathing.

1. What immediate assessment of Z.H. do you need to perform?

2. What intervention has the greatest priority?
   a. Obtaining a STAT toxicology screen
   b. Connecting her to the portable ECG monitor
   c. Establishing an IV line with 0.9% normal saline
   d. Supporting respirations by manually ventilating her

3. What assessment finding would lead you to suspect an opioid overdose is the reason for Z.H.'s condition?
   a. Hypertension
   b. Fever and tachycardia
   c. Constricted pupils and bradypnea
   d. Diaphoresis and cool, clammy skin

4. Z.H.'s respiratory rate is 8 and shallow. The respiratory therapist intubates her and continues to ventilate her manually. You attach ECG leads to her chest and find the results shown in the figure. What is your interpretation of Z.H.'s rhythm?

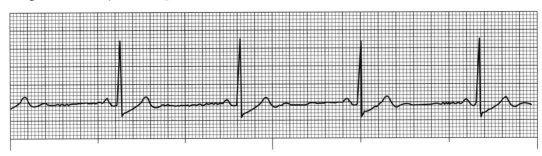

CASE STUDY PROGRESS

Z.H. is given an ampule of 50 mL D50W, 1 mg naloxone (Narcan), and 0.5 mg atropine IV push. Her respirations improve slightly, and her pulse increases to 56 beats/min. She is transported to the ED.

5. Describe the purpose of administering the combination of D50W, atropine, and naloxone.

6. What treatment will Z.H. require in the ED?

7. Within 30 minutes of receiving the naloxone, Z.H. is starting to respond. Why do you need to continue to observe her closely? Select all that apply.
   a. Z.H. may develop pulmonary edema after receiving naloxone.
   b. A common adverse effect of naloxone is the onset of atrial fibrillation.
   c. The duration of action of the drugs taken may exceed that of naloxone.
   d. The risk of developing diabetic ketoacidosis is high after receiving naloxone and D50W.
   e. Rapidly reversing the effects of the drug overdose will cause a rebound decline in level of consciousness.

8. The physician orders an additional 0.6 mg naloxone IV STAT. The vial in the accompanying illustration is available. How many milliliters will Z.H. receive?

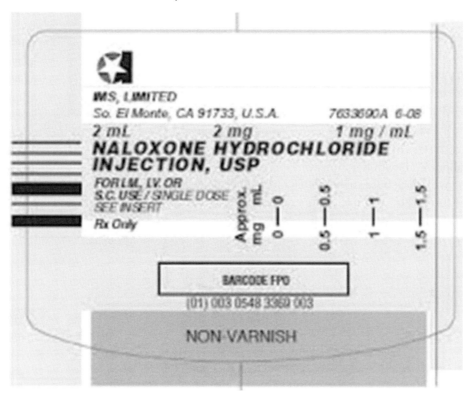

CASE STUDY PROGRESS

After the additional dose of naloxone, Z.H.'s level of consciousness and respiratory effort significantly improve, allowing her to be extubated.

9. What information do you need to obtain from Z.H.?

10. In response to your questions, Z.H. tells you that she took fentanyl and that she has been using fentanyl she has taken from the hospital "periodically" for the past several months. How does the Health Insurance Portability and Accountability Act (HIPAA) apply given that Z.H. is a nurse?

11. What is a chemically impaired nurse?

12. One of Z.H.'s colleagues calls on the phone to ask how she is. You convey that you cannot talk about Z.H. with her; however, she goes on to tell you that she thought something was wrong with Z.H. because her behavior had been so erratic, but "I had no idea it was drugs. I didn't think Z.H. would ever do anything like that!" What are the visible signs of a chemically impaired nurse?

13. State four problems associated with impaired nurses who are practicing.

14. Z.H. asks what is going to happen to her career. What are the regulatory issues related to impaired nurses that will guide your response?

15. She then asks you to call a friend to come stay with her. What information would you give her friend over the phone?

16. The friend asks you what is wrong. How do you respond?

CASE STUDY PROGRESS

Once stabilized, Z.H. is admitted to the chemical dependency unit. She successfully completes a rehabilitation treatment program and continues to practice as a nurse. She is now serving as a sponsor for another nurse undergoing treatment for chemical dependency.

11 Emergency Situations

Case Study **104**

Name _____ Class/Group _____ Date _____

Group Members _____

▶ **Scenario**

You are the nurse on a medical unit taking care of a 50-year-old man, A.A., who was admitted 18 hours ago with peptic ulcer disease secondary to suspected chronic alcoholism. You enter A.A.'s room and find him having a generalized convulsive (tonic-clonic) seizure.

1. What is your immediate concern for A.A.?

2. List five things you would do in order of priority.

3. Given A.A.'s history, state three possible causes for his tonic-clonic seizure.

CASE STUDY PROGRESS

The rapid response team is called, and the attending physician gives the orders shown in the chart.

Chart View

Medication Administration Record

Thiamine (vitamin B$_1$) 100 mg IM now
50% glucose, 1 50-mL IV bolus now
Lorazepam (Ativan) 4 mg IV now over 2-5 minutes

11 Emergency Situations

4. Indicate the expected outcome for A.A. associated with each medication.

5. In what order would you give A.A.'s medications? Defend your rationale.
   _____ Thiamine (vitamin B$_1$)
   _____ Glucose
   _____ Lorazepam (Ativan)

6. List one thing you would be particularly alert for when giving lorazepam intravenously.

7. The lorazepam is supplied in a single-use vial. How many milliliters will A.A. receive? Shade in the dose on the syringe.

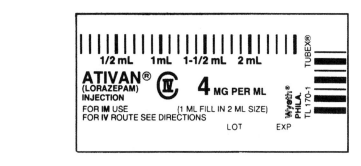

ATIVAN® (LORAZEPAM) INJECTION   Ⓒ Ⓘ𝐕   **4** MG PER ML
FOR IM USE   (1 ML FILL IN 2 ML SIZE)
FOR IV ROUTE SEE DIRECTIONS
LOT   EXP
TUBEX®
Wyeth® PHILA. TL 170-1

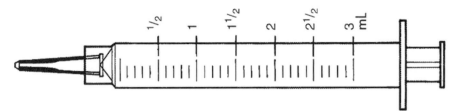

8. What assessments do you need to make during his ongoing seizure activity?

CASE STUDY PROGRESS

A.A.'s seizure activity does not subside. The physician orders an additional 4 mg of IV lorazepam without effect. Twenty minutes have now elapsed since you initially found A.A. having seizure activity.

9. What is the significance of this time lapse?

10. Define status epilepticus (SE).

11. The physician decides to administer propofol (Diprivan) and intubate A.A. to support his airway. What is propofol, and why is it being administered to A.A.?

12. The physician orders phenytoin (Dilantin) 15 mg/kg IV loading dose to be given at a rate of 50 mg/min. What is the rationale behind administering phenytoin?

13. A.A. weighs 143 pounds. How much phenytoin will you administer?

14. As you prepare to administer the phenytoin, you see that A.A. has D5W infusing at 75 mL/hr. Why does this concern you and what are your options?

11 Emergency Situations

15. You accompany A.A. as the rapid response team transfers him to the ICU. During the transport, his seizure activity ceases. What information would you provide to the ICU nurse?

16. What are the main complications of status epilepticus that the nurse will monitor for?

17. Identify nursing interventions that are appropriate for A.A. at this time.

CASE STUDY PROGRESS

A.A.'s seizure is successfully treated with lorazepam and phenytoin, and he has no further seizure activity. After his acute care needs are resolved, A.A. decides to enter a detoxification program on discharge. He successfully completes the program and remains free of drug and alcohol use.

Case Study **105**

Name _____ Class/Group _____ Date _____

Group Members _____

▶ **Scenario**

You are the charge nurse on the intermediate cardiac care unit in a large hospital. One of the patients on the unit is R.J., who was admitted at 1300 after an auto accident in which he sustained a chest contusion and fractures of the fourth and fifth ribs on his left side. At about 2000 hours, his wife runs up to you at the nurses' station and says, "I think my husband just had a heart attack. Come quick!" She follows you into his room, where you find him face down on the floor. He is breathing and is cyanotic from the neck up. His pulse is rapid but very weak.

1. What will your first action be?

2. What immediate care will you provide to R.J.?

3. Given R.J.'s admitting diagnosis, what differential diagnoses do you consider?

4. Suddenly you remember R.J.'s wife, who is anxiously hovering over you in the room. What are you going to do?

CASE STUDY PROGRESS

The code team arrives. R.J.'s trauma surgeon is making rounds on your unit when the code is called, and he runs into the room. R.J. is intubated, and the normal saline lock is changed to an IV of lactated Ringer's at "wide open." The trauma surgeon recognizes Beck's triad and calls for a cardiac needle and syringe. He inserts the needle below the xiphoid process and aspirates 75 mL of unclotted blood.

5. What is Beck's triad, and what causes it?

11 Emergency Situations

6. Explain the rationale for the surgeon performing a pericardiocentesis.

7. What is the significance of the surgeon aspirating unclotted blood?

8. The physician orders IV dopamine to "begin at 4 mcg/kg/min and titrate to maintain a systolic BP over 100 mm Hg." What is the rationale for this order?

9. Describe how you will titrate the dopamine infusion.

10. Identify four assessment findings that would indicate that R.J. is responding to the immediate actions.

CASE STUDY PROGRESS

R.J. is transferred to the surgical intensive care unit (SICU) for observation.

11. As the team prepares R.J.'s transfer, you go to find R.J.'s wife to thank her for alerting you to the emergency so promptly and to tell her what has happened. Briefly, and in lay terms, how would you explain what happened to her husband?

12. As you both get up to leave, Mrs. J. suddenly turns pale and says she feels very dizzy. What are you going to do?

11 Emergency Situations

Case Study **106**

Name _____ Class/Group _____ Date _____

Group Members _____

▶ **Scenario**

You are on duty in the intermediate care unit and scheduled to take the next admission. The emergency department (ED) nurse calls to give you the following report: "This is Barb in the ED, and we have a 62-year-old man, K.L., with lower GI bleeding. He is a sandblaster with a 12-year history of silicosis. He is taking 40 mg of prednisone per day. During the night, he developed severe diarrhea. He was unable to get out of bed fast enough and had a large maroon-colored stool in the bed. His wife 'freaked' and called the paramedics. He is coming to you. His vital signs (VS) are stable—110/64, 110, 28, Spo$_2$ 93%—and he's a little agitated. His temperature is 98.2° F (36.8° C). He has not had any stools since admission, but his rectal examination was guaiac positive and he is pale but not diaphoretic. We have him on 5 L O$_2$/NC. We started a 16-gauge IV with LR at 125 mL/hr. He has an 18-gauge Salem Sump to continuous low suction; that drainage is also guaiac positive. We have done a CBC with differential, chem panel, coagulation times, a T&C for 4 units, ABGs, and a UA. He's all ready for you."

1. How do you prepare for this patient's arrival?

2. Given K.L.'s history, what do you think significantly contributed to the GI bleeding?

CASE STUDY PROGRESS

K.L. arrives on your unit. As you help him transfer from the ED stretcher to the bed, K.L. becomes very dyspneic and expels 800 mL of maroon stool.

3. What immediate complication concerns you most?

4. What are the first three actions you should take?

CASE STUDY PROGRESS

K.L. reports that he is feeling nauseated. VS are 92/58, 116, 32, Spo$_2$ 93%. The physician orders an IV fluid bolus of 500 mL 0.9% normal saline and 2 units packed red blood cells stat.

5. What additional interventions do you need to institute?

6. What assessment indicators would you monitor in K.L.?

7. In caring for K.L., which of these activities can be safely delegated to the UAP? Select all that apply.
   a. Applying a pulse oximetry monitor
   b. Measuring his VS every 15 minutes
   c. Assessing K.L.'s peripheral circulation
   d. Monitoring K.L.'s hemoglobin and hematocrit levels
   e. Emptying the Foley catheter collection bag each hour
   f. Obtaining consent from K.L. for the blood transfusions

Chart View

Arterial Blood Gases (ABGs)

pH	7.47
$Paco_2$	33 mm Hg
Pao_2	65 mm Hg
HCO_3	23 mmol/L
Spo_2	91%

Complete Blood Count (CBC)

WBCs	4300/mm³
RBCs	4.0 million/mm³
Hemoglobin (Hgb)	7.8 g/dL
Hematocrit (Hct)	23%
Platelets	208,000/mm³

8. K.L.'s ED laboratory results are sent to you. Interpret his ABGs. What do they tell you?

9. Discuss K.L.'s hemoglobin and hematocrit results.

CASE STUDY PROGRESS

The physician discusses K.L. with the gastroenterologist, who schedules K.L. for an immediate colonoscopy. You accompany K.L. to the endoscopy suite and assist the endoscopy nurse in giving him IV midazolam (Versed) and morphine sulfate during the procedure.

10. Why is K.L. receiving midazolam (Versed) and morphine sulfate?

11. What is your priority nursing responsibility during the procedure?
    a. Reorienting K.L. as needed
    b. Monitoring K.L.'s IV fluid intake
    c. Assessing K.L.'s VS and oxygen saturation
    d. Documenting K.L.'s response to the procedures

11 Emergency Situations

CASE STUDY PROGRESS

During the colonoscopy, K.L. begins passing large amounts of bright red blood. He becomes paler and more diaphoretic and begins to have an altered level of consciousness.

12. Identify five immediate interventions you should initiate.

13. You are preparing to administer the first of two units of packed RBCs. Evaluate each of the following statements about the safe administration of blood. Enter *T* for true or *F* for false. Discuss why the false statements are incorrect.
    _____ 1. Prime the correct tubing and filter with normal saline
    _____ 2. Verify K.L.'s identification with the secretary in the endoscopy suite
    _____ 3. Obtain baseline vital signs before starting the transfusion
    _____ 4. Begin the transfusion at a rate of 125 mL/hr
    _____ 5. Take K.L.'s vital signs 30 minutes after starting the transfusion
    _____ 6. Complete the transfusion within 6 hours of receiving the unit

CASE STUDY PROGRESS

The physician is able to find the site of the bleeding and cauterize the affected vessels. There is no further evidence of active bleeding. K.L. is transferred back to the unit. His condition is stabilized with fluids, blood, and fresh frozen plasma. He received IV esomeprazole (Nexium) and is placed on twice-daily oral therapy.

14. Later, when he seems to be feeling better, K.L. tells you he is really embarrassed about the mess he made for you. How are you going to respond to him?

CASE STUDY OUTCOME

The physician concludes that the GI hemorrhage was prednisone induced. Because the prednisone was being used to suppress the progression of silicosis, the physician will attempt to decrease his maintenance dose of prednisone while monitoring his respiratory status.

Case Study **107**

Name _____ Class/Group _____ Date _____

Group Members _____

▶ **Scenario**

J.R. is a 28-year-old man who was doing home repairs. He fell from the top of a 6-foot stepladder, striking his head on a large rock. He experienced a momentary loss of consciousness. By the time his neighbor got to him, he was conscious but bleeding profusely from a laceration over the right temporal area. The neighbor drove him to the emergency department of your hospital. As the nurse, you immediately apply a cervical collar, lay him on a stretcher, and take J.R. to a treatment room.

1. What steps will you take to assess J.R.?

2. List at least five components of a neurologic examination.

3. What types of injuries may J.R. have sustained?

4. What complication common to each of these diagnoses concerns you most?

5. Identify at least six findings that would indicate this complication is occurring.

6. What is the most sensitive indicator of neurologic change?

You complete your neurologic examination and find the following: Glasgow Coma Scale (GCS) score of 15; pupils equal, round, reactive to light; and full sensation intact. J.R. complains of a headache and is somewhat drowsy. His vital signs (VS) are 120/72, 114, 30, 98.7 °F (37.1 °C) and Spo_2 94%. As the radiology technician performs a portable cross-table lateral cervical spine x-ray examination, J.R. begins to speak incoherently and appears to drift off to sleep.

7. What are the next actions you will take?

CASE STUDY PROGRESS

While waiting for the physician to arrive, you find that J.R. has become unresponsive to verbal stimuli. The right pupil is larger than the left and does not respond to light. J.R. responds to painful stimuli in the manner shown in the illustration.

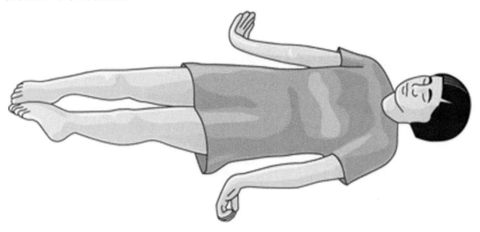

8. What is this response called and what does it signify?

9. Calculate J.R.'s GCS score. Describe the clinical implications of this score.

10. What is the likely cause of the change in J.R.'s neurologic status?

11. What are your nursing priorities at this time?

12. What immediate actions will you take?

13. His vital signs are now 160/72, 64, 10, 98.7 ° F (37.1 ° C), and Spo$_2$ 94%. What is your concern and why?

CASE STUDY PROGRESS

The physician arrives and gives the orders shown in the chart.

Chart View

Physician's Orders

Insert Foley catheter

Insert nasogastric tube to continuous low wall suction

Intubate: Vent settings assist-control 16, V$_T$ 900 mL, Fio$_2$ 0.5, PEEP (positive end-expiratory pressure) 3 cm

IV fluid 0.9% normal saline at 100 mL/hr

160 g Mannitol IV STAT over 30 minutes

Phenytoin (Dilantin) 1360 mg IV STAT over 30 minutes, then 100 mg IV tid

STAT CT scan

STAT trauma labs: CBC, CMP, UA, type and cross, PT/INR and PTT, ABGs, toxicology screen

14. Outline a plan for implementing these orders.

15. What is Mannitol, and why is it being administered to J.R.?

16. What is the expected outcome associated with administering phenytoin to J.R.?

CASE STUDY PROGRESS

J.R. is transported to radiology for a CT scan; he is found to have a large epidural hematoma on the right with a hemispheric shift to the left. He is taken straight to the operating room for evacuation of the hematoma. While he is in surgery, J.R.'s family arrives with their faith healer. They ask that their faith healer anoint J.R. and pray over him.

11 Emergency Situations

17. How should you respond?

Postoperatively J.R. is admitted to the neurologic ICU.

18. What assessment indicators will be closely monitored in J.R.?

19. Identify eight independent nursing interventions and the rationale for each that would be used to prevent increased intracranial pressure (ICP) in the first 48 postoperative hours.

Case Study **108**

Name _____ Class/Group _____ Date _____

Group Members _____

11 Emergency Situations

▶ Scenario

You are working in an outpatient clinic when a mother brings in her 20-year-old daughter, C.J., who has type 1 diabetes mellitus (DM) and has just returned from a trip to Mexico. She has had a 3-day fever and diarrhea with nausea and vomiting. She has been unable to eat and has tolerated only sips of fluid. Because she was unable to eat, she did not take her insulin as directed. You note C.J. is unsteady, so you take her to the examining room in a wheelchair. While assisting her onto the examination table, you note her skin is warm and flushed. Her respirations are deep and rapid, and her breath is fruity and sweet smelling. C.J. is drowsy and unable to answer your questions. Her mother states, "She keeps telling me she's so thirsty, but she can't keep anything down."

1. List four pieces of additional information you need to elicit from C.J.'s mother.

CASE STUDY PROGRESS

The mother tells you the following:

"Blood glucose monitor has been reading 'high.'"

"C.J. has had sips of ginger ale, but that's all."

"She has been vomiting about every other time she drinks."

"When she first got home, she went [voided] a lot, but yesterday she hardly went at all, and I don't think she has gone today."

"She went to bed early last night, and I could hardly wake her up this morning. That's why I brought her in."

2. Describe the pathophysiology of diabetic ketoacidosis (DKA).

Chart View

Vital Signs (VS)

Blood pressure	90/50 mm Hg
Heart rate	124 beats/min
Respiratory rate	36 and deep
Temperature	101.3° F (38.5° C) (tympanic)

Laboratory Test Values

Glucose	777 mg/dL
Potassium	5.8 mEq/L

3. Interpret C.J.'s VS, relating your discussion to the underlying pathophysiology.

4. Explain the rationale for C.J.'s other presenting signs and symptoms.

5. A decision is made to transport C.J. by ambulance to the local emergency department (ED). After evaluating C.J., the ED physician writes the following orders. Carefully review each order. Mark with an *A* if the order is appropriate; mark with an *I* if inappropriate. For each order you mark as *I*, explain why it is inappropriate, and correct the order.

   _____ 1. 1000 mL lactated Ringer's (LR) IV stat

   _____ 2. 36 units NPH (Humulin N) and 20 units regular (Humulin R) insulin subcut now

   _____ 3. CBC with differential; CMP; blood cultures×2 sites; clean-catch urine for UA and C&S; stool for ova and parasites, *Clostridium difficile* toxin, and C&S; serum lactate, ketone, and osmolality; ABGs on room air

   _____ 4. 1800-calorie, carbohydrate-controlled diet

   _____ 5. Bed rest

   _____ 6. Acetaminophen (Tylenol) 650 mg orally q4h as needed

   _____ 7. Furosemide (Lasix) 60 mg IV push now

   _____ 8. Urinary output every hour

   _____ 9. VS every shift

6. List five additional interventions that need to be performed for C.J. and the rationale for the use of each.

7. Which of these ABG results would you expect to see in C.J.?
    a. pH 7.40, Pao_2 88, $Paco_2$ 34, HCO_3 23
    b. pH 7.48, Pao_2 90, $Paco_2$ 30, HCO_3 28
    c. pH 7.27, Pao_2 90, $Paco_2$ 50, HCO_3 20
    d. pH 7.26, Pao_2 94, $Paco_2$ 23, HCO_3 18

8. When you attach C.J. to the cardiac monitor, which of the following would you expect to see on the ECG tracing?
    a. Peaked P waves and a shortened PR interval
    b. Presence of a U wave and ST segment depression
    c. Tall, peaked T waves and widened QRS complexes
    d. Narrow QRS complexes and shortening of the QT interval

11 Emergency Situations

All orders have been corrected and initiated. C.J. receives fluid resuscitation and sliding-scale insulin drip via infusion pump. After several hours, her latest laboratory findings are as shown in the chart.

Chart View

Laboratory Test Results

Na	149 mmol/L
K	3.0 mmol/L
Cl	119 mmol/L
Total CO_2	21 mmol/L
BUN	12 mg/dL
Creatinine	1.2 mg/dL
Glucose	307 mg/dL

9. Based on C.J.'s laboratory results, what changes in her IV fluids do you anticipate, and why?

10. The physician orders a change in the insulin drip infusion, decreasing it from 6 units to 4 units per hour. The label on the bag infusing reads, "100 units regular (Humulin R) insulin in 250 mL of normal saline." At how many milliliters per hour will you set the infusion pump?

11. What is the rationale behind using an infusion pump for the insulin drip?

12. True or False? A second registered nurse or physician must verify the IV infusion rate for the insulin dose change. State your rationale.

13. C.J. is ready for transport to the medical intensive care unit (ICU). C.J.'s mother is beginning to realize that C.J. is more acutely ill than she thought. She leaves the room and begins to cry. How would you handle this situation?

C.J. is transported in slightly improved condition. She continues to improve and is discharged from the hospital 3 days later. C.J. and her mother agree to attend an outpatient class offered by the diabetes education department to assist C.J. with better managing her diabetes.

11 Emergency Situations

Case Study **109**

Name _____ Class/Group _____ Date _____

Group Members _____

▶ Scenario

T.R. is a 22-year-old college senior who lives in the dormitory. His friend finds him wandering aimlessly about the campus appearing pale and sweaty. He engages T.R. in conversation and walks him to the campus medical clinic, where you are on duty. The friend explains to you how he found T.R. and says T.R. is "diabetic" and takes insulin. T.R. is not wearing a medical warning tag. It is 1015.

1. What do you think is going on with T.R.?

2. What is the first action you would take?

3. Which assessment findings would support the premise that T.R. is experiencing a hypoglycemic reaction?
   a. Extreme thirst and nausea
   b. Nervousness and tachycardia
   c. Hypertension with bounding pulses
   d. Fruity breath with deep, rapid respirations

4. If no glucose meter were available, would you treat T.R. on the assumption he is hyperglycemic or hypoglycemic? Explain your rationale.

5. It is 1025. T.R.'s glucose reading is 50 mg/dL. What should your next action be?

6. When you enter the room to administer the juice, T.R. is not responsive enough to drink the juice safely. What should you do?

7. T.R. is breathing at 16 breaths/min and has a pulse of 112 beats/min and regular. Because outpatient resources vary, describe your next actions if (1) your clinic is well equipped for emergencies or (2) your clinic has no emergency supplies.

CASE STUDY PROGRESS

A few minutes after administering 2 mg glucagon, T.R. begins to awaken. He becomes alert and asks where he is and what happened to him. You orient him and then explain what has transpired.

8. What questions would you ask to find out what precipitated this event?

9. What further action do you need to take at this time?

10. At 1045, you recheck T.R.'s glucose and the reading is 64 mg/dL. His vital signs are 120/72, 18, 92. Has his status improved or not? Defend your response.

11. What would your next action be?

12. At 1110, you recheck T.R.'s glucose and the reading is 104 mg/dL. What should you do now?

CASE STUDY PROGRESS

T.R. tells you he took 35 units glargine (Lantus) insulin and 12 units of regular (Humulin R) insulin at 0745. He says he was late to class, so he just grabbed an apple on the way.

13. Based on this information, why did T.R. experience this episode of hypoglycemia?

14. Based on your knowledge of the types of insulin T.R. is receiving, when would you expect T.R. to experience a hypoglycemic reaction?

11 Emergency Situations

15. He says he had two similar low-blood sugar episodes recently. He treated them by eating a candy bar. He says he is on a 2000-calorie, carbohydrate-controlled diet but has been checking his blood glucose levels every "couple of days" only. What common mistake in previously treated episodes of hypoglycemia did T.R. make?

16. List at least four important points that you would stress in a teaching plan with T.R.

17. You instruct him to check his blood glucose at 1230 then eat lunch at the normal time. He is to follow up with you in 1 week to discuss how he is managing. You will determine that T.R. understands your teaching regarding hypoglycemia if he states:
    a. "I need to eat within 30 minutes of taking the regular insulin."
    b. "If I am too sick to eat, I will not take any insulin until I feel better."
    c. "Only certain kinds of alcoholic drinks will affect my blood glucose levels."
    d. "I will exercise just before eating and taking insulin so I do not get cramps."

18. Write a sample documentation note for the encounter with T.R.

11 Emergency Situations

Case Study **110**

Name _____ Class/Group _____ Date _____

Group Members _____

▶ Scenario

S.K., a 51-year-old roofer, was admitted to the hospital 3 days ago after falling 15 feet from a roof. He sustained bilateral fractured wrists and an open fracture of the left tibia and fibula. He was taken to surgery for open reduction and internal fixation (ORIF) of all of his fractures. He is recovering in your orthopedic unit. You have instructions to begin getting him out of bed and into the chair today. When you enter the room to get S.K. into the chair, you notice that he is agitated and dyspneic. He says to you, "My chest hurts really badly. I can't breathe." You auscultate S.K.'s breath sounds and find they are diminished in the left lower lobe. S.K. is diaphoretic and tachypneic and has circumoral cyanosis. His apical pulse is irregular and 110 beats/min.

1. Identify five possible reasons for S.K.'s symptoms.

2. What is your primary nursing goal at this time?

3. List in order of priority three actions you should take next.

4. Using SBAR, what information will you provide to the physician?

11 Emergency Situations

CASE STUDY PROGRESS

The physician orders the following: STAT arterial blood gases (ABGs), chest x-ray (CXR) examination, ECG, and a helical (spiral) CT of the lungs.

Chart View

Arterial Blood Gases (ABGs)

pH	7.49
$Paco_2$	30.6 mm Hg
Pao_2	52 mm Hg
HCO_3	24.2 mmol/L
Sao_2	83%
A-a oxygen gradient	32 mm Hg

5. Interpret S.K.'s ABG results and give the rationale for your interpretation.

6. Based on the ABGs and your assessment findings, what complication do you think S.K. is experiencing?

7. Why is S.K. at risk for developing this complication?

8. The resident writes the following orders for S.K. Review each order. Mark with an *A* if the order is appropriate; mark with an *I* if the order is inappropriate. Correct all inappropriate orders, and provide rationales for your decisions.

    _____ 1. Albuterol (Proventil) metered-dose inhaler (MDI), two puffs q6h

    _____ 2. Heparin 20,000 units IV now, then 20,000 units in 1000 mL/D5W to run at 1000 units/hr

    _____ 3. PT/INR and PTT q4h; call house officer with results

    _____ 4. 3 L oxygen by nasal cannula

    _____ 5. Patient-controlled analgesia (PCA) pump with morphine sulfate: loading dose 4 mg; dose 2 mg; lock-out time 15 minutes; maximum 4-hour dose 30 mg

    _____ 6. Streptokinase 250,000 IU IV over 30 minutes, then 100,000 IU/hr for 24 hours

    _____ 7. Prednisolone (Solu-Cortef) 1 g IV push now

    _____ 8. Warfarin (Coumadin) 7.5 mg PO daily × 2 days

    _____ 9. CBC daily

9. S.K. asks why he is being put on heparin. Your best response is:
   a. "It will stop any blood clots from going to your lungs."
   b. "The heparin will dissolve any other blood clots you have."
   c. "Heparin will prevent any new blood clots from developing."
   d. "The heparin will thin your blood so you will be able to breathe better."

CASE STUDY PROGRESS

All the orders are corrected. S.K.'s helical CT scan confirms the diagnosis of pulmonary embolism (PE) in the left lower lobe and heparin therapy is initiated. Two hours later, repeat ABGs show the values shown in the chart.

Chart View

Arterial Blood Gases (ABGs)	
pH	7.45
$Paco_2$	35 mm Hg
Pao_2	82 mm Hg
HCO_3	24.1 mmol/L
Sao_2	90%
A-a oxygen gradient	28 mm Hg

10. What do these ABGs indicate?

11. The physician orders furosemide (Lasix) 20 mg IV push now. What is the expected outcome associated with administering furosemide to S.K.?

12. Because S.K. is being treated with heparin therapy, he has the potential for bleeding. What interventions will be part of his plan of care to reduce this risk? Select all that apply.
   a. Assess vital signs every 4 hours.
   b. Use a central line to obtain blood specimens.
   c. Apply direct pressure to any venipuncture site for 5 minutes
   d. Do not administer any IM medications unless absolutely necessary.
   e. At least once a shift, check stool, urine, sputum, and vomitus for occult blood.

13. List four independent nursing interventions that would be implemented for S.K. and the rationale for each.

14. What instructions would you give to the UAP who is assisting with S.K.'s care? Select all that apply.
    a. Use an electric razor when shaving S.K.
    b. Immediately report any signs of bleeding.
    c. Inflate the BP cuff only as high as needed to obtain a reading.
    d. Position S.K. with the head of the bed elevated, on his left side
    e. Use a sponge-toothed applicator when helping S.K. with oral care.
    f. Be careful when repositioning S.K.; make sure you have adequate help.

Chart View

Laboratory Test Values

Prothrombin time (PT)	12.1 sec
Partial thromboplastin time (PTT)	60 sec
INR	1.4

15. Coagulation times are rechecked after S.K. has been on heparin therapy for 4 hours. What changes, if any, do you anticipate, based on your interpretation of these values?

CASE STUDY PROGRESS

S.K. is watched closely for the next several days for the onset of pulmonary edema. Anticoagulant therapy, oxygen, pulse oximetry, daily CXR studies and ABG analysis, and pain management are continued.

16. On postoperative day 8, S.K. suddenly becomes very angry and throws the physical therapist out of his room. He yells, "I'm sick and tired of having everyone tell me what to do." How are you going to deal with this situation?

11 Emergency Situations

Case Study **111**

Name _____ Class/Group _____ Date _____

Group Members _____

▶ Scenario

D.V. is a 34-year-old woman who had a ruptured appendix 10 days ago with subsequent peritonitis. She was discharged to home care yesterday, on postoperative day 9, with a left peripherally inserted central catheter (PICC) for IV antibiotic therapy. You work for the home care department of the hospital. You have been assigned to D.V.'s case, and this is your first home visit. You are to do a full assessment on D.V. During the assessment you notice a large ecchymotic area over the right upper arm. You ask her whether she fell and hit her arm. She tells you, "The nurses took my blood pressure so many times it bruised."

1. Do you accept D.V.'s explanation? Why or why not?

2. In examining D.V. further, you find a fine, nonraised, dark red rash over her trunk (petechiae). What questions would you ask D.V. to elicit additional information?

CASE STUDY PROGRESS

D.V. had not noticed the petechiae before you pointed it out. She states that the rash does not itch or cause pain and that she has never had one like it before. She denies any other bleeding.

3. What other information would you want to gather?

CASE STUDY PROGRESS

Her vital signs are within normal limits except for a temperature of 99.8°F (37.7°C). The abdominal wound is not discolored or draining; however, her abdomen is tender to light palpation. The rash is confined to the trunk. There is slight oozing of serosanguineous fluid around the PICC insertion site. She has no other signs of bleeding. You make a decision to call the physician regarding your findings.

11 Emergency Situations

4. Using SBAR, what information will you relay to the physician?

5. The physician orders blood to be drawn for coagulation studies and a CBC with differential. What tests would you expect to see performed in coagulation studies?

6. You give D.V. a dose of her antibiotic and draw her blood. You tell her that you will return in 6 hours to give her another dose of antibiotics. She asks you, "What is going on?" How would you respond?

CASE STUDY PROGRESS

You drop the blood off at the hospital and proceed to your next visit. When you return to the car, you see that D.V. sent you a text wanting you to "come back now." When you return to D.V.'s home, she greets you at the door. She is upset and ushers you to the bathroom, where you find blood in the toilet. She tells you that she went to the bathroom and urinated blood. She also shows you a tissue in which she has bloody-appearing sputum and some bloody drainage from the blood draw 2 hours earlier. You call 911 immediately to have D.V. taken to the emergency department (ED) and notify the physician of your actions. You call the ED and give your report to the triage nurse on duty.

7. What are you going to tell the triage nurse?

Chart View

Laboratory Test Values

PT	19 sec
aPTT	96 sec
INR	1.8
D-dimer	4.8 mcg/mL
Fibrinogen	56 mg/dL
WBC	12,500/mm^3
Platelet count	46,000/mm^3

8. Interpret D.V.'s laboratory values.

9. D.V. is diagnosed with disseminated intravascular coagulation (DIC). What would be the most likely cause of DIC in D.V.'s case?
   a. Acute liver failure
   b. Presence of an undetected pregnancy
   c. Development of toxic shock syndrome
   d. Presence of infection in the abdominal cavity

10. Are D.V.'s presenting signs and symptoms consistent with DIC? Explain.

11. What are the goals of care for D.V.?

12. What medical interventions do you anticipate for D.V. and why?

11 Emergency Situations

13. List six nursing actions and the rationale for the use of each that nurses implement in patients with DIC.

CASE STUDY OUTCOME

D.V. is stabilized with oxygen, fluids, and blood products, and medication therapy is initiated. She is transferred to the intensive care unit (ICU) in guarded condition.

Case Study 112

Name _____ Class/Group _____ Date _____

Group Members _____

▶ **Scenario**

You are the trauma nurse working in the emergency department (ED) of a busy tertiary care facility. You receive a call from the paramedics that they are en route with the victim of gunshot wounds to the chest and abdomen. They started two large-bore IV lines with lactated Ringer's and oxygen by mask at 15 L/min. The patient has a sucking chest wound on the left and a wound in the right upper quadrant of the abdomen. Vital signs in the field are 80/36, 140, and 42. The patient is diaphoretic, very pale, and confused. The estimated time of arrival is 4 minutes.

1. To determine the possible extent of the patient's injuries, the most important information the nurse needs to ask the paramedics is:
   a. "How long ago was the patient shot?"
   b. "Do you have the weapon that was used?"
   c. "What was the reason this incident occurred?"
   d. "Where are the assumed entry and exit wounds?"

2. List at least six things you will do to prepare for this patient's arrival.

3. Prioritize the actions of the physicians and nurses in the trauma situation.

4. Who usually responds to a trauma code, and what are the functions of the people from other disciplines?

5. What are your basic responsibilities regarding gathering forensic evidence?

CASE STUDY PROGRESS

On arrival, your patient, B.W., is cyanotic and in severe respiratory distress. When he is transferred to the trauma stretcher, you notice that there is an occlusive dressing over the chest wound. It is taped down on all sides.

6. Is taping the occlusive dressing on all sides appropriate? Explain.

7. Based on B.W.'s vital signs and condition, what are the priority interventions at this time?

CASE STUDY PROGRESS

Treatments aimed toward stabilizing B.W.'s respiratory and volume statuses are started. You begin the secondary survey.

8. Describe the actions that you will perform as part of the secondary survey.

9. You note the following ecchymotic area on B.W.'s abdomen. What might this signify?

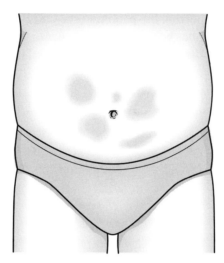

10. B.W.'s abdomen has become distended and rigid. What are the possible reasons for the abdominal distention and rigidity?

11. You report your findings to the physician, who orders a focused abdominal sonography for trauma (FAST). Why would this procedure be appropriate for B.W.?

CASE STUDY PROGRESS

The FAST is positive, and B.W. is sent for a CT of the abdomen, which shows a large liver laceration. The surgeon needs to take B.W. to the operating room (OR) for an exploratory laparotomy with repair of the liver laceration.

12. Because B.W. is not currently able to give consent for surgery, how will consent be obtained?

13. When you return from transporting the patient to the OR, B.W.'s wife is in the ED, upset and frightened. The social worker has been called to another emergency. What information do you need to obtain from B.W.'s wife?

14. How would you support her?

Pediatric Disorders

Case Study 113

Name _____ Class/Group _____ Date _____

Group Members _____

▶ **Scenario**

A.P. is an 8-year-old who is sent to the nurse's office because she has had a 2-day history of scratching her head so badly that she complains that her "head hurts." You complete a general examination of A.P.'s head and notice that she has red, irritated areas with several scratch marks; a few open sores; and sesame seed–sized, silvery white and yellow nodules (bugs) that are adhered to many of her hair shafts. You determine that A.P. has pediculosis capitis.

1. What is pediculosis capitis?

2. What will be your next steps in A.P.'s care?

3. What should be included in the educational plans for A.P. and her parents?

4. The parents take A.P. home to treat her. Which statement by A.P.'s mother would help make A.P. the most comfortable during this treatment period? Explain.
   a. "Here is the shampoo. Be sure to scrub your head for several minutes."
   b. "We can pretend you're at the beauty parlor! Lean back while I wash your hair."
   c. "I sure hope this works. I never thought this would happen!"
   d. "It might be best to go ahead and cut your hair. It will grow back quickly."

5. Why would head lice occur in school-aged children?

6. What possible complications can occur as a result of failing to treat head lice?

7. What nursing actions would you take regarding A.P.'s classmates?

8. A.P.'s mother calls you to ask what complications may occur with the head lice infestation. Which answer is correct?
   a. "Head lice may transmit certain viral illnesses."
   b. "Head lice are not known to transmit disease."
   c. "Head lice are common carriers of impetigo."
   d. "It is common to have a ringworm infection after a case of head lice."

CASE STUDY PROGRESS

Ten days later, A.P.'s mother calls you and states, "I think she has lice again! We worked so hard to get rid of them and clean everything. Is there something else we can use to treat her? What do we do now?"

9. What would you tell A.P.'s mother at this time?

12 Pediatric Disorders

Case Study **114**

Name _____ Class/Group _____ Date _____

Group Members _____

▶ Scenario

Z.O. is a 3-year-old boy with no significant medical history. He is brought into the emergency department by the emergency medical technicians after experiencing a seizure lasting 3 minutes. His parents report no previous history that might contribute to the seizure. On questioning, they state that they have noticed that he has been irritable, has had a poor appetite, and has been clumsier than usual over the past 2 to 3 weeks. Z.O. is admitted for diagnosis and treatment for a suspected brain tumor. A magnetic resonance imaging (MRI) scan of the brain shows a 1-cm mass in the posterior fossa region of the brain, and Z.O. is diagnosed with a cerebellar astrocytoma grade II. The tumor is contained, and the treatment plan will consist of a surgical resection followed by chemotherapy.

1. Which of these are common presenting symptoms of a brain tumor? Select all that apply.
   a. Headaches, especially on awakening
   b. Vomiting with eating
   c. Diarrhea
   d. Ataxia
   e. Seizures
   f. Pallor

2. Outline a plan of care for Z.O., describing at least two nursing interventions that would be appropriate for managing fluid status, providing preoperative teaching, facilitating family coping, and preparing Z.O. and his family for surgery.

12 Pediatric Disorders

CASE STUDY PROGRESS

Z.O. returns to the pediatric intensive care unit after surgery. He is arousable but cannot answer questions. His pupils are equal and reactive to light. He has a head dressing covering the entire scalp with small amount of serosanguineous drainage. His IV is intact and infusing as ordered through a new central venous line. His breath sounds are equal and clear, and SpO$_2$ is 98% on room air. You get him settled in his bed and leave the room.

3. You check the postoperative orders, which are listed in the chart. Which orders are appropriate, and which would you question? State your rationale.

Chart View

Postoperative Orders

1. Vital signs every 15 minutes×4, and then every 15 to 30 minutes until stable
2. Contact healthcare provider for temperature less than 36° C or over 38.5° C (96.8° F to 101.3° F)
3. Maintain NPO until fully awake; may offer clear liquids as tolerated
4. Maintain Trendelenburg position
5. Reinforce bandage as needed
6. Neuro checks every 8 hours
7. Elbow restraints if needed

4. You return to the room later in the shift to check on Z.O. Which of these assessment findings would cause concern? Select all that apply.
   a. Blood pressure 90/55 mm Hg
   b. Increased clear drainage on dressing

   c. Decreased responsiveness
   d. Facial edema
   e. Heart rate 120 beats/min

5. Discuss some of the emotional issues Z.O.'s parents will experience during the immediate postoperative period.

6. Which of these actions are appropriate ways to assist the family during this time? Select all that apply.
   a. Reassure them that everything will be fine
   b. Ensure that they have as much privacy as possible
   c. Encourage them to talk about their feelings, if they can
   d. Tell them you understand how they are feeling.
   e. Ask them if they would like to talk with the hospital chaplain and/or social worker
   f. Remind them that they need to care of themselves to be able to care for their child

CASE STUDY PROGRESS

Z.O.'s wound and neurologic status are monitored and he continues to improve. Z.O. is transferred to the oncology service on postoperative day 7 for initiation of chemotherapy.

7. Outline a plan of care that addresses common risks secondary to chemotherapy, describing at least two nursing interventions that would be appropriate for managing risks for infection, bleeding, dehydration, altered growth and nutrition, altered skin integrity, and body image.

12 Pediatric Disorders

8. The nursing assistive personnel (NAP) is in the room caring for Z.O. Which of these safety observations would you need to address? Explain your answer.
   a. NAP encourages Z.O. to use a soft toothbrush for oral care.
   b. NAP applies the disposable probe cover to the rectal thermometer.
   c. NAP applies hand gel before and after assisting Z.O. to the restroom.
   d. NAP assists Z.O. out of bed to prevent a fall.

CASE STUDY PROGRESS

On day 10 after initiation of chemotherapy, you receive the laboratory results shown in the chart.

Chart View

Laboratory Test Results

Hemoglobin (Hgb)	12.5 g/dL
Hematocrit (Hct)	36%
White blood cells (WBCs)	7.5×10^3 cells/mm^3
Red blood cells (RBCs)	4.0 million/mm^3
Platelets	$80,000 \times 10^3$/mm^3
Albumin	2.5 g/dL
Absolute neutrophil count (ANC)	75/mm^3

9. Which of the laboratory results would you be concerned about, and why?

10. Z.O. has a 5-year-old sister. She has been afraid of visiting at the hospital because her "brother might die." Discuss a preschooler's concept of death and strategies to help cope with the illness of a sibling.

CASE STUDY PROGRESS

Postoperatively, Z.O. completed his initial course of chemotherapy. Now, 4 months later, he is experiencing new symptoms, including behavior changes and regression in speech and mobility. His tumor has recurred. After a long discussion with Z.O.'s parents, the physician suggests hospice care.

11. List at least four of the goals of hospice care for this patient and family.

12 Pediatric Disorders

12. Pain control, supplemental nutrition and hydration, and resuscitation are common ethical dilemmas nurses face when caring for terminally ill children. List the common reasons for providing and withholding care in each situation.

Rationale for Providing Care	Rationale for Withholding Care
Pain Control	
Supplemental Nutrition and Hydration (IV, Enteral Feeding)	
Resuscitation	

CASE STUDY OUTCOME

Z.O. dies at home just before his fourth birthday. The hospice nurse and chaplain help the family by providing support and comfort for all family members and assistance in dealing with funeral arrangements. In addition, they offer the family ongoing bereavement resources and services.

12 Pediatric Disorders

Case Study **115**

Name _____ Class/Group _____ Date _____

Group Members _____

▶ **Scenario**

S.G. is a 6-month-old girl who is scheduled for sequential repair of her cleft lip (cheiloplasty) and palate (palatoplasty). She has recently been adopted from China and her past medical history is unknown. S.G. is scheduled for her cleft lip repair, and Mrs. G. brings her to the same-day surgery unit the week before for her preoperative workup. As you do her workup, you recognize that care of the child with clefting uses a multidisciplinary approach.

1. Discuss additional health problems for which these patients are at risk and who on the craniofacial team would address each issue:

2. S.G. weighs 6.5 kg. Plot this finding on the Centers for Disease Control and Prevention (CDC) growth chart (see www.cdc.gov/growthcharts/data/set1clinical/cj41l018.pdf). Which of these statements best summarizes your findings?
   a. S.G. falls below the 5th percentile.
   b. S.G.'s weight is at or near the 25th percentile.
   c. S.G.'s weight is at or near the 75th percentile.
   d. S.G.'s weight is above the 95th percentile.

3. What information regarding her health history is important to obtain from her mother to plan her perioperative care? Select all that apply and explain your rationale.
   a. Current known health status
   b. Current method of feeding
   c. Parent's employment status
   d. Immunization status
   e. Adoption status
   f. Gross motor milestones

4. Choose the laboratory tests that you expect to be obtained preoperatively, and discuss the rationale for your choices.
   a. CHEM-7
   b. Urinalysis
   c. Stool sample for fat content
   d. ABGs (arterial blood gases)
   e. Complete blood count (CBC) with differential

CASE STUDY PROGRESS

The laboratory test results and findings of S.G.'s preoperative workup are normal, and she is scheduled for her cheiloplasty.

5. What will you include in your preoperative teaching to S.G.'s parents?

6. Determine S.G.'s daily fluid maintenance requirements. How can her parents ensure this intake and determine adequate hydration status?

S.G returns to the unit after her cheiloplasty. The surgeon notes on the chart that surgical glue was used to close the incision. You note standing postoperative orders to clean with normal saline and apply antibiotic ointment three times per day.

7. True or False: You would call the surgeon to question this order. Explain your answer.

8. S.G.'s parents are advised that S.G. will return 6 months later for the palatoplasty. They are concerned about the delay between surgeries. What will your response be?

S.G. returns to your unit 6 months later for her cleft palate repair (palatoplasty).

9. Which of these nursing interventions are appropriate as you plan her care? Select all that apply, and explain why or why not.
   a. Position patient side-lying or on abdomen postoperatively.
   b. Use elbow restraints as needed.
   c. Clear fluids; advance as tolerated. Patient may use a straw.
   d. Administer pain medications as ordered.
   e. Oral suction with a Yankauer catheter as needed.
   f. Maintain strict intake and output.

12 Pediatric Disorders

10. S.G. has a normal recovery and is being discharged. When giving her parents discharge instructions, what will you advise them concerning diet and signs and symptoms to report?

CASE STUDY OUTCOME

S. G. is discharged to home with instructions for follow-up with the surgeon and multidisciplinary team.

12 Pediatric Disorders

Case Study **116**

Name _____ Class/Group _____ Date _____

Group Members _____

▶ **Scenario**

Mr. and Mrs. B. arrive in the emergency department (ED) with their 6-week-old infant, S.B. As the triage nurse, you ask the couple why they have brought S.B. to the ED. Mrs. B. states, "My baby breastfed well for the first couple of weeks but has recently been throwing up all the time, sometimes a lot and really forcefully. He looks skinny and is hungry and fussy all the time." You determine that the couple is homeless and has been living out of their car for the past month. S.B. has had no primary care since discharge after delivery.

1. What additional information will you need to obtain from Mr. and Mrs. B.?

CASE STUDY PROGRESS

Your primary assessment of the infant reveals the following: S.B is alert and fussy and consoles with a bottle of Pedialyte (per physician orders). His anterior fontanel is slightly depressed and posterior fontanel cannot be palpated. You auscultate regular breath sounds at a rate of 18 breaths/min. No adventitious sounds. Pulse oximetry is 98% on room air. Heart rate is 140 beats/min with regular rate and rhythm. Brachial and pedal pulses are +3 and equal. Abdomen is round and nontender to palpation. Positive bowel sounds. Diaper is dry. S.B. moves all extremities and there are no rashes noted. Rectal temperature is 98.9°F (37.2°C). There is a quarter-sized flat red area on occiput that "has been there since he was born" according to the mother. Slight "tenting" noted.

You transport S.B. to radiology and he vomits a large amount of clear fluid. Patient returns to the room in his mother's arms, awake and alert. The mother appears anxious and states, "I don't know what's wrong with my baby! Why can't you people tell me anything?"

2. Your institution uses electronic charting. Based on the assessment described, which of the following systems would you mark as abnormal as you document your findings? Mark abnormal findings with an "X" and provide a brief narrative note.

   X Abnormal
   ☐ Neurologic:
   ☐ Respiratory:
   ☐ Cardiovascular:
   ☐ Gastrointestinal:
   ☐ Genitourinary:
   ☐ Musculoskeletal:
   ☐ Skin:
   ☐ Psychosocial:
   ☐ Pain:

3. The emergency physician orders a complete blood count, complete metabolic profile, urinalysis, blood pH, and x-rays. The physician suspects dehydration and metabolic alkalosis secondary to hypertrophic pyloric stenosis. Which of these laboratory findings would you expect with metabolic alkalosis?

   a. Na: 128 mEq/L, K: 2.6 mEq/L, Cl: 90 mEq/L, HCO_3: 28 mEq/L
   b. Na: 130 mEq/L, K: 5.7 mEq/L, Cl: 94 mEq/L, HCO_3: 22 mEq/L
   c. Na: 130 mEq/L, K: 3.9 mEq/L, Cl: 98 mEq/L, HCO_3: 17 mEq/L
   d. Na: 148 mEq/L K: 4.1 mEq/L, Cl: 108 mEq/L, HCO_3: 13 mEq/L

4. What is the underlying cause of S.B.'s diagnosis of metabolic alkalosis?

5. Which of these clinical manifestations might you find with metabolic alkalosis? Select all that apply.
   a. Increased respiratory rate
   b. Tetany
   c. Increased risk for seizures
   d. Hyperthermia
   e. Neuromuscular irritability

6. What additional assessment findings might reflect the consequences of frequent prolonged vomiting in the infant?

CASE STUDY PROGRESS

S.B. is diagnosed with hypertrophic pyloric stenosis, admitted to the pediatric unit, and scheduled for surgery.

7. S.B.'s parents are concerned that their living situation contributed to S.B.'s diagnosis. How would you respond to their concerns?

8. Mr. and Mrs. B. have questions about the necessity of surgery and question what is going to be done next. What are your responsibilities as you respond to Mr. and Mrs. B.'s concerns?

12 Pediatric Disorders

9. Which of these preoperative orders would you question?

Chart View

Preoperative Orders

Vital signs q4h
Strict intake and output (I&O)
30 mL Pedialyte q3h PO
Place IV and begin $D_5\frac{1}{3}NS$ at 50 mL/hr
Nasogastric (NG) tube placed to low continuous wall suction
Daily weights

---

10. Which of these interventions can be delegated to nursing assistive personnel (NAP)? Select all that apply.
    a. Teaching parents the rationale for NG tube insertion
    b. Reminding parents to save diapers to be weighed
    c. Obtaining VS every 4 hours and reporting any abnormal findings to the RN
    d. Assisting parents in holding infant without removing NG tube
    e. Assessing for NG tube placement every shift

11. You note that your patient was hypokalemic and the fluids you hung per orders do not include potassium. You contact the surgeon to clarify. You receive the following order: "Discontinue $D_5\frac{1}{3}NS$ at maintenance and hang $D_5\frac{1}{3}NS$ with 20 mEq KCl at maintenance." You obtain the new fluids and hang per orders. True or False: This is an appropriate nursing action. Explain your answer.

CASE STUDY PROGRESS

S.B. returns to your unit after a pyloromyotomy. Mrs. B. is concerned about when she will be able to resume breastfeeding and what they need to do for their baby.

12. What postoperative teaching would you provide to them?

CASE STUDY OUTCOME

S.B. progresses well and is tolerating normal breastfeeding within 48 hours with minimal vomiting. He is discharged with follow-up in 2 weeks with the parents' new primary care provider. A social worker has helped Mr. and Mrs. B. obtain temporary housing and apply for available insurance.

12 Pediatric Disorders

Case Study **117**

Name _____ Class/Group _____ Date _____

Group Members _____

▶ ### Scenario

K.B. is a 16-year-old who fell while skiing. She briefly lost consciousness but is now alert and oriented. She was transported down the hill by the ski patrol after being stabilized and then was flown to the hospital. She has a fractured right femur and humerus. She will be admitted to your unit after an open reduction and internal fixation (ORIF) of the femur fracture and casting of her leg and arm.

1. You are taking the report from the postanesthesia care unit (PACU) nurse. K.B. is awake and taking ice chips. What information will you document on the patient admission form?

2. How will you use this information in planning your immediate assessment and care of K.B. on admission?

12 Pediatric Disorders

Chart View

Physician's Orders

1. Vital signs per routine
2. Neurologic checks every 4 hours
3. Turn, cough, and deep breathe and incentive spirometer every 2 hours while awake
4. Heat pack and elevate right lower extremity and right upper extremity
5. Neurovascular checks every 1 hour
6. NPO
7. IV fluids $D_5\frac{1}{2}NS$ at 100 mL/hr
8. Morphine sulfate 5 mg IV every 4-6 hours prn

3. For each order listed in the chart, state whether the order is appropriate or not and state why.

K.B. is settled into her room and begins to complain of pain (7 of 10) in her leg and arm. She weighs 65 kg. You note that the ordered dose of morphine sulfate was given 4 hours ago. Your drug reference states that the appropriate dose is 0.05 to 0.1 mg/kg every 4 to 6 hours.

4. Is this dose safe for your patient?

5. The morphine for injection comes in a concentration of 2 mg/mL. How much will you draw up and have a second RN double-check? Indicate the amount on the syringe.

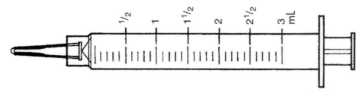

After K.B. has been on the unit for 6 hours, you identify the following changes in her assessment data: K.B. is difficult to arouse, but when awake she is able to identify who and where she is; PERRLA 1+ with slower reaction time than earlier; color pale, pink; skin cool and clammy; heart rate 126 beats/min, respiratory rate 28 breaths/min, temperature (oral) 99°F (37.2°C); Spo$_2$ 90%. The findings of the neurovascular checks of the affected extremities are unchanged.

6. What will your immediate nursing interventions include?

7. K.B.'s Glasgow Coma Scale score begins to decline from 15 to 11. What are possible reasons for changes in her neurologic status?

8. What would you document about this incident?

CASE STUDY PROGRESS

K.B. is transferred to the pediatric intensive care unit (PICU) and treated for changes in her neurologic status. The next day her primary care provider determines that her condition is stable and has her transferred back to the pediatric unit. It is now 36 hours after surgery. K.B. suddenly begins to complain of extreme pain in her lower right leg. She had pain medication 2 hours ago and rates her pain as a 10 of 10.

9. Which of these findings are early signs of compartment syndrome? Select all that apply.
   a. Diminished pedal pulse
   b. Macular rash
   c. Edema
   d. Paresthesia
   e. Capillary refill less than 2 seconds
   f. Increased pain

12 Pediatric Disorders

10. You page the orthopedic surgeon. Use SBAR (situation, background, assessment, recommendation) to address patient status.

11. K.B.'s cast is split and her foot pulses are restored. K.B. and her parents are extremely anxious. What education and support will be provided to K.B. and her parents?

CASE STUDY PROGRESS

K.B.'s status continues to improve. Physical and occupational therapists work with her on transfers and performing activities of daily living. She has many questions about how she will be able to go to school and resume her normal routine.

12. Recognizing K.'s developmental and cognitive stage, which of the following statements best supports your approach to discharge teaching?
    a. Adolescents are capable of thinking in concrete terms only.
    b. Adolescents are preoccupied with the immediate situation rather than future events.
    c. Adolescents can anticipate future implications of current decisions.
    d. Family acceptance is more important than peer acceptance.

13. The multidisciplinary team is made aware of K.B.'s progress in discharge rounds. Discuss how the following disciplines will be incorporated into her follow-up care after discharge.
    Discharge planning
    Education
    Physical and occupational therapy
    Nutrition

CASE STUDY OUTCOME

K.B. is discharged to home on postoperative day 5 with homebound schooling ordered and follow-up with orthopedics in 2 weeks.

12 Pediatric Disorders

Case Study **118**

Name _____ Class/Group _____ Date _____

Group Members _____

▶ **Scenario**

J.R., a 13-year-old with cystic fibrosis (CF), is being seen in the outpatient clinic for a biannual evaluation. J.R. lives at home with his parents and 7-year-old sister, C.R., who also has CF. J.R. reports that he "doesn't feel good," explaining that he has missed the last week of school, doesn't have any energy, is coughing more, and is having "a hard time breathing."

1. Discuss additional data that should be obtained from J.R. and his parents.

2. CF is a multisystem disorder. Describe the condition and its physiologic effect on the following systems: respiratory system, gastrointestinal system, reproductive system, and skin and electrolyte balance. Focus on factors that place J.R. at risk for developing respiratory infections.

CASE STUDY PROGRESS

J.R. is admitted to the hospital for a suspected respiratory infection and CF exacerbation. His mother helps get him settled into the room. Your assessment includes the following: vital signs: 115/76, 85, 28, 101.8° F (38.8° C) (oral) and SpO_2: 88% on room air. J.R. weighs 30 kg. Color: pale and dry with bluish-tinged nail beds and clubbing; capillary refill 3 seconds. Respiratory effort labored; coarse productive cough; rhonchi noted throughout; states he has pain of 3 to 4 of 10 with coughing. Thorax has a barrel-chest appearance; patient appears thin with decreased muscle mass. Last void and bowel movement this morning, no problems. Patient anxious and answers questions in short phrases.

3. Your institution uses electronic charting. Based on the assessment just described, which of the following systems would you mark as abnormal as you document your findings? Mark abnormal findings with an "X" and provide a brief narrative note.
   X Abnormal

   ☐ Neurologic:
   ☐ Respiratory:
   ☐ Cardiovascular:
   ☐ Gastrointestinal:
   ☐ Genitourinary:
   ☐ Musculoskeletal:
   ☐ Skin:
   ☐ Psychosocial:
   ☐ Pain:

4. What are the common microorganisms that cause respiratory infections in children with CF?

Chart View

Medication Orders

Ceftazidime (Fortaz) 2 g IV q8h
Gentamicin (Gentak) 100 mg IV q8h
Vancomycin (Vancocin) 450 mg IV q8h

5. You review the drugs that have been ordered to treat J.R.'s suspected infection. You are orienting a new nurse. Which of the following statements would you question as you review the ordered medications with her?
   a. "I will verify dosage and medication compatibility with the pharmacy."
   b. "I have assessed for possible allergies or hypersensitivities."
   c. "I will obtain a blood glucose level before administering the medications."
   d. "I will need to monitor serum levels for some of these medications."

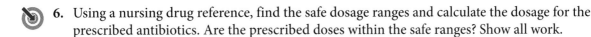

6. Using a nursing drug reference, find the safe dosage ranges and calculate the dosage for the prescribed antibiotics. Are the prescribed doses within the safe ranges? Show all work.

7. You are reviewing the physician orders for respiratory care. State whether you would expect to perform each of the following interventions, and give your rationale.
   a. Administer aerosolized albuterol (AccuNeb) 0.042%
   b. Administer chest physiotherapy (CPT) before administering the albuterol
   c. Monitor continuous pulse oximetry
   d. Administer aerosolized dornase alfa (Pulmozyme) after administration of bronchodilator
   e. Administer nebulized NS (normal saline)
   f. Administer tobramycin (TOBI) via JET nebulizer
   g. Limit fluid intake

12 Pediatric Disorders

8. J.R.'s weight is below the 5th percentile. He has been on a high-calorie, high-protein diet at home; J.R. reports that he hasn't been hungry and really hasn't been eating much. Describe the link between malnutrition and CF.

9. Which of the following actions can be delegated to the nursing assistive personnel (NAP)?
   a. Charting daily weights and intake and output
   b. Instructing the parents on correct administration of NS nebulizers
   c. Administering pancreatic enzymes from the home supply with each snack
   d. Increasing O_2 during an episode of desaturation

10. Which of these strategies are appropriate to manage GI dysfunction that CF patients often experience? Select all that apply.
    a. Administer fat-soluble vitamins daily.
    b. Administer pancreatic enzymes with meals and snacks.
    c. Restrict fat intake.
    d. Encourage a high-protein diet.
    e. Breastfeeding is contraindicated in infants with CF.
    f. Encourage snacks between meals.

11. What clinical sign assists in determining the effective dosage of pancreatic enzymes?

12. Which of the following GI comorbidities might you see in a patient with CF? Select all that apply.
    a. Celiac disease
    b. Meconium ileus
    c. Rectal prolapse
    d. Chronic vomiting
    e. Constipation

CASE STUDY PROGRESS

J.R. will be spending 14 to 21 days in the hospital for treatment of his pulmonary infection.

13. List interventions that would foster development while J.R. is hospitalized.

14. J.R. asks you, "Will I be able to have children when I grow up?" Keeping his age in mind, your best response would be:
   a. "You should discuss this with your parents. I will let them know you asked."
   b. "Most males have a significant chance of being sterile and you won't need to consider use of contraception."
   c. "Although nearly 95% of males are sterile, you should discuss this with your physician and family."
   d. "CF does not affect the male reproductive system; however, it does affect the female reproductive tract."

CASE STUDY OUTCOME

J.R.'s condition improves with antibiotic therapy and he is being discharged to home.

15. As you provide your discharge teaching, discuss health promotion points to reinforce with J.R. and his parents.

Case Study **119**

Name _____ Class/Group _____ Date _____

Group Members _____

▶ Scenario

J.H. is a 5-week-old infant brought to the emergency department (ED) by his mother, who speaks little English. Her husband is at work. She is young and appears frightened and anxious. Through a translator, Mrs. H. reports that J.H. has not been eating, sleeps all of the time, and is "not normal."

1. What are some of the obstacles you need to consider, recognizing that Mrs. H. does not speak or understand English well?

2. You perform your primary assessment and question Mrs. H. with a translator. Which of these findings are abnormal and need to be reported? Select all that apply and state rationale.
   a. Anterior fontanel palpable and tense
   b. Pupils equal and +3
   c. Temperature 96.8° F (36° C) rectally
   d. Heart rate: 85 beats/min
   e. Positive Babinski reflex
   f. High-pitched cry
   g. Refusal of PO intake per mother

3. Place an X where you would assess the Babinski reflex on an infant.

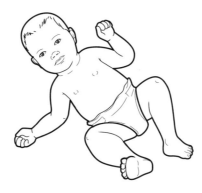

12 Pediatric Disorders

569

CASE STUDY PROGRESS

J.H. is admitted to the medical unit with the diagnoses of meningitis and rule out sepsis. The ED physician gives the orders shown in the chart.

Chart View

Emergency Department Orders

CBC with differential
Blood culture
CMP
UA
Cerebrospinal fluid (CSF) for culture, glucose, protein, cell count (following lumbar puncture)
Ceftriaxone (Rocephin) 260 mg IV now (loading dose)
Acetaminophen (Tylenol) 50 mg suppository per rectum for irritability

4. Prioritize the order of your interventions, with 1 being your first action and 7 being your last action.
   _____ Administer ceftriaxone (Rocephin)
   _____ Place IV
   _____ Straight catheterization for urine specimen
   _____ Place on contact isolation and droplet precautions
   _____ Assist with lumbar puncture
   _____ Administer Tylenol
   _____ Obtain blood culture, CMP

5. You have a difficult time placing the IV line and the physician writes an order to give the Rocephin IM while you wait for the vascular access team to place the IV. Name the appropriate site for an IM injection for an infant.

6. Before administering the ceftriaxone (Rocephin), you must verify the dose with another RN. The therapeutic range is 100 mg/kg loading dose and then 80 mg/kg daily. J.H. weighs 3.5 kg. Is the loading dose ordered safe? Is it therapeutic? Show your work.

7. Interpret J.H.'s laboratory findings, and explain the rationale for abnormal results.

Chart View

Laboratory Test Results

Urinalysis

pH	7.2
Color	Clear
Leukocytes	Negative

Complete Blood Count

Hct	32%
HgB	10.5 g/dL
WBC	22,000/mm^3
Sodium	6 mEq/L

8. Interpret the CSF findings. Would you suspect bacterial or viral meningitis? Why?

Chart View

Cerebrospinal Fluid Analysis

CSF	Clear
Gram stain	Pending
Protein	300 mg/dL (elevated)
Leukocytes	1030 cells/mcL (elevated)
Glucose	40 mg/dL (decreased)

9. What are the most common pathogens in this age group?

12 Pediatric Disorders

> **CASE STUDY PROGRESS**

J.H. is diagnosed with *Escherichia coli* meningitis. His medical care plan will include 14 to 21 days of antibiotic therapy. You are developing his nursing plan of care.

10. Outline a plan of care for J.H., describing nursing interventions that would be appropriate for managing pain and infection, maintaining hydration, assisting with increased intracranial pressure (ICP), and teaching to review with his parents.

> **CASE STUDY PROGRESS**

Mrs. H., through her translator, asks you what could have caused her baby to be sick, given that he had an immunization when he was born. She asks whether he should get "more shots" so this won't happen again. You reinforce to Mrs. H. that infants have immature immune systems, and they are vulnerable to infections until they have been fully immunized. Mrs. H. asks when J.H. will get more shots and what will they be?

11. According to the CDC immunization schedule, which of the following immunizations will J.H. receive at 2 months? You can refer to the current immunization schedules posted at www.cdc.gov/vaccines/schedules/index.html
    a. Hib
    b. MMR
    c. OPV
    d. IPV
    e. Rotavirus

    f. DTaP
    g. Varicella
    h. Hep B
    i. Pneumococcal

12. What is the impact of hospitalization on J.H.'s growth and development?

13. J.H. is being discharged after 3 weeks of IV antibiotic therapy. What educational topics will be important to discuss with J.H.'s parents when he is discharged?

14. You are providing developmental teaching to Mrs. H. with your translator. Which of the following milestones would be appropriate to anticipate.at 2 months? Select all that apply.
    a. Able to see an object 4 to 5 feet away
    b. Coos and gurgles
    c. Able to roll from stomach to back
    d. Able to purposely reach for toys
    e. Develops a social smile

CASE STUDY OUTCOME

J.H. is discharged to home with his parents. He will continue antibiotics by mouth for 1 week and receive a home health visit for infant care follow-up. The parents are to return him to his primary care provider in 1 week or call with any concerns.

12 Pediatric Disorders

Case Study **120**

Name _____   Class/Group _____   Date _____

Group Members _____

▶ Scenario

L.S. is a 7-year-old who has been brought to the emergency department (ED) by his mother. She immediately tells you he has a history of ED visits for his asthma. He uses an inhaler when he wheezes, but it ran out a month ago. She is a single parent and has two other children at home with a babysitter. Your assessment finds L.S. alert, oriented, and extremely anxious. His color is pale, and his nail beds are dusky and cool to the touch; other findings are heart rate (HR) 136 beats/min, respiratory rate (RR) 36 breaths/min regular and even, oral temperature 99.1° F (37.3° C), Spo$_2$ 89%, breath sounds decreased in lower lobes bilaterally and congested with inspiratory and expiratory wheezes, prolonged expirations, and a productive cough. As you ask L.S.'s mother questions, you note that L.S.'s RR is increasing; he is sitting on the side of the bed, leaning slightly forward, and is having difficulty breathing. You are concerned that he is experiencing status asthmaticus.

1. You check the orders and need to decide which interventions are the priority at this time. Select all that apply and explain the rationale.
   a. Monitor HR and RR every 2 hours
   b. Administer oxygen via face mask to keep Spo$_2$ above 90%
   c. Have L.S. lie flat
   d. Administer albuterol (Proventil) and ipratropium bromide (Atrovent) via hand-held nebulizer (HHN) STAT
   e. Reassess in 20 minutes, and if no improvement, administer salmeterol (Serevent Diskus) via dry-powder inhaler (DPI)
   f. Start IV normal saline (NS) at 15 mL/hr and administer methylprednisolone 2 mg/kg IV STAT × 1 dose
   g. Have L.S. perform incentive spirometry
   h. Encourage PO fluids as tolerated

2. Identify the nursing responsibilities associated with giving albuterol.

12 Pediatric Disorders

CASE STUDY PROGRESS

You give L.S. the albuterol and Atrovent. His O_2 saturation does not improve and remains at 88% with oxygen at 6 L/min via facemask. He says he "does not feel any better." He is retracting and RR rate remains 34 breaths/minute. You have started his IV infusion and administered the methylprednisolone. L.S.'s mother is pacing and tells you she very upset and worried. You overhead page the attending ED resident to assess, and you notify the patient-family advocate. The ED resident, Dr. S., arrives within 2 minutes to assess L. and to speak to L.'s mother. New orders are pending.

3. Chart your actions and the patient's response in the DAR (Data, Action, Response) format.

CASE STUDY PROGRESS

L.S. is admitted to the pediatric intensive care unit (PICU) for close monitoring. His condition improves, and 24 hours later is transferred to the floor. Asthma teaching is ordered. You assess Ms. S.'s understanding of asthma and her understanding of the disorder.

4. Which of these statements by Ms. S. would indicate a need for further teaching?
   a. "He should go to the doctor regularly to make sure his asthma is being treated correctly."
   b. "If he takes medications for a while, he will outgrow his asthma."
   c. "Part of his treatment should be avoiding things that irritate his lungs."
   d. "If I recognize early warning signs, he might be able to take medicine and not go to the ED."

5. You are educating L.S. and his mother on possible asthma triggers in their environment. They live in public housing in an apartment without air conditioning. Which of these statements indicate possible asthma triggers? Select all that apply, and discuss strategies to avoid these triggers.
   a. "The building has copper pipes."
   b. "He coughs when we have cold nights after a warm day."
   c. "We have a pet fish."
   d. "There are hardwood floors."
   e. "L. collects stuffed animals."
   f. "Our visitors smoke outside."
   g. "There are dark stains in our bathroom."
   h. "The housing authority puts a foam down for bugs."

CASE STUDY PROGRESS

The following day, L.S. gets the discharge orders shown in the chart.

Chart View

Discharge Orders

Discharge to home

Follow up with primary care provider in 3 days for evaluation

Albuterol (Proventil HFA) MDI: 2 puffs with spacer every 4 hours prn

Prednisolone (Prelone) 1 mg/kg PO every day for 5 days (L.S. weighs 23 kg.)

Fluticasone (Flovent HFA) MDI: 1 puff twice a day

Montelukast (Singulair) 5 mg every evening PO

Provide peak flow meter

Regular diet

6. Ms. S. asks why she will use the spacer with the medicine L.S. breathes in. Explain the purpose of a metered-dose inhaler (MDI and spacer.

7. Place the steps of using the MDI with the spacer in the correct order (1 = first step, 5 = last step)
   a. Depress the top of the inhaler to release medication, and breathe in slowly for 3 to 5 seconds, holding the breath for 5 to 10 seconds at the end of inspiration.
   b. Shake the inhaler and attach to the spacer.
   c. Wait 1 to 2 minutes between puffs if more than 1 puff of the same medication is ordered.
   d. Remove and exhale through the nose.
   e. At the end of expiration, place mouthpiece into the mouth, forming an airtight seal.
   f. Tilt the head back and exhale completely.

12 Pediatric Disorders

8. During your medication teaching session with Ms. S. and L.S., Ms. S. makes this statement: "So, if he has to take both inhalers at the same time, he should take the Flovent first, then the albuterol. Right?" Is this statement true or false? Explain your answer.

9. Ms. S. then asks, "How long should we wait between giving the two inhalers if they are both due at the same time? Can we just give them one after the other?" What is your response?

10. As you continue your medication teaching, you explain the difference between controller and reliever medications. Place a *C* beside the controller medication(s) and an *R* beside the reliever medication(s).
    _____ a. Albuterol
    _____ b. Prelone
    _____ c. Flovent
    _____ d. Singulair

11. After L.S. takes a dose of the inhaled corticosteroid Flovent, what is the most important action he should do next?
    a. Hold his breath for 45 seconds
    b. Rinse out his mouth with water
    c. Repeat the dose in 5 minutes if he feels short of breath
    d. Check his PFM reading for an improvement of function

12. Ms. S. comes back from the pharmacy with the Prelone and asks you to show her how much to give. Prelone is dispensed as 15 mg/5 mL. You give her a 10-mL oral dosage syringe. How much will she draw up for this dose? (Round to tenths.)

13. During the teaching session, you give L.S. a peak flow meter (PFM) and provide teaching for him and Ms. S. But L. looks puzzled and asks you, "Is this another medicine I have to take?" How would you explain the purpose of a peak flow meter to L.?

14. L.S. tells you that he loves to play basketball and football and asks you whether he can still do these activities. How will you respond?

15. Discuss the points to include in your discharge teaching regarding prevention of acute asthmatic episodes and symptom management,

CASE STUDY OUTCOME

L.S. is discharged to home and has a follow-up appointment scheduled in 2 weeks. He plans to try out for his school's swim team.

Case Study 121

Name _____   Class/Group _____   Date _____

Group Members _____

▶ ## Scenario

E.M., a 5-month-old girl, is brought to the emergency department (ED) with respiratory distress, hypoxia, and fever. Her parents state that she has had mild cold symptoms for a few days. She has breastfed poorly over the last few days, with a decreased number of wet diapers. You take her vital signs and complete an initial assessment.

Chart View

Vital Signs

Blood pressure	130/72 mm Hg
Respiratory rate	83 breaths/min
Heart rate	188 beats/min
Temperature	38.4° C (101.1° F)
Spo_2	88% on room air
Weight	8 kg

Initial Assessment

Neurologic	Alert, fussy; consoles briefly; anterior fontanel soft and slightly depressed
Cardiovascular	Tachycardia; capillary refill less than 3 seconds
Respiratory	Upper airway congestion; coarse cough; tachypnea, transient bilateral wheezing; coarse rhonchi and slightly decreased breath sounds at bases; mild intercostal retractions
Gastrointestinal	Positive bowel sounds; last bowel movement yesterday
Genitourinary	Decreased urine output (per history); no urine output in last 4 hours
Skin	No rashes; slightly flushed
Other	Mucous membranes "sticky"; decreased tearing

Emergency Department Orders

Acetaminophen (Tylenol) 80 mg PO for fever × 1 dose
Start IV and administer normal saline (NS) bolus 20 mL/kg IV bolus over 30 minutes
Oxygen to keep saturation greater than 93%
Nebulizer trial of albuterol (Proventil) 2.5 mg STAT × 1 dose

12 Pediatric Disorders

1. Review the standing ED orders. Prioritize your interventions and give rationales.

2. Based on E.M.'s vital signs and assessment, what diagnostic tests would you anticipate?

3. Calculate how much NS E.M. will receive as a bolus.

CASE STUDY PROGRESS

E.M. begins coughing and has copious nasal secretions. You provide nasopharyngeal suctioning and obtain a large amount of thick secretions. She is allowed to recover and is reassessed. The respiratory rate and retractions have not changed significantly. Her breath sounds are less coarse but are diminished in the bases. The Spo_2 is now 92% to 93% on 1.5 L oxygen. After E.M. settles, her mother asks whether she can feed her because she has not eaten much for the past few days. You tell her that with a current respiratory rate of greater than 65 breaths/min, she should not be fed.

4. What is the rationale for holding feedings?

5. When E.M.'s respiratory rate decreases, what teaching would you provide the parents concerning feeding?

Chart View

Medication Administration Record

Normal saline drops to nares q3h with suctioning
Acetaminophen (Tylenol) 80 mg PO q4h prn for fever
Amoxicillin (Amoxil) 45 mg/kg/day PO tid×7 days

6. You are reviewing the medication administration record. Which order(s) would you question? Explain.

CASE STUDY PROGRESS

E.M.'s mother calls you to the room because her baby is "not right." You note E.M.'s respiratory rate is 23 breaths/min, and the retractions have increased. The Spo_2 is 89% on 1.5 L of oxygen. She is pale and listless and does not cry with stimulation.

7. Why is the respiratory rate significantly lower even though other signs of respiratory distress have increased?

CASE STUDY PROGRESS

You are concerned and call the rapid response team. You check her Spo_2 again with results of 88%. The senior resident orders a portable chest x-ray (CXR) examination and capillary blood gas (CBG). The CXR is consistent with bronchiolitis with atelectasis.

Chart View

Capillary Blood Gas (CBG)	
pH	7.31
$Paco_2$	72 mm Hg
HCO_3	29 mEq/L
Pao_2	57 mm Hg

8. Interpret E.M.'s CBG results.

CASE STUDY PROGRESS

E.M. is transferred to the pediatric intensive care unit (PICU) and placed on a continuous positive airway pressure (CPAP) machine. You know from experience that patients are usually on CPAP for a couple of days before they are ready to be taken off and continue to improve until they are ready for discharge. You explain this to the parents, who are very distressed.

9. What resources might you seek for E.M.'s parents during this unanticipated change in status?

12 Pediatric Disorders

CASE STUDY PROGRESS

After 2 days in the PICU, E.M. is transferred back to your unit. You note that she is taking increased oral fluids and requiring less suctioning. Her Spo_2 is 96% to 98% on room air. As you are preparing the parents for discharge, they want to know how they can prevent this in the future. They ask whether there is a "shot" E.M. can get to avoid getting this again.

10. How would you address their concerns?

11. E.M.'s parents ask you for instructions about the treatment of cold symptoms if E.M. develops them again. Which answer is your best reply?
    a. "Over-the-counter cough suppressants may be safely administered at night."
    b. "If a fever is present, you can treat the fever with baby aspirin."
    c. "Saline nose drops and bulb suctioning can be done before feedings."
    d. "You do not need to worry if she is not drinking; intake should improve in a day or so."

Case Study **122**

Name _____ Class/Group _____ Date _____

Group Members _____

▶ **Scenario**

You admit L.M., a 2-month-old girl with a history of hydrocephalus and ventriculoperitoneal (VP) shunt placement 1 month earlier. Her parents report that she has been more irritable than usual and for the past 3 days has fed poorly and has had emesis five or six times every day.

1. Explain the pathophysiology of hydrocephalus and cerebrospinal fluid (CSF) imbalance.

2. Explain how the placement of a VP shunt helps the patient.

CASE STUDY PROGRESS

You get L.M. settled on the unit and promptly perform her admission assessment.

3. A nursing student is assisting you with L.'s admission. Assessment of growth and development is an important part of patient assessment. Which of the nursing student's statements is correct?
   a. "We will assess her anterior fontanel because it should be closed."
   b. "We should not see any head lag."
   c. " I do not need to do a frontal occipital circumference (FOC) measurement because her sutures have fused.
   d. " L. should be able to focus on objects that are near."

12 Pediatric Disorders

4. Your assessment includes the following findings. Select the abnormal findings and state a possible rationale for each.

System	Assessment and Vital Signs	If Abnormal, State Rationale
Weight	4.5 kg	
Neurologic	Irritable, awake, and fussy; difficult to console	
	FOC: 44 cm, "increased 2 cm from measurement yesterday" per mother	
	Anterior fontanel slightly bulging	
	Unable to palpate posterior fontanel	
	Pupils equal and reactive	
Respiratory	Bilateral breath sounds equal and clear	
	SpO$_2$ 95% on room air	
	Respiratory rate: 40 breaths/min	
Cardiovascular	Rectal temperature: 38.8° C	
	Heart rate (HR): 182	
	Blood pressure (BP): 111/70	
	Pulses 2+ and equal bilaterally	
Gastrointestinal	Positive bowel sounds	
	Emesis during examination	
	Last feeding 6 hours ago	
Genitourinary	Last urine output 2 hours ago	
Musculoskeletal	Moves all extremities well	
	Head lag noted	
Skin	Diaper rash noted	

5. The doctors order a CT scan and lumbar puncture with a cell count, culture, Gram stain, glucose, and protein run on the CSF. What is the rationale for each procedure?

CASE STUDY PROGRESS

It is determined that the VP shunt is infected and must be temporarily removed. L.M. is taken to surgery to have a left extraventricular drain (EVD) placed. She returns to your unit in stable condition. You get her settled back into her room and perform her assessment. You note that her EVD is intact and draining CSF. The dressing is clean and dry and intact under a sterile dressing.

6. True or False: The position of the EVD should be maintained at the level of the auditory meatus. Explain your answer.

Chart View

Medication Administration Record (MAR)

    Acetaminophen (Tylenol) 15 mg/kg PO q4h

    Morphine sulfate 0.05 mg/kg IV q4h

    Enalapril (Vasotec) 5 mcg/kg q24h

    Cefotaxime (Claforan) 150 mg/kg/day IV in divided doses q8h

    Baclofen (Lioresal) 10 mg/kg/day PO q8h

    Ondansetron (Zofran) 0.1 mg/kg IV now

7. Which of these medications are appropriate for L.M.'s diagnosis? Select all that apply and state the rationale for the ones you chose. Then, give a reason for those you feel are not appropriate.

8. You are preparing to give the first dose of antibiotic that is ordered. Referring to L.M.'s medication administration record, calculate the amount of the antibiotic that you will administer per dose.

9. L.M. is very fussy, and you decide to medicate her for pain. Calculate the amount of morphine L.M. will receive for pain per dose (do not round). Then calculate the amount you will draw up for the required dose, and mark the syringe appropriately (round to hundredths). The morphine is available in an injection solution of 2 mg/mL.

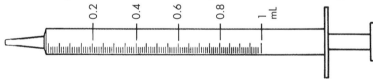

10. Which of these tasks can be appropriately delegated to the nursing assistive personnel?
    a. Performing the every-2-hour neurologic check
    b. Obtaining a complete set of VS and charting
    c. Instructing the parents on changes in neurologic status
    d. Changing the dressing on the surgical site

11. In which of the following positions should L.M. be placed immediately postoperatively?
    a. Flat, left side-lying
    b. Flat, right side-lying
    c. Supine, head of bed (HOB) 45 degrees
    d. Supine, Trendelenburg

12. What points will you address while teaching the parents about the EVD system?

CASE STUDY PROGRESS

Several days later, L.M.'s mother is changing L.M.'s diaper and she tells you that she is worried because L.M. has started having diarrhea recently, and it is getting worse.

13. Based on the medications that L.M. is receiving, what is the most likely cause of the diarrhea? What is a possible concern you should consider, and what should your care plan include?

CASE STUDY PROGRESS

L.M. responds well to the antibiotics, and her shunt is internalized 2 weeks later. She is released from the hospital after observation for 2 days.

14. While you are giving your discharge instructions, L.M.'s mother states that she normally gives L.M. 1 mL of acetaminophen (Tylenol Elixir), 160 mg/5 mL, and asks whether this is the correct dose. L.M.'s current weight is 4.5 kg and the therapeutic range of acetaminophen dosage is 10 to 15 mg/kg q4-6 h. Which of these statements would be your best response?
   a. "This is a safe amount; you should continue to give that dose every 4 hours."
   b. "You can continue to give her that amount; you can give her a dose every 2 hours."
   c. "You should give 1.4 to 2.1 mL every 4 to 6 hours based on her current weight."
   d. "Tylenol should not be given to a child her age."

CASE STUDY OUTCOME

L.M. returns for her postoperative checkup 2 weeks later and is playful and alert. The neurologist will continue to monitor her closely with follow-up visits.

12 Pediatric Disorders

Case Study **123**

Name _____ Class/Group _____ Date _____

Group Members _____

▶ **Scenario**

The charge nurse tells you that you will be admitting a 1-hour-old infant, Baby Girl R., to the neonatal intensive care unit (NICU) with a myelomeningocele that was discovered in utero. Her aunt and father arrive shortly after her admission while the mother remains at the local medical center recovering from a cesarean delivery.

1. What is the rationale for doing a cesarean delivery for babies with myelomeningocele?

CASE STUDY PROGRESS

While you are getting vital signs, the father tells you that he has been trying to research myelomeningocele on the Internet, but he is still confused, especially about the difference between myelomeningocele and meningocele.

2. Using lay terms, what would you tell the father about the pathophysiology of myelomeningocele? What is the difference between myelomeningocele and meningocele?

3. After your discussion with the family, which of the father's statements would indicate a need for more teaching?
   a. "My baby's malformation can also be referred to as *spina bifida cystica.*"
   b. "My baby will probably not require surgery until she is a year old."
   c. "My baby will need to lie on her stomach in her incubator."
   d. "I need to wash my hands carefully to prevent spread of germs."

12 Pediatric Disorders

4. The father asks questions about the infant's condition but does not look at his newborn. Which of these statements are correct? Select all that apply.
   a. Most new fathers are not interested in looking at their newborns.
   b. Even though the meningomyelocele was diagnosed in utero, seeing the congenital anomaly or physical defect on his infant is very difficult.
   c. People grieve for the loss of a "normal newborn" differently.
   d. This is an abnormal reaction for a parent of a child born with a very visible physical defect.
   e. It is apparent that he does not care about his newborn's condition.

CASE STUDY PROGRESS

R. is in an open warmer. You document the information shown in the chart.

Chart View

Admission Data

Blood pressure	67/33 mm Hg
Pulse	173 beats/min
Respirations	52 breaths/min
Axillary temperature	37.1° C (98.8° F)
Spo$_2$	95%
Weight	3.5 kg
Frontal occipital circumference (FOC)	37 cm

5. Which of the these assessment and monitoring data are abnormal for a 1-hour-old infant? Select all that apply.
   a. Fontanelles soft and flat
   b. Pupils 2 cm, brisk reaction
   c. No reaction when pulse oximeter is placed on right foot
   d. Sleepy, squirms and fusses during pupil check
   e. Breath sounds clear
   f. Pulses 2+ and capillary refill time less than 2 to 3 seconds
   g. Bilateral clubfeet
   h. Sac in sacral region covered with sterile gauze that is moistened with saline
   i. Acrocyanosis

6. You are carefully assessing the sutures and fontanelles. True or False? The posterior fontanel is joined by the temporal and parietal bones.

7. Explain the rationale for each of the orders in the table.

Orders	Rationale
1. Open warmer	
2. Place in prone position	
3. Use appropriate positioning aids such as diaper rolls, pads, pressure-reducing mattress	
4. Maintain sterile gauze with normal saline (NS) to sac and monitor q2-4 h	
5. Place peripheral IV with $D_{10}W$ at 15 mL/hr	
6. Administer IV antibiotics as ordered.	
7. NPO	
8. Keep clean padding under diaper area; check frequently	
9. Assess for urine output every 2 to 4 hours; if none, assess for retention	
10. Clean intermittent catheterization (CIC) as needed	
11. Measure FOC every shift	
12. Physical therapy (PT) consultation	
13. Orthopedic consultation	
14. Maintain latex free environment	

CASE STUDY PROGRESS

The next day Baby Girl R. is taken to the operating room. The anesthesiologist orders cefazolin (Ancef) 140 mg IV to be given 30 minutes before the surgery begins.

8. You add 10 mL of sterile water to the 1-g vial for a concentration of 100 mg/1 mL. Calculate how many milliliters you will draw up for this dose. Shade in the dose on the syringe.

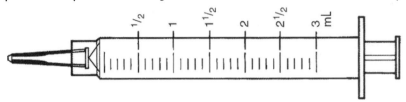

CASE STUDY PROGRESS

Postoperatively, the postanesthesia care unit (PACU) nurse tells you Baby Girl R.. did well during surgery and is ready to return to your unit. When she arrives, you and the nursing assistive personnel start putting on the monitors. R.'s father is present, and he asks you to give the baby some pain medication. The open warmer starts alarming because the infant's skin temperature is reading 35° C (95° F). You look to see whether the temperature probe has fallen off. You see that it is still on, but you notice that the suture from surgery is no longer intact. The oxygen monitor reads 71% saturation with an accurate waveform, and the pulse oximeter probe is correctly placed. The respiratory rate is 25 breaths/min and heart rate is 102 beats/min.

9. Which of the issues should you address first? Give rationale.

CASE STUDY PROGRESS

Baby Girl R.'s condition stabilizes. Her temperature is 36.7° C (98.1° F) per skin probe. Respiratory rate and heart rate improve and her Spo_2 is 98% on ¼ L of oxygen per minute via nasal cannula. The surgeon is at the bedside and opts to return her to the OR for revision of the incision.

Two nights later, you are caring for Baby Girl R.. In report, you hear that the parents really want to hold their baby, but they have not yet done so because they are afraid of causing the suture to open again. They are currently at the bedside, and the infant is due for a feeding.

10. How can you help the parents become comfortable with holding their baby?

11. When you take the bottle into the room, you notice a growth chart next to the bed tracking the FOC measurement at least once per shift. Baby Girl R.'s FOC has increased to 38.5 cm. Using the appropriate CDC growth chart (www.cdc.gov/growthcharts/data/who/grchrt_girls_24hdcirc-l4w_9210.pdf), is the following statement true or false? The FOC is close to the 95th percentile and can be monitored less frequently because this is a normal finding. (Explain your answer)

CASE STUDY PROGRESS

Discharge teaching is an essential part of Baby Girl R.'s care. Teaching and preparation of the family have been done since the diagnosis in utero and are ongoing issues.

12. Which of these topics would be important to include in discharge teaching for Baby Girl R.? Select all that apply.
   a. Specialized feeding techniques
   b. Positioning
   c. Appropriate stimulation such as sitting in an infant seat or swing
   d. Skin care and wound care
   e. Maintenance of the Foley catheter
   f. Range-of-motion (ROM) exercises as appropriate per PT
   g. Comfort measures and pain control
   h. Signs and symptoms of when to call the physician
   i. Importance of multidisciplinary follow-up

CASE STUDY OUTCOME

Baby Girl R. is followed closely in the Level 2 nursery/NICU. She stabilizes and is able to be discharged to home in 2 weeks with intensive discharge teaching and close multidisciplinary follow-up.

12 Pediatric Disorders

Case Study **124**

Name _____   Class/Group _____   Date _____

Group Members _____

▶ **Scenario**

R.O. is a 12-year-old girl who lives with her family on a farm in a rural community. R.O. has four siblings who have recently been ill with stomach pains, vomiting, diarrhea, and fever. They were seen by their primary care provider (PCP) and diagnosed with viral gastroenteritis. A week later, R.O. woke up at 0200 crying and telling her mother that her stomach "hurts really bad!" She had an elevated temperature of 37.9° C (100.2° F). R.O. began to vomit over the next few hours, so her parents took her to the local emergency department (ED). R.O.'s vital signs, complete blood count, and complete metabolic panel were normal, so she was hydrated with IV fluids and discharged to home with instructions for her parents to call their PCP or to return to the ED if her condition did not improve or if it worsened. Over the next 2 days, R.O.'s abdominal pain localized to the right lower quadrant, she refused to eat, and she had slight diarrhea. On the third day, she began to have more severe abdominal pain, increased vomiting, and fever that did not respond to acetaminophen. R.O. has returned to the ED. Her VS are 128/78, 130, 28, 39.5° C (103.1° F). R.O. is guarding her lower abdomen, prefers to lie on her side with her legs flexed, and is crying. IV access is established, and morphine sulfate 2 mg IV is administered for pain. An abdominal CT scan confirms a diagnosis of appendicitis. R.O.'s white blood count is 12,000 mm³.

1. Which of the following are common clinical manifestations of appendicitis? Select all that apply.
   a. Diarrhea
   b. Vomiting
   c. Left lower quadrant abdominal pain
   d. Constipation
   e. Arthralgia
   f. Diffuse rash
   g. Fever

2. Discuss why R.O.'s presenting clinical manifestations make diagnosis more difficult. Identify two other possible diagnoses.

CASE STUDY PROGRESS

The abdominal CT scan confirms that R.O. has appendicitis. The ED physician has written orders.

3. Note whether the orders are appropriate or inappropriate and give rationale.

Chart View

Emergency Department (ED) Orders

    a. Make patient NPO

    b. Place a peripheral IV and begin D5½NS at 80 mL/hr

    c. Administer Fleet Enema now to rule out impaction

    d. Administer morphine sulfate 2 mg IV q2h for pain

    e. Obtain surgical consent from patient

    f. Administer cefotaxime (Claforan) IVPB, at 150 mg/kg/day q6h

4. R.O.'s weight is 42 kg, and her height is 155 cm. Calculate her maintenance fluid needs and discuss how these will be met.

5. R.O.'s parents give informed consent, and R.O. assents to the surgery after the procedure is explained to her. Why is it important for R.O. to provide her assent for the procedure?

6. What should be included in the preoperative teaching for R.O. and her parents?

CASE STUDY PROGRESS

R.O. undergoes an appendectomy; the appendix has ruptured. The peritoneum is inflamed and abscesses are seen near the colon and small intestine. R.O. is admitted to the surgical unit; she is NPO, has a nasogastric tube (NGT), Foley catheter, IV line, abdominal dressing, and a Penrose drain.

7. Identify the priority nursing considerations. Select all that apply.
    a. Reduced bowel function
    b. Pain
    c. Skin integrity changes
    d. Cardiac output changes
    e. Changed family processes
    f. Potential hypothermia
    g. Potential fluid and electrolyte imbalance

CASE STUDY PROGRESS

On postoperative day 2, R.O. continues to improve and is tolerating ice chips. Breath sounds are clear, and she is performing her pulmonary hygiene. NGT has minimal drainage. The Foley catheter and Penrose drain have been removed, and her urine output is adequate. Her IV line is saline locked. The incision is well approximated with no drainage or redness. Her pain is 4 to 6 out of 10 with pain medication every 4 hours.

Later that evening your assessment shows that R.O. is pale and listless; bowel sounds are absent; abdomen is distended and tender to the touch; the NGT is draining an increased amount of dark, greenish black fluid. Her lung sounds are moist bilaterally, and her temperature has spiked to 40.2° C (104.4° F), O_2 saturation is 97% on room air. She rates her pain at 10 out of 10 and is having difficulty taking deep breaths because of the pain, which she says "hurts over my whole stomach."

8. What actions would you take?

9. Using SBAR, what would you communicate to the surgeon?

12 Pediatric Disorders

10. What will you consider as part of your nursing management of R.O.'s pain?

CASE STUDY PROGRESS

The surgeon assesses R.O. and orders an immediate return to the operating room. R.O. returns to surgery, where she has lysis of adhesions, removal of necrotic bowel, and drainage of an abscess. The surgeon has left her abdominal wound open and has ordered wound packing changes twice daily and abdominal irrigation with normal saline. R.O. cries and becomes agitated when you go to perform the procedure.

11. Which of the following pain and coping concepts would you question as you assist R.O to prepare for the procedure?
    a. R. may fear loss of control during the dressing change.
    b. R. may fear separation from family members during painful experiences.
    c. R. is concerned about privacy during the dressing change.
    d. Prior coping strategies can be used to prepare for the dressing change.

12. In anticipation of R.O.'s discharge, identify expected outcomes that must be achieved before discharge from the hospital.

CASE STUDY PROGRESS

After a week, R.O. continues to meet expected outcomes, with her wound healing well. Her discharge to home is planned for the next day. You provide discharge teaching to R.O. and her parents.

13. Which of these statements would indicate that more teaching is required?
    a. "We need to return if R.O. begins vomiting again or develops a fever."
    b. "R.O. should wait 1 week before returning to her gymnastics program."
    c. "We will keep the incision clean and call if we see redness or drainage."
    d. "R.O. can advance her diet to the regular foods that she likes to eat."

CASE STUDY OUTCOME

R.O. is discharged to home with her parents and has an uneventful recovery. She is scheduled for a follow-up visit with the surgeon in 2 weeks.

Case Study 125

Name _____   Class/Group _____   Date _____

Group Members _____

▶ Scenario

T.M. is a 3-year-old boy with cerebral palsy (CP) who has been admitted to your unit. He is scheduled for surgery tomorrow morning for a femoral osteotomy and tendon lengthening to stabilize hip joints and to help reduce spasticity. You are orienting the parents to the unit and have a nursing student assisting you.

1. After getting the family settled, you return to the nurses' station and the nursing student asks you to explain what CP is and what might have caused it in this patient. How would you answer the student's question?

2. The nursing student asks what the family might have noticed that would indicate CP in T.M. when he was a baby. Which of these findings will you include in your discussion with the student? Select all that apply, and state your rationale.
   a. Head lag at 5 months
   b. Ability to sit unassisted at 7 months
   c. Positive Moro (startle) reflex at 2 months
   d. Leg scissoring
   e. Right hand preference at 12 months
   f. Use of pincer grasp at 9 months
   g. Increased irritability

CASE STUDY PROGRESS

You and the nursing student finish a health history with the family and determine that T.M. has impaired vision corrected with glasses, a speech impairment, and a seizure disorder and has had poor weight gain and feeding issues since birth. He has a skin-level feeding device (Mic-Key button) and receives supplemental tube feedings in addition to oral intake. He is not able to ambulate without braces and wears ankle-foot orthotics. He receives physical, occupational, and speech therapy on an outpatient basis. T.M. is verbal and able to answer questions with simple phrases and responds to commands. T.M. weighs 12 kg.

3. The admitting physician orders the following. Explain the rationale for each order.

Chart View

Admission Orders

    Baclofen (Lioresal) 5 mg every 8 hours PO
    Diazepam (Valium) 2 mg twice a day PO
    Lamotrigine (Lamictal) 60 mg twice a day PO
    Diet as tolerated; NPO for solids and hold tube feedings at midnight; clear fluids until 4 AM
    Place IV on admission and begin D5½NS at 45 mL/hr
    VS every 4 hours

---

4. Calculate T.M.'s maintenance fluid requirements. Do the IV fluids ordered meet this requirement? Show your work.

5. You ask T.M.'s mother about his history of seizures. She states that he has not had seizures since his medication doses were adjusted several months ago. With this knowledge, which of the admission orders would you question?

T.M. returns to your unit the next afternoon from the postanesthesia care unit (PACU). He is in a bilateral spica cast, has a Foley catheter, and has a family-controlled patient-controlled analgesia (PCA) device for pain control. You assess T.M. and chart the following findings.

Chart View

Postoperative Assessment

Neurologic	Awake and alert, verbalizes and responds to commands. Periods of agitation and restlessness.
Respiratory	RR 25 breaths/min. Bilateral breath sounds, equal, clear, good air exchange. O_2 saturation 98% on room air.
Cardiovascular (CV)	Peripheral IV line to right forearm infusing D5 ½ normal saline (NS) at 45 mL/hr. HR 85 beats/min. Temperature 36.8° C (98.2° F) (axillary).
Gastrointestinal (GI)	Positive bowel sounds; taking sips of juice PO; Mic-Key button to abdomen clamped. Mic-Key site clean, no signs of breakdown.
Genitourinary (GU)	8 French Foley catheter intact and secured, draining yellow clear urine to collection bag. Diaper to spica cast opening.
Neuromuscular	Bilateral spica cast to legs with hip abductor bar intact. Toes warm to touch; able to move, unable to palpate pedal pulses. Cap refill less than 2 seconds.
Pain	T.M. occasionally whines and frowns but is comforted by parents. PCA is Y-connected to IV and infusing morphine at 0.01 mg/kg continuous and 0.015 mg/kg PCA with 15-minute lockout.
Psychosocial	Parents at bedside active in care.

6. What are your top five priorities while providing nursing care to T.M. postoperatively? How will you address these areas?

7. Score T.M. on the FLACC pain scale. Why is the FLACC scale an appropriate tool?

Category	Score		
	0	**1**	**2**
Face	No particular expression or smile	Occasional grimace or frown, withdrawn, disinterested	Frequent-to-constant quivering chin, clenched jaw
Legs	Normal position or relaxed	Uneasy, restless, tense	Kicking, or legs drawn up
Activity	Lying quietly, normal position, moves easily	Squirming, shifting back and forth, tense	Arched, rigid, or jerking
Cry	No cry (awake or asleep)	Moans or whimpers, occasional complaint	Crying steadily, screams or sobs, or frequent complaints
Consolability	Content, relaxed	Reassured by occasional touching, hugging, or being talked to, distractible	Difficult to console or comfort

Each of the five categories–(F) Face, (L) Legs, (A) Activity, (C) Cry, (C) Consolability–
is scored from 0-2, which results in a total score between 0 and 10.

8. Which of these nonpharmacologic interventions would be age appropriate for T.M.? Select all that apply.
    a. Encourage "positive self-talk"—statements such as, "I will feel better when the cast comes off."
    b. Offer a favorite DVD or video.
    c. Use bubbles to "blow the hurt away."
    d. Educate T.M. on pain and relationship to the procedure.
    e. Read a favorite book.
    f. Use guided imagery.

CASE STUDY PROGRESS

T.M.'s condition is stable throughout the day, and the physician writes the following orders:
    Patient can PO ad lib. Resume home schedule of 520 mL PediaSure via G-tube from 10 PM to 6 AM. Remove Foley catheter.

9. Place the steps for setting up a feeding with a Mic-Key button in the correct order. Calculate the hourly rate at which you will set the pump.
    1. Clean the skin-level device with alcohol
    2. Wash hands and apply gloves
    3. Place the correct amount of PediaSure in the feed bag with overfill for priming
    4. Start the feeding
    5. Attach the feeding bag to the pump and continue with "auto prime"
    6. Attach tubing to patient

10. The physician orders the Foley catheter discontinued. What nursing interventions and teaching will you include for T.M. and his family as you implement this order?.

T.M.'s condition continues to improve, and you provide discharge education. T.M.'s mother asks how she will care for his cast when he gets home. You discuss with her the care of a synthetic spica cast.

11. Which of these statements by T.M.'s mother would indicate that further education is needed? Select all that apply.
    a. "I need to check the toes on his feet several times a day for the first week or so to see if they are warm and he is able to wiggle them."
    b. "I need to keep his feet elevated when I get him home."
    c. "It is okay if I give him a tub bath. Because it is a synthetic cast, I can dry it with a blow dryer."
    d. "Because T. uses pull-up diapers, I will need to use plastic tape to protect the cast opening."
    e. "If he has an itch, it is okay to use a knitting needle to scratch under the cast."

12. What additional information should be included in your discharge teaching?

13. The nursing assistive personnel offers to review the hospital "home medication" form with Mrs. M to review prior medications taken at home. True or False: This is an appropriate delegation of tasks. Explain your answer.

T.M.'s parents verbalize understanding of the discharge instructions, and T.M. is discharged to home with a wheelchair and a home-health follow-up. He will return to the orthopedic surgeon in 2 weeks.

12 Pediatric Disorders

Case Study **126**

Name _____ Class/Group _____ Date _____

Group Members _____

▶ **Scenario**

Three-week-old J.T. and her parents arrive at the cardiac cath lab for her cardiac catheterization. She was born at term with Down syndrome and her pediatrician is concerned because of lack of weight gain and poor feeding. You are getting her and her parents prepared for the procedure.

1. As you obtain her history and take vital signs, which statements or findings would be concerning and suggestive of heart failure (HF)? Select all that apply.
   a. "J. takes 30 to 40 minutes to take 2 to 3 ounces of formula."
   b. Rectal temperature: 36.6° C
   c. "J. gets damp and sweaty when she feeds."
   d. Heart rate: 195 at rest
   e. Peripheral pulses +3
   f. "J. seems to have fewer wet diapers than when we brought her home from the hospital."

2. You are preparing J.T.'s parents for the procedure. Describe the points you would address in your teaching.

CASE STUDY PROGRESS

After the catheterization, J.T. returns to the unit in a crib. The orders shown in the chart have been written.

12 Pediatric Disorders

Chart View

Physician's Orders

Daily weights: Current weight 4 kg

Strict intake and output

O_2 per nasal cannula as needed to maintain O_2 saturation greater than 93%

VS every 15 minutes × 4, then every 1 hour × 4, then every 4 hours

Digoxin (Lanoxin) 60 mcg PO now, then 20 mcg PO every 12 hours

Furosemide (Lasix) 4 mg PO now, then 4 mg PO every 12 hours

3. What will you document in your postprocedure assessment? Include rationale.

4. You are reviewing J.T.'s medications. J.T's mother states the following rationale for starting J.T. on digoxin (Lanoxin): "I need to give this to J. to decrease her blood pressure so her heart doesn't have to work so hard." Is this true or false? Explain your answer.

5. You have a student nurse working with you, and the student asks why the first ordered dose is high. What would be a possible explanation for this?

6. The student nurse asks whether there are any precautions to observe when giving digoxin to an infant. Describe medication safety precautions that should be observed when giving this medication.

You administer the ordered medication and proceed with your assessment.

7. Which of these are possible complications to monitor for after a cardiac catheterization? Select all that apply.
   a. Hemorrhage
   b. Hematoma
   c. Hyperglycemia
   d. Dysrhythmia
   e. Decreased pulse in unaffected leg
   f. Vasospasm

 8. You are preparing to administer J.T.'s furosemide. Your drug reference gives the following therapeutic range: 0.5 to 1 mg/kg/dose every 8 to 24 hours. Is the ordered dose of 4 mg a safe dose for J.T?

You note the following serum metabolic panel results for J.T.

Chart View

Laboratory Results

Glucose	85 mg/dL
Calcium	9.1 mg/dL
Sodium	142 mEq/L
Potassium	3.3 mEq/L
Chloride	101 mEq/L

9. Which laboratory finding would concern you, and why?

12 Pediatric Disorders

10. The cardiologist is present and tells J.T.'s parents that J.T. has a ventricular septal defect (VSD). On the diagram, circle the area affected by this defect.

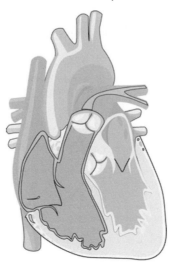

11. True or False: This defect would create decreased pulmonary flow. Explain your answer.

CASE STUDY PROGRESS

The cardiologist consults with the family, and it is decided that J.T. will be discharged to home the following day with medications and close monitoring. J.T. will return in several months for surgical repair of the VSD.

12. You begin your discharge teaching. Describe the information you will include in teaching.

12 Pediatric Disorders

Case Study **127**

Name _____   Class/Group _____   Date _____

Group Members _____

▶ **Scenario**

Three-year-old C.E. is admitted to the emergency department (ED) fast track clinic. Her mother tells the nurse that C.E. has had a low-grade fever for 2 days and is complaining of ear pain and a sore throat. C.E.'s mother states that C.E.'s appetite has been "off," but she has been drinking and using the bathroom as usual. As you get C.E. settled in the exam room, you suspect C.E may have otitis media (OM).

1. Place an arrow where you suspect fluid would be found.

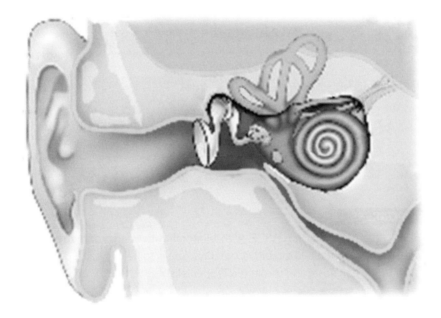

2. What routine information regarding risk factors for OM would you want to obtain from C.'s mother?

3. C.'s mother asks, "Why does C. keep getting ear infections? Is there something I should do?" Explain the etiology of ear infections.

12 Pediatric Disorders

CASE STUDY PROGRESS

You continue to obtain a history from C.'s mother and learn C.E. has had "ear problems" and throat infections since she was a baby. She is in day care each weekday, the father smokes outside of the house, and there is a family history of seasonal allergies. C.E. is allergic to penicillin. Her weight is 14 kg.

4. Describe what you will include in your physical examination with rationales.

CASE STUDY PROGRESS

The primary care provider (PCP) diagnoses C.E. with bilateral otitis media and strep pharyngitis. C.E. is given a prescription for Augmentin 600 mg bid PO × 7 days. She is to be discharged to home with instructions to follow-up with the ear, nose, and throat (ENT) specialist.

5. You review the orders before completing discharge teaching. What is your first action?

CASE STUDY PROGRESS

C.'s mother is given a new prescription for azithromycin (Zithromax) PO 160 mg daily × 5 days. Azithromycin is dispensed as 200 mg/5 mL.

6. Calculate the dose for C.'s mother to administer to C.E., and mark it on the oral syringe below.

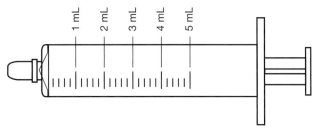

7. You are providing C.'s mother with information on medication administration. Which of these statements by C.'s mother indicates need for further teaching? Select all that apply.
   a. "I will place the correct amount of antibiotic in the ear canal once a day."
   b. "I will monitor for vomiting, diarrhea, or stomachaches because this might be a side effect of the medication."
   c. "If C. refuses to take her medication, I will tell her it tastes like the candy we get at the movies."
   d. "This medicine can be given with or without food."
   e. "I don't have to finish the medication if she feels better after a few days."

8. C.'s mother asks when C. can return to day care. Which of these statements is your best response?
   a. "She should be able to return in about a week."
   b. "She can return 24 hours after her last documented normal temperature."
   c. "She can return 24 hours after she starts her antibiotics and is free of fever."
   d. "She can return 48 hours after her last documented normal temperature."

12 Pediatric Disorders

CASE STUDY PROGRESS

C.'s mother takes C.E. to an ENT specialist. It is determined that her enlarged tonsils might be contributing to the frequent throat and ear infections, and a tonsillectomy and adenoidectomy (T&A) is scheduled. She is admitted postoperatively for 24-hour observation. After the surgery, the postoperative nurse receives C.E. in the short-stay unit from the postanesthesia care unit (PACU). C.E. is awake and alert, bilateral breath sounds are clear, and her oxygen saturation is 98% on room air. She has tolerated sips of clear fluids, and her parents are with her.

9. Which of these orders would you expect to see in her postoperative orders? Select all that apply, and discuss the rationales for each of your choices.
   a. Vital signs q4h
   b. Clear liquids; advance to regular toddler diet
   c. Methylprednisolone (Solu-Medrol) 2.3 mg IV q8h × 3 doses
   d. Acetaminophen (Tylenol) 210 mg (15 mg/kg) PO q4h prn for pain
   e. Home prescription for amoxicillin (Amoxil) 120 mg PO q8h
   f. Maintain peripheral IV with $D_5\frac{1}{2}NS$ at 50 mL/hr; saline lock when taking PO well
   g. Aggressively gargle and swish with water after eating or drinking

10. State at least two nursing interventions for each of these commonly encountered nursing problems during the postoperative phase of care.
    a. Airway
    b. Pain
    c. Fluid and electrolyte balance
    d. Bleeding risk

11. C. is able to verbalize discomfort to you and her mother. Which of these pain rating scales would be most appropriate?
     a. 1-10 scale
     b. Neonatal Infant Pain Scale (NIPS)
     c. Face, Legs, Activity, Cry, Consolability (FLACC) scale
     d. Oucher

 12. You are reviewing discharge instructions with C.'s mother She asks, "How would I know if we need to come back?" Discuss common findings and when C.'s mother would need to seek immediate medical attention for C.E.

CASE STUDY OUTCOME

C.'s mother indicates an understanding of discharge instructions and follow-up care. C.E. continues to take oral fluids well and meets discharge criteria and is discharged to home to follow up with the ENT physician in 2 weeks.

12 Pediatric Disorders

Maternal and Obstetric Care

Case Study 128

Name _____ Class/Group _____ Date _____

Group Members _____

▶ **Scenario**

T.N. delivered a healthy male infant 2 hours ago. She had a midline episiotomy. This is her sixth pregnancy. Before this delivery, she was para 4014. She had an epidural block for her labor and delivery. She is now admitted to the postpartum unit.

1. What is important to note in the initial assessment?

2. You find a boggy fundus during your assessment. What corrective measures can be instituted?

3. The patient complains of pain and discomfort in her perineal area. How will you respond?

4. The nurse reviews the hospital security guidelines with T.N. The nurse points out that her baby has a special identification bracelet that matches a bracelet worn by T.N., and reviews other security procedures. Which statement by T.N. indicates a need for more teaching?
   a. "If I have a question about someone's identity, I can ask about it."
   b. "If someone comes to take my baby for an examination, that person will carry my baby to the examination room."
   c. "Nurses on this unit all wear the same purple uniforms."
   d. "Each staff member who takes my baby somewhere will have a picture identification badge."

5. An hour after admission, you recheck T.N.'s perineal pad and find that there is a very small amount of drainage on the pad. What will you do next?
   a. Ask T.N. to change her perineal pad
   b. Check her perineal pad again in 1 hour
   c. Check the pad underneath T.N.'s buttocks
   d. Document the findings in T.N.'s medical record

6. That evening, the nursing assistive personnel assesses T.N.'s vital signs. Which vital signs would be of concern at this time?

Chart View

Vital Signs

Temperature	99.9° F (37.7° C) oral
Pulse rate	120 beats/min
Blood pressure	100/50 mm Hg
Respiratory rate	16 breaths/min

7. What will you do next?

8. After your prompt intervention, you need to document what happened. Write an example of a documentation entry describing this event.

9. Two hours later, you perform another perineal pad check and note the findings in the diagram. How will you describe the amount of drainage in your note?

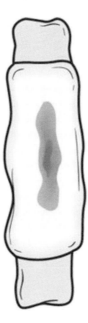

    a. Scant
    b. Light
    c. Moderate
    d. Heavy

10. T.N.'s condition is stable and you prepare to provide patient teaching. What patient teaching is vital after delivery?

13 Maternal and Obstetric Care

11. T.N. tells you she must go back to work in 6 weeks and is not sure she can continue breastfeeding. What options are available to her?

CASE STUDY OUTCOME

T.N. is discharged to home and plans to consult a lactation specialist before returning to work.

Case Study 129

Name _____   Class/Group _____   Date _____

Group Members _____

▶ Scenario

P.M. comes to the obstetric (OB) clinic because she has missed two menstrual periods and thinks she might be pregnant. She states she is nauseated, especially in the morning, so she completed a home pregnancy test and the result was positive. As the intake nurse in the clinic, you are responsible for gathering information before she sees the physician.

1. What are the two most important questions to ask to determine possible pregnancy?

2. You ask whether she has ever been pregnant, and she tells you she has never been pregnant. How would you record this information?

3. What additional information would be needed to complete the TPAL record?

4. It is important to complete the intake interview. What categories will you address with P.M.?

CASE STUDY PROGRESS

According to the clinic protocol, you obtain the following for her prenatal record: complete blood count, blood type with Rh factor, urine for urinalysis (protein, glucose, blood), vital signs, height, and weight. Next, the nurse-midwife does a physical examination, including a pelvic examination and confirms that

P.M. is pregnant. P.M. has a gynecoid pelvis by measurement, and the fetus is at approximately 6 weeks' gestation.

Chart View

Vital Signs

Blood pressure	116/74 mm Hg
Heart rate	88 beats/min
Respiratory rate	16 breaths/min
Temperature	98.9° F (37.2° C)

---

5. Do any of these vital signs cause concern? What should you do?

6. P.M. tells you that the date of her last menstrual period (LMP) was February 2. How would you calculate her due date? What is her due date?

7. What is the significance of a gynecoid pelvis?

8. What specimens are important to obtain when the pelvic examination is done?

CASE STUDY PROGRESS

Nursing interventions focus on monitoring the woman and fetus for growth and development; detecting potential complications; and teaching P.M. about nutrition, how to deal with common discomforts of pregnancy, and activities of self-care.

9. A psychological assessment is done to determine P.M.'s feelings and attitudes regarding her pregnancy. How do attitudes, beliefs, and feelings affect pregnancy?

10. P.M. asks you whether there are any foods that she should avoid while pregnant. She lists some of her favorite foods. Which foods, if any, should she avoid eating while she is pregnant? Select all that apply.
   a. Hot dogs
   b. Sushi
   c. Yogurt
   d. Deli meat
   e. Cheddar cheese

11. As the nurse, you know that assessment and teaching are vital in the prenatal period to ensure a positive outcome. What information is important to include at every visit and at specific times during the pregnancy?

13 Maternal and Obstetric Care

12. After her examination, P.M. states that she is worried because her sister had an ectopic pregnancy and had to have surgery. She asks you, "What are the signs of an ectopic pregnancy?" Which of these are correct? Select all that apply.
    a. Fullness and tenderness in her abdomen, near the ovaries
    b. Pain, either unilateral, bilateral, or diffuse over the abdomen
    c. Nausea
    d. Dark red or brown vaginal bleeding
    e. Increased fatigue

13. P.M. asks the nurse about what should be reported to her doctor. List at least six of the danger signs during pregnancy.

14. Changes in the body caused by pregnancy include relaxation of joints, alteration to center of gravity, faintness, and discomforts. These changes can lead to problems with coordination and balance. In teaching P.M. about safety during pregnancy, what will you include in your teaching?

15. P.M. asks, "Is a vaginal examination done at every visit?" Select the best response and explain your answer.
    a. "Yes, an examination is done with each visit because it allows the examiner to note any possible infections that may be developing."
    b. "Yes, an examination is done with each visit because it offers vital information about the status of the pregnancy."
    c. "No, a vaginal examination will not be done again until you go into labor."
    d. "No, vaginal examinations are not routinely done until the final weeks of your pregnancy."

CASE STUDY OUTCOME

P.M. makes an appointment for her next checkup. You tell her that an ultrasound may be done at about 8 to 12 weeks' gestation to check fetal growth.

13 Maternal and Obstetric Care

Case Study **130**

Name _____   Class/Group _____   Date _____

Group Members _____

▶ Scenario

You are the charge nurse working in labor and delivery at a local hospital. D.H. comes to the unit having contractions and feeling somewhat uncomfortable. You take her to the intake room to provide privacy, have her change into a gown, and ask her three initial questions to determine your next course of action—that is, whether to do a vaginal examination or to continue asking her more questions.

1. What three initial questions will you ask, and why?

2. D.H. has contractions 2 to 3 minutes apart and lasting 45 seconds. It is her third pregnancy (gravida 3, para 2002). Her bag of waters is intact at this time. You determine that it is appropriate to ask for further information before a vaginal examination is done. What information do you need?

3. What assessment should you make to gain further information from D.H.?

13 Maternal and Obstetric Care

4. On examination, D.H. is 80% effaced and 4 cm dilated. The fetal heart rate (FHR) is 150 beats/min and regular. She is admitted to a labor and delivery room on the unit. What nursing measures should be done at this time?

5. As part of your assessment, you review the fetal heart strip pictured here. What will you do?

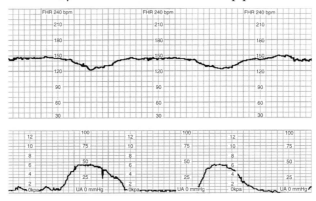

6. List the stages of labor. D.H. is in what stage of labor?

7. D.H. states that she is feeling discomfort and asks you whether there is alternative therapy available before taking medication. List at least four alternative methods to assist D.H. with controlling her discomfort.

8. As you assess both D.H. and the fetus during the active stage of labor, you will look for abnormalities. Which of these are potential abnormalities during labor? Select all that apply.
   a. Unusual bleeding
   b. Brown or greenish amniotic fluid
   c. Contractions that last 40 to 70 seconds
   d. Sudden, severe pain
   e. Increased maternal fatigue

CASE STUDY PROGRESS

Although D.H. continues to use alternative therapies for discomfort, she asks for pain medication and receives a dose of meperidine (Demerol). Three hours later, D.H. is lying on her back, and during contractions you notice a few late decelerations of the FHR. You stay with D.H. to monitor her and her fetus and immediately call for someone to notify the primary care provider.

9. Put these actions in order of priority:
_____ a. Discontinue the oxytocin infusion.
_____ b. Turn D.H. onto her left side and elevate her legs.
_____ c. Increase the rate of the maintenance IV fluids.
_____ d. Administer oxygen at 8 to 10 L/min by facemask.

10. Decelerations occur in an early, variable, or late pattern. What is the significance of these patterns? State what the nurse should do for each type.

11. As you monitor D.H., you observe for prolapse of the umbilical cord. Describe what this is and what can happen to the fetus if this occurs.

12. What would be done if you were to note that D.H. has a prolapsed cord?

629

CASE STUDY PROGRESS

The decelerations stop, and the remainder of the labor is uneventful; D.H. has an episiotomy to allow more room for the infant to emerge and delivers a male infant.

13. What is involved in the immediate care of the newborn?

14. As you assess the newborn, you observe for central nervous system (CNS) depressant effects that might result because the mother received an opioid during labor. What drug would be helpful to reverse signs of CNS depression in the infant?
    a. Carbamazepine (Tegretol)
    b. Nalbuphine (Nubain)
    c. Midazolam (Versed)
    d. Naloxone (Narcan)

15. D.H. has her episiotomy repaired and the placenta delivered. What are the signs that the placenta has released from the uterine wall?

16. What assessments are important for D.H. after delivery?

CASE STUDY OUTCOME

D.H. and her newborn baby boy are taken to the maternity unit where she begins to breastfeed him.

13 Maternal and Obstetric Care

Case Study **131**

Name _____ Class/Group _____ Date _____

Group Members _____

▶ **Scenario**

Baby H. was just born in a hospital that provides single-room maternity care (SRMC). SRMC allows the infant to remain with the parents after birth. H.'s mother was in labor for 12 hours and gave birth vaginally. Baby H. is the first baby born to these parents. The nurse will complete the physical assessment and observe for physiologic changes in the infant's transition from intrauterine to extrauterine life.

1. Name the three phases that occur during this transition period and state an approximate time frame for each.

2. What care is specific to the first period of reactivity?

3. The sleep phase and second reactive phase might occur in the SRMC or in the nursery. Identify eight assessments or tasks that the nurse needs to do during the transitional care period.

13 Maternal and Obstetric Care

4. You are preparing to give the injection of vitamin K (AquaMEPHYTON). The order is to give 0.5 mg subcutaneously on arrival in the nursery. The medication comes in a solution of 1 mg/0.5 mL. Calculate how much medication you will draw up into the syringe.

5. Erythromycin ointment is instilled in both eyes to prevent which of these infections?
   a. Chlamydia
   b. Herpes simplex virus infection
   c. Gonorrhea
   d. Human papillomavirus (HPV) infection

6. Once the transitional care and documentation are completed, the infant might be transferred to the normal newborn nursery if the hospital does not use SRMC. The newborn nursery nurse is responsible for what ongoing care of the newborn infant?

13 Maternal and Obstetric Care

7. The laboratory performs a Coombs test on Baby H. What is the purpose of the Coombs test?
   a. It is done to identify the infant's blood type.
   b. It tests for damage to the red blood cells (RBCs) from maternal antibodies.
   c. It checks the RBCs for anemia.
   d. It is a test for immunity to the hepatitis virus.

8. True or False: A phenylketonuria (PKU) blood test can be done any time before an infant is discharged to home. If false, explain your rationale.

CASE STUDY PROGRESS

Baby H.'s mother has decided to breastfeed her infant. She asks for assistance.

9. Identify six important points to include in your teaching plan.

10. H.'s mother calls you to tell you that her baby seems too sleepy and is not feeding well. What will your next action be?

CASE STUDY PROGRESS

You are meeting with Baby H.'s mother to review discharge instructions. She has many questions.

11. Baby H.'s mother asks you about cord care and circumcision care for her infant. What will you tell her?

12. Baby H.'s mother asks you how she can keep her infant from catching a cold or some other type of infection. What is the most important measure to teach her?

13. After discharge, it is important for Baby H. to receive follow-up care. What should you teach the mother to help her understand the importance of regular visits?

14. You realize that Baby H.'s mother needs information about safety issues before being discharged. After a review of safety issues, which statement by Baby H.'s mother indicates that she needs further instruction?
    a. "I have a car seat and will use it for my baby every time we use the car."
    b. "I can leave him on the infant table for just a few moments while he is a newborn."
    c. "I will not drink hot coffee while holding my baby."
    d. "I will check the bath water temperature before bathing him."

CASE STUDY OUTCOME

Baby H. is discharged to home with his parents.

Case Study **132**

Name _____ Class/Group _____ Date _____

Group Members _____

▶ **Scenario**

P.T. is a married 30-year-old gravida 4, para 1203 at 28 weeks' gestation. She arrives in the labor and delivery unit at a level 2 hospital complaining of low back pain and frequency of urination. She states that she feels occasional uterine cramping and believes that her membranes have not ruptured.

1. You are the charge nurse and admit P.T. to the unit. Based on the information you have been given, identify the two most likely diagnoses for her.

2. You need additional information from P.T. to determine what you will do next. What important questions do you need to ask to differentiate what is going on with P.T.?

3. What actions would you take to help identify her underlying problem before calling the health care provider?

4. Early recognition of preterm labor is essential to successfully implement interventions. The diagnosis of preterm labor is based on what three major diagnostic criteria?

5. What is the significance of misdiagnosing preterm labor?

6. What other problems might be going on with P.T. that you should consider?

CASE STUDY PROGRESS

P.T.'s history reveals that she had one preterm delivery 4 years ago at 31 weeks' gestation. The infant girl was in the neonatal intensive care unit (NICU) for 3 weeks and discharged without sequelae. The second preterm infant, a boy, was delivered 2 years ago at 35 weeks' gestation and spent 4 days in the hospital before discharge. She has no other risk factors for preterm labor. Vital signs are normal. Her vaginal examination findings were essentially within normal limits: cervix long, closed, and thick; membranes intact. Abdominal examination revealed that the abdomen was nontender, with fundal height at 29 cm, fetus in a vertex presentation.

7. While you are waiting for laboratory results, what therapeutic measures do you consider?

8. If P.T. is in preterm labor, the nurse can expect that her provider will initiate medication therapy to stop the uterine contractions. Which class of medication is useful in stopping uterine contractions?
   a. Tocolytics
   b. Antianxiety medications
   c. Cervical ripening agents
   d. Antibiotic therapy

9. The provider orders indomethacin (Indocin) 100 mg now, followed by 50 mg every 8 hours PO for 3 days. In addition, she is to receive sucralfate (Carafate). Explain the purpose of each drug in this situation.

10. When caring for a woman with symptoms of preterm labor, it is important to question the woman about whether she has symptoms when she is engaged in certain activities that might require lifestyle modifications. You should assess for which activities?

CASE STUDY PROGRESS

While waiting for laboratory results, you consider that if P.T. is experiencing preterm labor, she would receive antenatal glucocorticoids.

11. What is the rationale for the administration of antenatal glucocorticoids for preterm labor?
    a. To accelerate fetal lung maturity
    b. To stop uterine contractions
    c. To soften the cervix
    d. To prevent maternal infection

12. How long do these drugs take to become effective?

13. Which of these situations are considered contraindications to antenatal glucocorticoids when a woman is in preterm labor? Select all that apply.
    a. Cord prolapse
    b. Chorioamnionitis
    c. Presence of twin fetuses
    d. Cervical dilation of 2.5 cm
    e. Abruptio placentae

13 Maternal and Obstetric Care

CASE STUDY OUTCOME

Two hours later, the laboratory results indicate a urinary tract infection (UTI). The contraction monitor indicates infrequent, mild contractions. Her physician discharges her to home on an antibiotic for the UTI.

14. What follow-up measures should be considered in providing P.T. with discharge instructions?

Case Study **133**

Name _____   Class/Group _____   Date _____

Group Members _____

▶ **Scenario**

J.F. is an 18-year-old woman, gravida 1 para 0, at 38 weeks' gestation. She felt fine until 2 days ago, when she noticed swelling in her hands, feet, and face. She complains of a frontal headache, which started yesterday and has not been relieved by acetaminophen (Tylenol) or coffee. She says she feels irritable and doesn't want the "overhead lights on." Her physician is admitting her for induction of labor. You begin to assess her.

Chart View

Assessment

  Vital signs: BP 152/84 mm Hg; HR 88 beats/min
  Oral temperature: 98.8° F (37.1° C)
  Weight: 131.4 kg (289 lb); height: 5 ft, 4 in
  Edema: noted in hands, feet, and face
  Deep tendon reflexes (DTRs) +2, no clonus
  Urine dipstick reveals proteinuria +3

1. Based on the assessment data you have obtained so far, what do you think is happening to J.F. at this time?

2. As you assess J.F. for edema in her ankles, you note that she is closest to letter B in the figure below, with edema at about 4 mm. How would you document this edema?

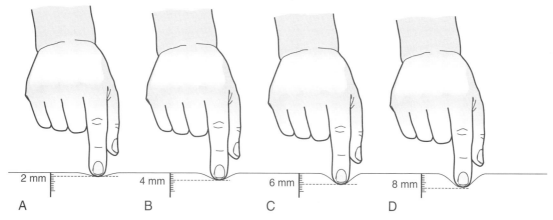

13 Maternal and Obstetric Care

3. What other assessment questions should you ask her at this time?

4. What information should you obtain from her obstetric record?

5. What laboratory values should be considered at this time?

6. Name at least three possible maternal and three possible fetal complications with J.F.'s diagnosis.

7. What risk factors does J.F. have that cause her to be at risk for this condition? Select all that apply.
   a. Obesity
   b. Nulliparity
   c. Single-fetus pregnancy
   d. Age younger than 20 years
   e. Coffee drinker

8. Identify eight measures that would likely be implemented.

CASE STUDY PROGRESS

The physician orders a magnesium sulfate infusion. You prepare the infusion and explain to J.F. what you are doing.

9. J.F. asks you, "Why am I getting magnesium now?" Explain your answer.

10. As you monitor J.F., you observe for signs of magnesium sulfate toxicity. What are potential signs of magnesium sulfate toxicity? Select all that apply.
    a. Absent DTRs
    b. Increased respiratory rate
    c. Oliguria
    d. Muscle rigidity
    e. Severe hypotension

11. Four hours later, a serum magnesium level is drawn, and the results show 7.8 mEq/L. Does this result need to be reported to the physician? If so, what would you prepare to do?

13 Maternal and Obstetric Care

12. Is there an antidote for magnesium sulfate?

The magnesium sulfate infusion rate is reduced. An oxytocin infusion has been ordered by the physician and is being given intravenously in increments to achieve an adequate contraction pattern. You notice on the fetal monitor strip that J.F. is experiencing seven uterine contractions in a 10-minute period over a 30-minute window, with a few fetal heart rate (FHR) decelerations noted.

13. What is happening at this time?

14. What are your priority actions?

15. After your prompt intervention, J.F.'s tachysystole resolves and you need to document what happened. Write an example of a documentation entry describing this event.

J.F. progresses in labor, and at 4-cm dilation her membranes spontaneously rupture. The small amount of amniotic fluid is green.

16. What does the green amniotic fluid indicate? What are the risks?

Four hours later, J.F. delivers a 6-pound, 8-ounce boy, with Apgar scores of 6 and 7.

17. What are your responsibilities at this time?

Case Study **134**

Name _____ Class/Group _____ Date _____

Group Members _____

▶ ## Scenario

You are working as a registered nurse (RN) in a large women's clinic. Y.L., a 28-year-old Asian woman, arrives for her regularly scheduled obstetric appointment. She is in her 26th week of pregnancy and is a primigravida. After examining the patient, the nurse-midwife tells you to schedule Y.L. for a glucose challenge test. You review Y.L.'s chart and note she is 5 feet, 3 inches tall and weighs 143 pounds; her pre-pregnancy body mass index (BMI) was 25. Her father has type 2 diabetes mellitus (DM), and both paternal grandparents had type 2 DM. You enter the room to talk to Y.L.

1. What is the purpose of a glucose challenge test?

2. When is a glucose challenge test performed?

3. What instructions would you provide Y.L. regarding the test?

Chart View

Laboratory Test Results

Time of Test	Value	Normal Range
0730	109 mg/dL	Less than or equal to 92 mg/dL
0830	213 mg/dL	Less than or equal to 180 mg/dL
0930	162 mg/dL	Less than or equal to 153 mg/dL

4. Interpret the results of Y.L.'s test.

5. Y.L. is diagnosed with gestational diabetes mellitus (GDM). What is GDM?

13 Maternal and Obstetric Care

6. List five risk factors for GDM. Place a star or asterisk next to those risk factors that Y.L. has.

CASE STUDY PROGRESS

Medical nutrition therapy is the primary treatment for the management of GDM. Because treatment must begin immediately, you call the dietitian to come see Y.L. You also schedule Y.L. to meet with other members of the DM management team later in the week.

7. What is the goal of medical nutrition therapy?

8. Describe the usual diet used in treating GDM.

9. Why is medical nutrition therapy for a woman with GDM higher in fat and protein than for a woman who is not pregnant?

10. Women with GDM cannot metabolize concentrated simple sugars without a sharp rise in blood glucose. Name five examples of simple sugars you would teach Y.L. to limit.

11. Complex carbohydrates (CHOs) do not cause a rapid rise in blood glucose when eaten in small amounts. Identify five foods from this group.

13 Maternal and Obstetric Care

CASE STUDY PROGRESS

During the meeting with the dietitian, Y.L. gives a diet history that is high in noodles and rice with little protein. She informs the dietitian she is lactose intolerant but can have dairy products occasionally in small portions.

12. Is it important that Y.L. take a calcium supplement along with her prenatal vitamins?

13. Y.L. is instructed to monitor her fasting blood glucose first thing in the morning and 2 hours after every meal. What are the purposes of this request?

14. Y.L. is instructed to complete ketone testing using the first-voided urine in the morning. What is the rationale for this request?

15. Y.L. asks whether having gestational diabetes will hurt her baby. How would you respond?

16. At the conclusion of the visit, you need to evaluate your teaching. Which statement made by Y.L. indicates that clarification is necessary?
    a. "I will stay on the diabetic diet described by the dietitian."
    b. "I will monitor my glucose levels at least four times each day."
    c. "I need to stop exercising because I will need more carbohydrates."
    d. "I should immediately report any ketones in my urine."

13 Maternal and Obstetric Care

17. Y.L. states that she plans to have another child soon and asks you if she will develop GDM with that pregnancy. Select the best response:
    a. "Yes, once you develop GDM during a pregnancy, you will develop it with any future pregnancies."
    b. "No, there is no further risk for development of GDM if you get pregnant again."
    c. "If you lose weight and do not eat any sweets before your next pregnancy, you will not develop GDM again."
    d. "There is a risk for recurrence of GDM in the next pregnancy. Let your health care provider know that you had GDM with this pregnancy."

13 Maternal and Obstetric Care

Women's Health Care

Case Study 135

Name _____ Class/Group _____ Date _____

Group Members _____

▶ Scenario

K.W. is an 18-year-old woman who comes to Planned Parenthood for a pregnancy test because a condom broke during intercourse the night before. Her last menstrual period (LMP) was 13 days ago and was normal. She always has a monthly menstrual cycle. She is extremely nervous about pregnancy because she is beginning college on a scholarship soon. She states there have been no other acts of unprotected intercourse since her LMP and declines a gynecologic examination.

1. As the nurse working in the clinic, should you run a pregnancy test?

2. K.W. asks whether she is at risk for pregnancy. How will you respond?

3. She asks if any options are available to her at this point. How will you answer?

4. K.W. says, "Are you talking about having an abortion?" Formulate a response.

CASE STUDY PROGRESS

There are four emergency contraceptive options: levonorgestrel (Plan B, Next Choice), uliptristal acetate (Ella), contraceptive pills containing estrogen and progesterone, and the copper intrauterine device (IUD).

5. She asks you to explain the differences among the various options. What will you tell her?

6. She asks you about the side effects of each. What will you tell her?

7. What past medical information do you need to obtain from K.W.?

8. You determine that K.W. has no contraindications to the use of hormones. Which of the EC methods do you feel would be the best option for K.W. and why?

9. What teaching will you provide K.W. based on this option?

14 Women's Health Care

Case Study **136**

Name _____ Class/Group _____ Date _____

Group Members _____

▶ **Scenario**

L.W., a 20-year-old college student, comes to the university health clinic for a pregnancy test. She has been sexually active with her boyfriend of 6 months, and her menstrual period is now "a few" weeks late. The pregnancy test result is positive. The patient begins to cry, saying, "I don't know what to do."

1. How will you begin to counsel L.W.?

2. What information do you need to obtain from L.W. and why?

3. What options does a woman experiencing a pregnancy have?

4. If your role is to assist her in making a choice, what information will you want L.W. to provide?

5. What are the nurse's moral and ethical obligations in this situation?

14 Women's Health Care

6. L.W. asks you to tell her about abortion. What will you tell her?

7. You tell L.W. there are two types of abortions, vacuum aspiration and medical abortion. How would you explain the difference to her?

8. What are the contraindications to using mifepristone (Mifeprex) for a medical abortion?

9. She tells you that she has heard that if a woman has an abortion, she might not be able to get pregnant again. How would you counsel her?

10. L.W. asks you, "Do you think abortion is killing?" What is your best response?
    a. "Good question. What do you think about it?"
    b. "A lot of people think this is what an abortion is."
    c. "Absolutely not. What happens with pregnancy is a woman's choice."
    d. "I am not able to answer that question. Are you uncertain about abortion as an option?"

11. What types of emotional reactions do women experience after an abortion?

12. L.W. wants to know about adoption. What will you tell her?

13. You ask L.W. if her boyfriend is aware of the possibility she was pregnant. She tells you that she did not tell him about her period being late or her visit to the clinic today. She asks you if she should tell him because she is afraid he will "freak out." How should you respond?

14. L.W. says she is uncertain as to what to do and wants to know how long she has to decide. How will you respond?

15. L.W. declines an examination and says she needs to "think about all this." She does make an appointment to return in 1 week. What teaching do you need to provide L.W. about how to care for herself in the meantime? How will you respond?

14 Women's Health Care

Case Study **137**

Name _____   Class/Group _____   Date _____

Group Members _____

▶ **Scenario**

You are working in a busy obstetrics/gynecology (OB/GYN) office, and the last patient of the day is P.B., a 35-year-old who is planning to get married soon. She wants to use birth control but is not sure what to choose. Her fiancé is in law school, and they do not have health insurance, so she is anxious not to get pregnant right away. She asks you to review the various methods and help her explore what is best for her.

1. What past medical information will you need to obtain from P.B. and why?

2. What other factors would influence the choice of a contraceptive method?

3. What lifestyle information will help you assist P.B. in choosing an appropriate method for her?

4. P.B. asks you about the effectiveness rating of available birth control methods. Describe the term *efficacy* and categorize the available methods according to the following efficacy ratings: most effective (more than 99%), highly effective (97% to 99%), and moderately effective (less than 90%).

5. P.B. asks you to explain the main advantages and disadvantages of the most effective methods.

658

6. What are the main advantages and disadvantages of the contraceptive methods in the highly effective category?

7. What about the moderately effective birth control methods? What are the main advantages and disadvantages?

14 Women's Health Care

8. She wants to know about cost with each method because she will be on a tight budget, with limited insurance coverage.

9. She asks you which method you would pick. What do you tell her?

CASE STUDY PROGRESS

P.B. comes back in a week and tells you that she can get a low-cost oral contraceptive (OC) through a local store. You convey this information to the nurse practitioner, who examines P.B. and writes a prescription for a biphasic 28-day pill pack containing ethinyl estradiol and norethindrone. You are asked to discuss the use of the pill with P.B.

10. What key factors should you address with P.B.?

11. Using the acronym *ACHES*, what symptoms should you teach K.B. to report?

12. A few months later, K.B. calls the clinic because she realized she missed a dose of her OC. What will you tell her? Select all that apply.
   a. "Throw that pill away. Restart taking your pills tomorrow."
   b. "It's okay; you're still protected from pregnancy if you take two now."
   c. "You should use a backup form of contraception until you start your menses."
   d. "Don't take any more pills. Begin a new pack when you start your next menses."
   e. "Take the missed pill now, along with today's pill, then resume the pack tomorrow."
   f. "Please make an appointment so we can insert a temporary intrauterine device (IUD)."

14 Women's Health Care

Case Study **138**

Name _____ Class/Group _____ Date _____

Group Members _____

▶ **Scenario**

You are working as the triage nurse in the emergency department at a busy tertiary care center. A woman comes in complaining of very heavy vaginal bleeding and extreme pain. S.K. is single, is 47 years of age, and has been bleeding for 24 hours, soaking a pad an hour. She works in a law firm as a paralegal and was embarrassed yesterday when she leaked around her pad and stained a chair in the conference room. She has two sexual partners currently and has been relying on condoms for birth control. She thinks her last menstrual period was 2 months ago, but they have been irregular and she is not sure. She has had some occasional spotting during the past 6 months. She states she is afraid of the amount of bleeding in the past 24 hours.

1. Identify three conditions that would require emergency care and could prove life-threatening.

2. She asks you, "Could I be pregnant?" How will you respond?

3. You ask her how she would feel if she was pregnant, and she says, "It would ruin my life." She states she is a single mother with two children in high school. What can you tell her to help her with her obvious distress?

4. Describe the assessment you would need to perform to differentiate what might be occurring with S.K.

14 Women's Health Care

Chart View

Laboratory Test Results

Hemoglobin (Hgb)	12.2 g/dL
Hematocrit (Hct)	44%
Red blood cells (RBCs)	4.2 dL

Vital Signs

Blood pressure (BP)	110/68 mm Hg
Heart rate	88 beats/min
Respiratory rate	22 breaths/min

5. Interpret S.K.'s laboratory results and vital signs.

CASE STUDY PROGRESS

You determine that S.K. is stable at the present; she is not diaphoretic or pale. The physician orders an ultrasound (US) to determine whether she is pregnant and to evaluate some possible causes of her bleeding. During her US, her BP drops to 90/42 mm Hg, and she complains of considerable cramping.

Chart View

Physician's Orders

Infuse 1 L of D5LR over 4 hours
Meperidine (Demerol) 5 mg IV now

6. Before administering the meperidine, what will you ask her?

7. What precautions do you need to take to safely administer meperidine? Select all that apply.
   a. Administer the medication undiluted
   b. Administer the dose over a minimum of 4 to 5 minutes
   c. Place her in semi-Fowler position with her head to the side
   d. Have oxygen equipment and naloxone (Narcan) at her bedside
   e. Monitor S.K.'s respiratory status every 15 minutes for 1 hour afterward

8. You are preparing to infuse the D5LR. The available intravenous (IV) tubing supplies 15 gtt/mL. At how many drops per minute will you regulate the infusion?

CASE STUDY PROGRESS

Thirty minutes later the UAP reports S.K.'s vital signs are 90/64, 118, 8, 97.6° F (36.4° C), and Spo_2 84% on room air.

9. What is your immediate concern and why?

10. What actions will you initiate?

CASE STUDY PROGRESS

With treatment, S.K. stabilizes within an hour. You administer a nonopioid analgesic the physician orders for pain and continue to monitor her status. The US results arrive and show she does not have an ectopic or intrauterine pregnancy. The US shows a very thick endometrial lining, even after 24 hours of bleeding.

11. S.K. is obviously relieved about not being pregnant, but she expresses fear that this could be cancer. What should you tell her to reassure her?

14 Women's Health Care

12. S.K. asks what she can do to keep this from happening again. Please respond.

13. What risk factors will you ask her about before discussing birth control pills as a treatment option?

CASE STUDY PROGRESS

You continue to monitor S.K. for the next few hours. Her respiratory status remains stable and she is feeling more comfortable. The physician prescribes birth control pills to control her bleeding. He tells her to take one pill four times a day for the next 5 days or until her bleeding stops. Once the bleeding has stopped, she should continue using the medication, one pill per day, for the rest of the cycle, then continue to use the pills for at least three cycles. She will need to follow up with her OB/GYN.

14. What warning signs and symptoms do you want to tell her about as she starts her contraceptive pills?

15. Which statements indicate that S.K. understands the discharge instructions? Select all that apply.
   a. "I can take 325 mg of aspirin every 6 hours for the cramping pain."
   b. "I will try to eat more beans and spinach over the next several days."
   c. "I will call if I continue to have heavy bleeding, soaking a pad an hour."
   d. "I will avoid sexual intercourse until the bleeding has completely stopped."
   e. "If I get dizzy or feel my heart beating funny, I will come back to the emergency room."

Case Study **139**

Name _____ Class/Group _____ Date _____

Group Members _____

▶ **Scenario**

You are the nurse in a walk-in clinic. A.P. is being seen this morning for a 2-day history of diffuse, severe abdominal pain. She has complaints of nausea without vomiting; she denies vaginal bleeding or discharge. A.P. reports having unprotected sex with several partners recently, two of whom had penile discharge. Her last menstrual period ended 3 days ago. She has no known drug allergies and denies previous medical or psychiatric problems. Vital signs are 108/60, 110, 20, 100.6° F (38.1° C). Physical examination reveals that her abdomen is very tender. The slightest touch of her abdomen causes her to wince with pain. Bowel sounds are normal. Pelvic examination reveals purulent material pooled in the vaginal vault, which appears to be coming from the cervix. A sample of the vaginal drainage is obtained and sent for culture. The result of a pregnancy test is negative; a rapid diagnostic test for chlamydial infection has a positive result.

1. Which of these assessment findings are significant and why?

2. What medical interventions can you anticipate?

3. What should you teach A.P. about chlamydial infection?

4. How would you provide emotional support to A.P. at this time?

CASE STUDY PROGRESS

The physician has the option of treating A.P. by one of two different methods. First, the physician could prescribe treatment over a period of 1 week. A.P. would be given the first dose of doxycycline (Monodox) 100 mg PO, and then she would be prescribed the same dose to be taken PO bid for 7 days. Second, the physician could prescribe a one-time dose of azithromycin (Zithromax) 1 g PO, which could be administered in the clinic.

5. Which choice is best for A.P.? Explain your reasoning.

6. You tell A.P. that chlamydial infection is a sexually transmitted infection (STI) that is mandated to be reported to the public health department. What is the purpose of reporting the infection, and what actions will be taken?

7. A.P. says she does not understand why her partners must be told about the infection. How would you respond?

8. Based on the information A.P. has given you, you determine that she is at risk for other STIs and unplanned pregnancy. What risk assessment questions do you need to ask A.P.?

9. You ask whether someone has talked with A.P. about "safe sex." She laughs and tells you there is nothing safe about sex. Undaunted, you ask if she would be willing for you to discuss the use of condoms with her sexual partners. She tells you that she is already careful; if she does not "know the guy," then she uses a condom. How are you going to respond?

10. You ask A.P. whether she has been tested for HIV. She says no, she does not know anyone with acquired immunodeficiency syndrome (AIDS) and she does not have sex with gay men. Now what are you going to say?

11. You ask her whether she would like to be tested for HIV. It will not cost her anything, no one will know the results but she, and it is completely confidential. She agrees to the test. What counseling will you provide A.P.?

12. You make an appointment for A.P. to return to the clinic in 1 week for her HIV test results. Describe the instructions you will give to A.P. before she leaves the clinic.

CASE STUDY PROGRESS

A.P. returns to the clinic in 1 week for her HIV test results, which are negative. Her culture results confirm the diagnosis of chlamydial infection.

13. What are your primary nursing concerns at this time?

14 Women's Health Care

14. A.P. has completed the course of antibiotic therapy and is no longer experiencing any symptoms. After counseling her on ways to reduce her risk of acquiring another STI, you determine that A.P. understood your teaching regarding safe sexual practices if she states that she will do which of the following? Select all that apply.
    a. Use a new application of spermicidal jelly before each sexual encounter
    b. Not worry about contacting an STI if the man states he has few partners
    c. Have her partner and her both wear a new condom with each sexual encounter
    d. Douche with an over-the-counter solution within 4 hours of having intercourse
    e. Inspect the genitalia of her partner before intercourse or other contact with perianal area

Case Study **140**

Name _____ Class/Group _____ Date _____

Group Members _____

▶ Scenario

T.C. is a 49-year-old woman who 3 weeks ago underwent a vaginal hysterectomy and right salpingo-oophorectomy for abdominal pain and endometriosis. Postoperatively, she experienced an intra-abdominal hemorrhage, requiring transfusion with 3 units of packed red blood cells (RBCs). After discharge, she continued to have abdominal pain, chills, and fever. She was readmitted twice: first for treatment of postoperative infection and second for evacuation of a pelvic hematoma. Despite treatment, T.C. continued to have abdominal pain, chills, fever, and nausea and vomiting.

T.C. has now been admitted to your unit from the postanesthesia care unit (PACU) after an exploratory laparotomy. Vital signs (VS) are 130/70, 94, 16, 99.7° F (37.6° C). Respirations are shallow and her Spo_2 is 93% with oxygen at 2 L by nasal cannula. She is easily aroused and oriented to place and person. She dozes between verbal requests. She has a low-midline abdominal dressing that is dry and intact and a Jackson-Pratt drain that is fully compressed and contains a scant amount of bright red blood. Her Foley to down drain has clear yellow urine. She is receiving an IV of 1000 mL D5.45NS at 100 mL/hr in her left forearm, with no swelling or redness. T.C. is receiving IV morphine sulfate for pain control through a patient-controlled analgesia (PCA) pump. The settings are dose 2 mg, lock-out interval 20 minutes, 4-hour maximum dose of 30 mg. When aroused, she states that her pain is an 8 on a scale of 1 to 10.

1. What concerns you most right now about T.C. and why?

2. Identify factors that are affecting T.C.'s respiratory status.

3. What interventions do you need to implement to promote T.C.'s respiratory status?

CASE STUDY PROGRESS

The unit is busy, and you are concerned about monitoring T.C. carefully enough. Your present patient load is six; of these, two patients are newly postoperative and one is getting ready for discharge. You have one experienced unlicensed assistive personnel (UAP) to help you. You are concerned that T.C.'s respiratory status may further decline.

4. Formulate a plan for the UAP and you to care for T.C. during your shift.

5. Which of T.C.'s vital sign values would be most important for the UAP to report to you immediately?
    a. Heart rate of 100 beats/min
    b. Temperature of 100° F (37.8° C)
    c. Respiratory rate of 9 breaths/min
    d. Blood pressure of 160/80 mm Hg

6. Identify three outcomes that you expect for T.C. as a result of your interventions.

CASE STUDY PROGRESS

Throughout the first postoperative day, it is difficult to balance T.C.'s need for pain medication and depression of her respiratory status.

7. Discuss how PCA devices are used for controlling pain.

8. During the past 24 hours, T.C. had 122 PCA demands and 31 doses delivered. How many total milligrams of morphine sulfate did she receive?

9. What adjustments could be made to her plan of care to better control her pain?

10. What other measures can you use to manage T.C's pain more effectively?

11. How do you best evaluate the effectiveness of the PCA therapy?
    a. Assess the time interval between doses received
    b. Have T.C. state her pain level on a scale of 1 to 10
    c. Determine how many doses of medication T.C. received
    d. Appraise whether T.C. understands the purpose of PCA therapy

CASE STUDY PROGRESS

The physician adjusts T.C.'s pain management regimen. By the end of the second postoperative day, her pain is better controlled, although she is still complaining of moderate abdominal and incisional pain. She is able to ambulate in her room with assistance, void after the Foley catheter removal, and tolerate oral fluids without nausea. As you perform your shift assessment, you note that her abdominal dressing is saturated with blood. You identify the need to assess T.C.'s wound.

12. Why do you need to assess the wound?

13. How should her wound appear at this time?

14. When you change T.C.'s dressing, you note a large amount of bloody drainage coming from the distal end of the wound. What other assessment do you need to obtain?

15. Her assessment findings are unremarkable and you place a new sterile dressing on the wound. What will you do next?

CASE STUDY PROGRESS

The physician comes and, after examining T.C., believes she is experiencing some internal bleeding. He takes her back to surgery where he isolates an area where the sutures have broken and cauterizes the affected vessels. T.C. returns to the unit, and her condition is quickly stabilized. The next evening you overhear T.C. and her husband saying that they are very dissatisfied with the care provided by the physician. They believe that he has mismanaged T.C.'s care. They are discussing getting an attorney. They ask you what you think.

16. What do you do and why?

17. You state, "Tell me what's going on with you right now. Maybe I can help you be more comfortable." What would be the benefit of taking this approach?

18. Mr. C. says, "No one is telling us anything. My wife came in here for a simple hysterectomy. She ends up with four surgeries. She still has pain, and she is worse off than when she started. Somebody has screwed up big time. Then they have the nerve to send me a bill. This morning they demanded $185,000. I'm not paying a dime until she gets better." How are you going to respond?

Case Study **141**

Name _____ Class/Group _____ Date _____

Group Members _____

▶ **Scenario**

You are the nurse working triage in the emergency department. This afternoon, a woman brings in her father, K.B., who is 74 years old. The daughter reports that over the past year she has noticed her father has progressively had problems with his mental capacity. These changes have developed gradually but seem to be getting worse. At times he is alert and at other times he seems disoriented, depressed, and tearful. He is forgetting things and doing things out of the ordinary, such as placing the milk in the cupboard and sugar in the refrigerator. K.B. reports that he has been having memory problems for the past year and at times has difficulty remembering the names of family members and friends. His neighbor found him down the street 2 days ago, and K.B. did not know where he was. This morning he thought it was night-time and wondered what his daughter was doing at his house. He could not pour his own coffee, and he seems to be getting more agitated. A review of his past medical history is significant for hypercholester-olemia and coronary artery disease. He had a myocardial infarction 5 years ago. K.B.'s vital signs today are all within normal limits.

1. What are some cognitive changes seen in a number of elderly patients?

2. You know that physiologic age-related changes in the elderly can influence cognitive functioning. Name and discuss one.

3. For each behavior listed, specify whether it is associated with delirium (DL) or dementia (DM).
   _____ a. Gradual and insidious onset
   _____ b. Hallucinations or delusions
   _____ c. A sudden, acute onset of symptoms
   _____ d. Progressive functional impairment
   _____ e. Inability to perform activities of daily living (ADLs)
   _____ f. Incoherent interactions with others
   _____ g. Possible wandering behavior
   _____ h. Behavioral disorders that often worsen at night

4. Based on the information provided by the daughter, do you think K.B. is showing signs of delirium or dementia? Explain.

5. You know that there are several types of dementia that result in cognitive changes. List two of these types of dementia.

6. How can the level or degree of the dementia impairment be determined?

7. A number of diagnostic tests have been ordered for K.B. From the tests listed, which would be used to diagnose dementia?

_____ Mental status examinations
_____ Toxicology screen
_____ Mini-Mental State Examination
_____ Electrocardiogram
_____ Electroencephalogram
_____ Complete metabolic panel
_____ Complete blood count with differential
_____ Thyroid function tests
_____ Colonoscopy
_____ Rapid plasma reagin (RPR) test
_____ Serum B_{12} level
_____ Bleeding time
_____ Human immunodeficiency virus screening
_____ Liver function tests
_____ Vision and hearing evaluation
_____ Magnetic resonance imaging (MRI)

After review of K.B.'s history and diagnostic test results, K.B. is diagnosed with Alzheimer's dementia. The physician calls a family conference to discuss the implications with K.B. and his daughter.

8. What neuroanatomic changes are seen in individuals with Alzheimer's disease?

9. List at least three interventions you would plan for K.B.

K.B. is discharged and sees his primary care physician 2 days later. K.B. receives a prescription for donepezil (Aricept) 5 mg PO per night. As you review the prescription with K.B.'s daughter, she tells you that she is "excited" because she did not know there were medications that could cure Alzheimer's disease.

10. How do you respond?

Two weeks later, K.B.'s daughter calls the physician's office and states, "I realize that the Aricept will not cure my dad, but there has been no improvement at all. Are we wasting our money?"

11. What is the best answer for her question?

12. K.B.'s daughter mentions that she has found him out in the front yard and once in the neighbor's yard. What are some interventions that you can suggest to promote safety for K.B.?

15 Psychiatric Disorders

Case Study **142**

Name _____ Class/Group _____ Date _____

Group Members _____

▶ **Scenario**

You are working the day shift on a medical inpatient unit. You are discussing discharge instructions with J.B., an 86-year-old man who was admitted for mitral valve repair. His serum blood glucose had been averaging 250 mg/dL or higher for the past several months. During this admission, his dosage of insulin was adjusted and he was given additional education in managing his diet. While you are giving these instructions, J.B. tells you his wife died 9 months ago. He becomes tearful when telling you about that loss and the loneliness he has been feeling. He tells you he just doesn't feel good lately, feels sad much of the time, and hasn't been involved in his normal activities. He has few friends left in the community because most of them have passed away. He has a daughter in town, but she is busy with her work and grandchildren. He tells you that he has been feeling so down the past few months that he has had thoughts about suicide.

1. What other information should you ask J.B. regarding his thoughts of suicide?

2. What characteristics of J.B. put him at high risk for suicide?

3. Which psychiatric disorders can result in suicidal ideations or gestures? Name at least three.

4. What questions would you ask J.B. to determine whether he is clinically depressed? Name at least six.

15 Psychiatric Disorders

5. Ill people often have trouble sleeping, experience a change in appetite, reduce their level of activity, and have thoughts of death. How can you tell the difference between old age with illness and depression?

6. List five of the most common signs of depression in the older adult.

CASE STUDY PROGRESS

You use the SAD PERSONS scale to assess J.B.'s potential for suicide and find that he is at a 4 on the 10-point scale. J.B. tells you that he has just had general thoughts of suicide, but has not really thought about how he would do it. You recall that there are two types of suicide methods based on lethality: higher-risk or hard methods, and lower-risk or soft methods.

7. Which of these would be considered soft methods of suicide? Select all that apply.
   a. Using a gun
   b. Slashing one's wrist
   c. Hanging
   d. Poisoning with carbon monoxide
   e. Ingesting pills
   f. Inhaling natural gas

8. What immediate interventions would you carry out for J.B.?

You decide to notify J.B.'s physician about your findings. The attending physician calls in a psychiatrist to evaluate J.B.

9. Identify two treatments that are available for depression.

10. Would J.B. be a candidate for electroconvulsive therapy (ECT)? Why or why not?

The psychiatrist on call comes in to evaluate J.B. After meeting with J.B., the psychiatrist writes an order for escitalopram (Lexapro) 10 mg daily at bedtime. J.B. is scheduled to see the psychiatrist the day after he is discharged from the hospital.

11. What special instructions will you give him regarding the Lexapro? Select all that apply.
    a. The full effects of the medication might not be seen for 4 to 6 weeks.
    b. The medication may cause nausea, dry mouth, sedation, and insomnia.
    c. There are no known food interactions.
    d. The herbal product St. John's wort will enhance the action of the Lexapro.
    e. Taking a glass of wine at bedtime will help him go to sleep.

12. Why do you think that a drug in the SSRI class was chosen over a tricyclic antidepressant or a monoamine oxidase inhibitor (MAOI)?

J.B.'s daughter visits him in the hospital, and they have a long talk. She is shocked when she realizes that her father is lonely to the point of considering suicide and tells you that she will do all she can to help him when he goes home.

15 Psychiatric Disorders

13. What important information needs to be conveyed to J.B.'s daughter about the first few weeks of therapy with the SSRI?

CASE STUDY OUTCOME

J.B. is discharged to home with a psychiatric home health nurse scheduled to visit him twice a week for 4 weeks. J.B.'s daughter also plans to check in on him daily and makes an effort to include him in more family activities. He also is considering a move to an assisted living facility.

15 Psychiatric Disorders

Case Study **143**

Name _____ Class/Group _____ Date _____

Group Members _____

▶ Scenario

You are the registered nurse case manager in an outpatient mental health clinic. S.T. is here today for her outpatient mental health appointment. She has a diagnosis of bipolar disorder and has been stable for the past year. Her last episode was one of mania that required hospitalization. She is 29 years old, married, with two children aged 2 and 4. She reports that her mood is better than it has been in a long time and she has lots of energy. When asked whether she thinks this is a recurrence of mania, she says *no,* she thinks that things are just finally getting better.

1. It is common for patients with bipolar illness to deny the onset of mania because it feels good. What other information would be important to ask S.T.?

2. What other information would help determine whether S.T. is experiencing the onset of a manic or hypomanic episode?

3. Bipolar disorder is a disorder of mood, characterized by episodes of depression, mania, or hypomania. What symptoms might you see if S.T. is experiencing mania or hypomania?

15 Psychiatric Disorders

4. How is hypomania different from mania?

Lithium (Eskalith) is commonly used to treat bipolar disorder. S.T. has been taking lithium for several years.

5. When S.T. first started taking lithium, she would have been cautioned to report side effects. Which are common side effects of lithium? Select all that apply.
   a. Thirst
   b. Nausea
   c. Constipation
   d. Tremor
   e. Dizziness

6. Lithium toxicity can occur in patients taking lithium. What are the symptoms of early lithium toxicity? Select all that apply.
   a. Vomiting
   b. Insomnia
   c. Dyspnea
   d. Diarrhea
   e. Lethargy

7. S.T.'s maintenance lithium level results are reported as 1.0 mEq/L. Interpret these results.

8. What other laboratory examinations should be routinely performed while S.T. is taking lithium?

9. What instructions should have been given to S.T. when she began lithium therapy?

10. Aside from lithium, what other medications are used to treat bipolar disorder?

11. Even though she has been taking lithium for a year, you review some teaching about drug therapy with S.T. Which statement by S.T. reveals a need for further education?
    a. "I will call my doctor if I have severe vomiting or diarrhea."
    b. "I need to be careful because lithium is addictive."
    c. "I take the lithium tablets with meals."
    d. I will keep my appointments to have my drug levels checked."

12. Given her history of bipolar disorder, what should you teach S.T. to minimize mood swings?

CASE STUDY OUTCOME

S.T. is told that her lithium level is within normal limits, and states, "I feel better than I've felt in ages!" She expresses hope that this will last a long time.

15 Psychiatric Disorders

Case Study **144**

Name _____ Class/Group _____ Date _____

Group Members _____

▶ **Scenario**

You are working on an inpatient psychiatric unit and need to do an initial assessment of R.B., who has just been admitted. He has a diagnosis of schizophrenia, paranoid type. He is 22 years old and has been attending the local university and living at home with his parents. He has always been a good student and has been active socially. Last semester his grades began declining and he became very withdrawn. He spends most of his time alone in his room. His grooming has deteriorated; he can go days without bathing. For several weeks before admission, he insisted on keeping all of the blinds and curtains in the house closed. He refuses to join family gatherings and games. For the past 2 days he has refused to eat, saying, "They have contaminated the food." As you approach R.B., you note that he appears to be carrying on a conversation with someone, but there is no one there. When you talk to him, he looks around and answers in a whisper but gives you little information. He states, "They are watching me and told me not to cooperate."

1. Explain what a negative symptom of schizophrenia is, and identify at least three negative symptoms of schizophrenia that R.B. might be experiencing.

2. Explain what a positive symptom of schizophrenia is, and identify at least two positive symptoms of schizophrenia that R.B. might be experiencing.

3. Give the definition of each of the following types of delusional thinking:
   a. Thought broadcasting
   b. Thought insertion
   c. Grandeur
   d. Ideas of reference
   e. Persecution
   f. Somatic delusions

4. What symptoms indicate that R.B. has paranoid schizophrenia?

5. Why is it important to know R.B.'s history before he is diagnosed with schizophrenia?

6. What diagnostic screenings are important in evaluating R.B.?

7. What are the most important initial interventions in treating R.B.?

CASE STUDY PROGRESS

After a full mental status assessment, the psychiatrist orders close monitoring in the inpatient setting and an antipsychotic medication.

8. Which class of antipsychotic medications is considered first-line therapy for schizophrenia?

9. K.B. will need to be monitored closely. How will this be done?

10. What types of psychosocial treatments may be used to treat R.B.'s schizophrenia? Name at least five.

CASE STUDY PROGRESS

R.B. is started on olanzapine (Zyprexa). You inform R.B. and his family about the common side effects of the atypical antipsychotics.

11. What are the common side effects of atypical antipsychotics such as olanzapine (Zyprexa)? Select all that apply.
    a. Tardive dyskinesia
    b. Drowsiness
    c. Dry mouth
    d. Palpitations
    e. Nausea
    f. Weight gain

CASE STUDY PROGRESS

As you go in to give R.B. his medication, he speaks to you in fragmented sentences. "Is that a bird? The little flowers jump up and down. What says the moon?" Before you can say anything, he asks, "Do you see that bird over my bed? She is telling me not to leave this room. If I move she will swoop down and try to peck at my eyes. Be careful!"

15 Psychiatric Disorders

12. Is he having a delusion or a hallucination? Explain your answer.

13. Which responses by the nurse are appropriate? Select all that apply.
   a. "I don't see a bird over your head, but I can understand how that would be upsetting to you."
   b. "There is no bird over your bed."
   c. "Tell me more about what you are seeing."
   d. "The voice you are hearing is part of your illness. It can't hurt you."
   e. "I'll come back to talk to you when you are settled down."

CASE STUDY OUTCOME

After 2 weeks of inpatient therapy, K.B. is discharged back to his parents' home and is enrolled in a day treatment program. He and his parents attend family therapy sessions twice a month. He hopes to move to a halfway house in the community.

Case Study **145**

Name _____   Class/Group _____   Date _____

Group Members _____

▶ ## Scenario

You are a nurse on an inpatient psychiatric unit. J.M., a 23-year-old woman, was admitted to the psychiatric unit last night after assessment and treatment at a local hospital emergency department for "blacking out at school." She has been given a preliminary diagnosis of anorexia nervosa. As you begin to assess her, you notice that she has very loose clothing, she is wrapped in a blanket, and her extremities are very thin. She tells you, "I don't know why I'm here. They're making a big deal about nothing." She appears to be extremely thin and pale, with dry and brittle hair, which is very thin and patchy, and she constantly complains about being cold. As you ask questions pertaining to weight and nutrition, she becomes defensive and vague, but she does admit to losing "some" weight after an appendectomy 2 years ago. She tells you that she used to be fat, but after her surgery she didn't feel like eating and everybody started commenting on how good she was beginning to look, so she just quit eating for a while. She informs you that she is eating lots now, even though everyone keeps "bugging me about my weight and how much I eat." She eventually admits to a weight loss of "about 40 pounds and I'm still fat."

1. Using *Diagnostic and Statistical Manual of Mental Disorders, Fifth Edition (DSM-V)* criteria, how is the diagnosis of anorexia nervosa determined?

2. Identify eight clinical signs or symptoms of anorexia nervosa. Place a star or asterisk next to those that J.M. has.

15 Psychiatric Disorders

3. What other disorders might occur along with anorexia nervosa? Name at least four.

4. How does bulimia nervosa differ from anorexia nervosa?

5. Name five behaviors that J.M. or any other patient with anorexia may engage in other than self-starvation.

6. What common family dynamics are associated with anorexia nervosa?

You review her admission laboratory studies. An electrocardiogram (ECG) has also been ordered.

Chart View

Admission Lab Work

Sodium	135 mEq/L
Potassium	3.4 mEq/L
Chloride	99 mEq/L
Magnesium	1.5 mEq/L
Blood urea nitrogen	18 mg/dL
Creatinine	1.0 mg/dL
Hemoglobin	11 g/dL
Hematocrit	35%

7. Which laboratory results might be of concern at this time? Explain your answers.

8. What clinical symptoms of anorexia nervosa, if present, should have the highest priority? Explain your answers.

J.M.'s ECG results show normal sinus rhythm with no ST segment or other changes. You meet with J.M. to formulate a plan of care.

9. Name at least four nutritional interventions.

10. List at least six psychological aspects of the plan of care for J.M.

15 Psychiatric Disorders

CASE STUDY PROGRESS

After 3 weeks, you are providing discharge teaching for J.M. You ask her whether she is ready to go home. J.M. states, "I'll be so glad to get out of this place. I'm so fat and ugly. I need to lose 10 pounds. I bet I can do it in just a couple of days. Otherwise, I don't want to live anymore."

11. What will you discuss with the physician before any further discharge teaching or plans?

12. You report J.M.'s statements to the physician. What actions do you expect the physician to take?

13. What medications would be indicated for J.M. to assist with resolution of both her anorexia nervosa and her depression?

14. Which statements by J.M. would indicate successful treatment? Select all that apply.
   a. "When you say I look 'healthy' I feel fat."
   b. "Lately I've been feeling a little better about things."
   c. "It's up to me to take care of my body by eating enough food."
   d. "I just have to stay skinny to feel good."
   e. "I am looking forward to going out with my friends again."

CASE STUDY OUTCOME

After 2 weeks, J.M. has gained 5 pounds and seems to be more willing to eat. She still expresses fears of "getting fat," but she states that she is ready to go home and back to school. The primary care physician arranges for J.M. to participate in an outpatient partial hospitalization program that specializes in eating disorders. J.M. expresses interest in meeting others with the same problems.

Case Study **146**

Name _____   Class/Group _____   Date _____

Group Members _____

▶ **Scenario**

You are working the afternoon shift in an inpatient psychiatric unit. The patients are in the day room watching a movie when suddenly someone starts yelling. You and other staff rush to the day room to find J.J., a 48-year-old male patient, crouched in the corner behind a chair, yelling at the other patients, "Get down. Get down quick." You and the other staff are able to calm J.J. and the other patients and take J.J. to his room. He apologizes for his outburst and explains to you that the movie brought back memories of the Gulf War. He had forgotten where he was and thought he was in combat again. He describes to you in detail the memory he had of being ambushed by the enemy and watching several of his comrades be killed. You remember hearing in report that J.J. is a Gulf War veteran admitted with posttraumatic stress disorder (PTSD).

1. What are common causes of PTSD, and what is the most likely cause of J.J.'s condition?

2. Name three criteria that must be present for a diagnosis of PTSD.

3. What is the difference between PTSD and acute stress disorder?

4. Which symptom(s) of PTSD did J.J. most likely experience?

15 Psychiatric Disorders

5. What therapeutic measures can be done to help J.J. during your shift this afternoon?

CASE STUDY PROGRESS

While you are in J.J.'s room, he states that he would like to rest for a while, and he requests something to "calm his nerves." You check his medical record see these PRN (as needed) medications listed.

Chart View

PRN Medications

Acetaminophen (Tylenol) 650 mg PO every 6 hours prn pain or fever
Alprazolam (Xanax) orally dissolving tablet, 0.5 mg by mouth every 4 hr prn anxiety
Zolpidem (Ambien) extended release, 12.5 mg PO at bedtime if needed

6. Which medication is most appropriate to administer at this time? Explain.

7. What are the adverse effects of long-term use of benzodiazepine anxiolytics?

8. You decide to notify J.J.'s physician about his reaction to the movie. The physician writes an order to start paroxetine (Paxil). How does this medication differ from alprazolam?

9. Which of these are potential side effects of paroxetine? Select all that apply.
    a. Nausea
    b. Constipation
    c. Postural hypotension
    d. Headache
    e. Tinnitus

J.J. asks you whether there are other things he can do, in addition to medications, to help his anxiety. He tells you that he's heard about relaxation therapy and wants to hear more about it.

10. What would you discuss with J.J. about relaxation therapy?

11. To what other treatment modalities could J.J. be referred after his hospitalization to help treat his PTSD and related problems?

CASE STUDY OUTCOME

Over the next 2 weeks, J.J. participates in individual and group therapy sessions and tells you that he is beginning to be able to face what happened to him years ago. He tells you that he feels "encouraged" and wants to help others with the same problems.

15 Psychiatric Disorders

Case Study 147

Name _____   Class/Group _____   Date _____

Group Members _____

▶ Scenario

J.G., a 49-year-old man, was seen in the emergency department 4 days ago, diagnosed with alcohol intoxication, and released after 8 hours to his brother's care. He was brought back to the ED 12 hours ago with an active gastrointestinal (GI) bleed and is being admitted to the intensive care unit (ICU); his diagnosis is upper GI bleed and alcohol intoxication.

You are assigned to admit and care for J.G. for the remainder of your shift. According to the ED notes, his admission vital signs (VS) were 84/56, 110, 26, and he was vomiting bright red blood. He was given IV fluids and transfused 6 units of packed red blood cells (PRBCs) in the ED. On initial assessment, you note that J.G.'s VS are blood pressure 154/90, 110, 24; he has a slight tremor in his hands, and he appears anxious. He complains of a headache and appears flushed. You note that he has not had any emesis and has not had any frank red blood in his stool or melena (black tarry stools) over the past 5 hours. In response to your questions, J.G. denies that he has an alcohol problem but later admits to drinking approximately a fifth of vodka daily for the past 2 months. He reports that he was drinking vodka when he got home from the ED the first time. He admits to having had seizures while withdrawing from alcohol in the past. He tells you that he "just can't help it" and has strong urges to drink, but that he never means "to drink very much." He has had trouble keeping a job over the past several months.

Chart View

Admission Lab Work	
Hgb	10.9 g/dL
Hct	23%
ALT (formerly SGPT)	69 units/L
AST (formerly SGOT)	111 units/L
GGT	75 units/L
ETOH	291 mg/dL

1. Which data from your assessment of J.G. are of concern to you?

2. What do the admission laboratory results indicate?

3. Which of the previous laboratory results specifically reflects chronic alcohol ingestion?

15 Psychiatric Disorders

4. What are the two most likely causes of J.G.'s symptoms?

5. What is the most likely time frame for someone to have withdrawal symptoms after abrupt cessation of alcohol?

CASE STUDY PROGRESS

You assess J.G.'s history of alcohol use by talking to J.G. and his brother and conclude that he is showing indications of alcohol use disorder.

6. Name the criteria for alcohol use disorder as outlined in the *Diagnostic and Statistical Manual of Mental Disorders,* Fifth Edition (DSM-V) and put an asterisk or star next to the ones J.G. demonstrates.

7. Based on the DSM-V criteria, how would you rate the severity of J.G.'s alcohol use? Explain your decision.
   a. No problem
   b. Mild
   c. Moderate
   d. Severe

8. What would be helpful for J.G.'s physician to know regarding J.G.'s substance abuse history?

CASE STUDY PROGRESS

J.G.'s physician comes to the ICU to assess J.G. and tells you to "watch out" because J.G. is about to go into alcohol withdrawal delirium. The physician writes several medication orders.

9. What medications are commonly prescribed for patients withdrawing from alcohol? Select all that apply.
   a. Benzodiazepines, such as chlordiazepoxide (Librium)
   b. Naltrexone (Revia), an opioid-reversal agent
   c. Acamprosate (Campral), an alcohol deterrent agent
   d. Clonidine (Catapres), an alpha-adrenergic blocker
   e. Antiepileptic drugs, such as carbamazepine (Tegretol)
   f. Disulfiram (Antabuse), an alcohol deterrent agent
   g. Atenolol (Tenormin), a beta-adrenergic blocker

10. Explain the rationale for each of the drugs used during acute alcohol withdrawal.

11. What chronic health problems are associated with alcoholism?

12. What laboratory tests might the physician order to assess for nutritional deficiencies or other medical problems J.G. is experiencing?

15 Psychiatric Disorders

J.G. experiences alcohol withdrawal delirium that lasts for 36 hours before subsiding. He did not experience any seizures this time. As his medical condition stabilizes, he is transferred out of the ICU to the hospital's psychiatric unit. He tells you that he is "ready to go home" and does not want to "touch another drink" but admits that he needs help.

13. What medications might be prescribed to J.G. to assist him with sobriety? What is the usual treatment regimen, and what side effects and precautions should you educate the patient about concerning each?

14. What types of education and referral will be done before J.G.'s discharge from the hospital?

15. J.G. is referred to the local Alcoholics Anonymous (AA) program. What strategy can be implemented to increase his likelihood of attendance at these meetings?

J.G.'s AA sponsor meets with him while J.G. was still in the hospital, and the meeting goes well. The day after his discharge from the hospital, J.G. attends his first AA meeting with his sponsor.

Case Study **148**

Name _____ Class/Group _____ Date _____

Group Members _____

▶ Scenario

It is 1000 hours in the emergency department (ED) when the ambulance brings in G.G., a 35-year-old man who is having difficulty breathing. He complains of chest pain and tightness, dizziness, palpitations, nausea, paresthesia, and feelings of impending doom and unreality; he is having trouble thinking clearly. He tells you, "I don't think I'm going to make it. I must be having a heart attack." He is diaphoretic and trembling. His vital signs are 184/92, 104, 28, 98.4° F (36.9° C). This episode began at work during a meeting at approximately 0920 and became progressively worse. A co-worker called 911 and stayed with him until medical help arrived. The patient has no history of cardiac problems.

1. What initial steps would you take and what orders would you expect to receive?

CASE STUDY PROGRESS

After a full medical workup, it is determined that G.G.'s condition is stable. His shortness of breath and anxiety resolve after he is given lorazepam (Ativan) 1 mg IV push (IVP). The lab work and ECG results are all within normal parameters and there is no evidence of any physical disorder. A diagnosis of panic attack is made. G.G. admits to having had three similar episodes in the past 2 weeks; however, they were not nearly as severe or long-lasting.

2. How do you think this diagnosis was determined?

3. G.G. asks whether there is something wrong with his memory because he has been having trouble remembering things. What effect does panic disorder have on memory?

15 Psychiatric Disorders

G.G. shares with the ED staff that he has been under severe stress at work and home. He tells them he is going through a divorce, he lost a child last summer in a motor vehicle accident, and his company is downsizing. He will probably be out of a job soon. He hasn't been sleeping well for the past couple of months and has lost about 20 pounds.

4. Identify five triggers that could cause anxiety to build to the point of panic.

5. G.G. has questions regarding the differences between panic attacks and panic disorder. According to the *Diagnostic and Statistical Manual of Mental Disorders*, Fifth Edition (DSM-V), what are the differences?

6. Has G.G. had an expected or unexpected panic attack? Explain your answer.

CASE STUDY PROGRESS

G.G.'s condition is stable and the ED physician discusses what has happened with G.G. The physician gives G.G. a prescription for a "week's worth" of medication and instructs G.G. to see his primary care physician for further treatment and evaluation.

7. The physician gives G.G. a prescription for alprazolam (Xanax) 0.5 mg tid to last 1 week and instructs G.G. to see his primary care physician for further treatment and evaluation. Why do you think the physician gave G.G. a prescription for only 1 week of Xanax?

8. What medications are used to treat panic attacks? What will your patient teaching include?

CASE STUDY PROGRESS

G.G. tells you all about his worries with his job and all that has happened to him in the past year. He tells you that he appreciates you listening to him. He expresses fear that the panic attacks will return.

9. What techniques to help him cope will you discuss with him? Name at least five.

10. What actions or interventions are most indicated in the treatment of panic disorder?

CASE STUDY OUTCOME

G.G. makes an appointment with his company's Employee Assistance Program to take advantage of the resources offered for counseling to help him work with his coping strategies. In addition, his primary care physician starts him on a low dose of an SSRI. After a few months, G.G.'s panic attacks have become very rare and he works on preparing a résumé to seek new employment before his company has another round of job cuts.

15 Psychiatric Disorders

Alternative Therapies

Case Study **149**

Name _____ Class/Group _____ Date _____

Group Members _____

▶ **Scenario**

J.B., a 45-year-old woman, is an office manager for a law firm and single mother of two children. While cleaning a shower stall on Friday afternoon, she experienced a sharp pain in her lower back. Over the next few hours, her lower back became increasingly more painful. By the time she picked up the children from school, she had sharp shooting pain into her right buttock. She went to the nearest walk-in medical clinic, where was diagnosed with acute musculoskeletal strain. The provider gave her a prescription for hydrocodone 5 mg/acetaminophen 500 mg (Lortab) every 6 hours as needed for severe pain with instructions to take a nonsteroidal anti-inflammatory medication such as ibuprofen (Motrin), rest for the next 24 hours, and follow up with her primary care physician in 1 week. Monday morning she called in sick to work because she could not think clearly because of the pain medication. She developed stomach pain, and her back pain had only slightly improved. She called a friend who had experienced a similar episode and who related a favorable outcome after treatment with acupuncture. J.B. comes to your alternative medicine clinic that afternoon for an acupuncture appointment.

1. As you complete her intake interview, she asks, "What is acupuncture?" What will you tell her?

2. J.B. wants to know how acupuncture works. How will you explain acupuncture to her?

3. J.B. asks how acupuncture can help her back pain. Explain how acupuncture differs from traditional Western medicine in the treatment of back pain.

4. J.B. asks, "What will happen during an acupuncture treatment?" What will you tell her?

5. J.B. asks, "Will it hurt?" How will you respond?

6. J.B. asks, "Does insurance cover the cost?" Provide a response.

7. What side effects and risks of acupuncture do you need to teach J.B.?

16 Alternative Therapies

8. Is there any screening you need to perform before J.B. receives acupuncture therapy?

9. J.B. asks if she should keep her follow-up appointment with her primary care physician and continue the medication therapy. How should you respond?

10. J.B. asks how acupuncture practitioners are licensed. What will you tell her?

11. Which response from J.B. indicates your teaching about acupuncture was effective?
    a. "It will likely take several treatments before I feel the full effects of therapy."
    b. "I will take ibuprofen beforehand so I will feel less pain during the treatment."
    c. "My primary care physician does not need to know I am receiving acupuncture."
    d. "There is only a slight risk of getting HIV infection from acupuncture treatment."

12. List three Internet sites to which you can refer J.B. for further information.

16 Alternative Therapies

Case Study **150**

Name _____   Class/Group _____   Date _____

Group Members _____

▶ **Scenario**

One month ago, J.P., a 50-year-old man, came to the outpatient clinic with complaints of mild shortness of breath and some mild intermittent chest pain. He described himself as a high-stress, type A personality who owns his own business and works long hours. He has smoked one pack of cigarettes per day for the past 30 years. He has tried to quit several times and was successful for as long as 6 months at a time, but when business became stressful, he started smoking again. J.P. said he has been trying to lose the extra 30 pounds he is carrying but stated it is difficult to exercise because of the long hours of work. The cardiac workup is negative for coronary artery disease, and he has returned for a follow-up visit. During the discussion about lifestyle changes, J.P. expresses interest in medical hypnosis for stress management and smoking cessation. He would like more information. You are the case manager for the clinic and meet with J.P. to discuss medical hypnosis.

1. J.P. asks, "What is hypnosis?" What will you tell him?

2. J.P. asks what you mean by *trance state*. Explain the term.

3. J.P. wants to know what you mean by *subconscious mind*. Explain the term.

4. J.P. asks, "How does hypnosis work to help someone change a subconscious belief?" How will you respond?

5. J.P. states he has seen TV shows where people did silly things on stage during hypnosis. He wants to know how medical hypnosis is different. Explain.

6. J.P. asks, "Is there a way to know if hypnosis will work?" Please respond.

7. J.P. wants to know what happens during a hypnosis session. You inform him that medical hypnosis has several components: patient preparation and education, establishing a rapport and a trusting relationship, induction and deepening, hypnotic suggestions, and reawakening from the trance state. Briefly explain each step.

8. J.P. asks, "How effective is hypnosis in helping someone stop smoking?" How will you respond?

9. J.P. asks whether hypnosis is contraindicated for anyone. What will you tell him?

10. J.P. apologizes for being full of questions but wants to know whether hypnosis has to be done with a hypnotist or if he can do it himself with a downloadable mp3 file. How will you respond?

11. J.P. asks you how he would go about finding a hypnotist. What will you tell him?

12. J.P. states he would like to read more about hypnosis on the Internet. List three credible websites you could give him.

16 Alternative Therapies

Appendix: Abbreviations and Acronyms

AAA	abdominal aortic aneurysm	CABG	coronary artery bypass graft
ABCs	airway, breathing, circulation check(s)	CAD	coronary artery disease
		C&DB	cough and deep breathe
ABGs	arterial blood gases	CAP	community-acquired pneumonia
A/C	assist-control	CBC	complete blood count
ACEI	angiotensin-converting enzyme inhibitor	CBC with diff	complete blood count with differential
ACTH	adrenocorticotropic hormone	CCU	coronary care unit
ADA	American Diabetes Association	CDC	Centers for Disease Control and Prevention
ADL	activities of daily living	CHO	carbohydrate(s)
ad lib	at one's leisure	CIC	clean intermittent catheterization
AIDS	acquired immunodeficiency syndrome	CK (CPK)	creatinine phosphokinase
Alk Phos	alkaline phosphatase	CK-MM	CK isoenzymes
ALP	alkaline phosphatase (serum)	Cl	chloride
ALS	amyotrophic lateral sclerosis	cm	centimeter
ALT (SGPT)	alanine transaminase (serum glutamic pyruvic transaminase)	CMP	complete metabolic panel (profile)
		CN	cranial nerve
AM	morning	CNS	central nervous system
ANA	antinuclear antibody	C/O	complaint(s) of, complaining of
ANC	absolute neutrophil count	CO_2	carbon dioxide
Anti-HAV	Anti–hepatitis A virus	COPD	chronic obstructive pulmonary disease
Anti-HCV	anti–hepatitis C virus		
aPTT	activated partial thromboplastin time	CP	cerebral palsy
		CPAP	continuous positive airway pressure
ARB	angiotensin II receptor blocker	CPK	Creatinine phosphokinase
ARDS	adult respiratory distress syndrome	CPP	cerebral perfusion pressure
ART	antiretroviral therapy	CPR	cardiopulmonary resuscitation
AST (SGOT)	aspartate transaminase (serum glutamic oxaloacetic transaminase)	CRP	C-reactive protein
		C&S	culture and sensitivity
AV	arteriovenous	CSF	cerebrospinal fluid
BAC	blood alcohol concentration	CT scan	computed tomography scan
BAL	blood alcohol level	CVA	cerebrovascular accident
bid	twice daily	CVC	central venous catheter
BiPAP	CPAP with mask over both mouth and nose	CVP	central venous pressure
		CWOCN	certified wound, ostomy, continence nurse
BMP	basic metabolic panel		
BNP	brain or b-type natriuretic peptide	CXR	chest x-ray
BP	blood pressure	D	Dextrose
BPH	benign prostatic hyperplasia	DBP	diastolic blood pressure
bpm	beats per minute	DEXA scan	duel-energy x-ray absorptiometry
BSA	body surface area	DIC	disseminated intravascular coagulation
BSF	basilar skull fracture		
BUN	blood urea nitrogen	DKA	diabetic ketoacidosis
Ca	calcium	DM	diabetes mellitus

DME	durable medical equipment	H/H	hemoglobin/hematocrit
DNA	deoxyribonucleic acid	Hib	Haemophilus influenzae type B
DO	doctor of osteopathy	HIPAA	Health Insurance Portability and Accountability Act
DOB	date of birth		
DOE	dyspnea on exertion	HIV	human immunodeficiency virus
DOT	directly observed therapy	HLA	human leukocyte antigen
DPT	diphtheria, pertussis, tetanus	HOB	head of bed
DRE	digital rectal examination	HPV	human papillomavirus
DTRs	deep tendon reflexes	HTN	hypertension
DVT	deep vein thrombosis	IBD	inflammatory bowel disease
EC	emergency contraception	IBS	irritable bowel syndrome
ECG	electrocardiogram	ICP	intracranial pressure
ECT	electroconvulsive therapy	ICU	intensive care unit
E. coli	*Escherichia coli*	IGT	impaired glucose tolerance
ED	emergency department	IM	intramuscular
EEG	electroencephalogram	INR	International Normalized Ratio
EF	ejection fraction	I&O	intake and output
ELISA	enzyme-linked immunosorbent assay	IPV	inactivated polio vaccine
EMG	electromyogram	IS	incentive spirometer
EMS	emergency medical system	IUD	intrauterine device
EOMs	extraocular movements	IV	intravenous
ERCP	endoscopic retrograde cholangiopancreatography	IVF	intravenous fluid
		IVP	intravenous push, intravenous pyelogram
ESR	erythrocyte sedimentation rate		
ETT	endotracheal tube	IVPB	intravenous piggyback
EVD	extraventricular drain	JNC	Joint National Committee on Prevention, Detection, Evaluation, and Treatment of High Blood Pressure
fb	fingerbreadths		
FBG	fasting blood glucose		
FDA	U.S. Food and Drug Administration		
FHR	fetal heart rate	JP	Jackson-Pratt
Fio_2	fraction of inspired oxygen	JVD	jugular venous distention
FLACC	Face, Legs, Activity, Cry, Consolability (scale)	K	potassium
		kcal	calorie(s)
FOC	frontal occipital circumference	KCl	potassium chloride
Fr	French	KS	Kaposi's sarcoma
GBS	Guillain-Barré syndrome	KUB	kidney, ureters, and bladder x-ray
GCS	Glasgow Coma Scale	KVO	keep vein open
GDM	gestational diabetes mellitus	L	liter
GERD	gastroesophageal reflux disease	lab(s)	laboratory; laboratory tests
GI	gastrointestinal	LAD	left anterior descending coronary artery
gtt	drops	lb	pound(s)
GU	genitourinary	LBBB	left bundle branch block
H_2O	water	LDH	lactate dehydrogenase
Hb A_{1c}	hemoglobin A_{1c}; glycosylated hemoglobin test	LDL	low-density lipoprotein
		LFTs	liver function tests
HBsAg	hepatitis B surface antigen	LH	luteinizing hormone
HBV	hepatitis B virus	LLL	left lower lobe (of lungs)
hCG	human chorionic gonadotropin	LMP	last menstrual period
HCO_3	bicarbonate ion	LOC	level of consciousness
Hct	hematocrit	LP	lumbar puncture
HCTZ	hydrochlorothiazide	LPN	licensed practical nurse
HDL	high-density lipoprotein	LR	lactated Ringer's or Ringer's lactate
HF	heart failure	LUQ	left upper quadrant (of abdomen)
Hgb	hemoglobin	LV	left ventricle
		LWS	low wall suction

718

MAOI	monoamine oxidase inhibitor
MDI	metered-dose inhaler
meds	medications
MG	myasthenia gravis
MI	myocardial infarction
mL	milliliter
MMR	measles, mumps, rubella
MNT	medical nutrition therapy
MOM	milk of magnesia
MRI	magnetic resonance imaging
MS	multiple sclerosis
MVA	motor vehicle accident
MVI	multivitamins
Na	sodium
NaCl	sodium chloride
NAP	nursing assistive personnel
NC	nasal cannula
NG	nasogastric
NICU	neonatal intensive care unit
NIHSS	NIH Stroke Scale
NKA	no known allergies
NKDA	no known drug allergies
NPO	nothing by mouth
NS	normal saline
NSAIDs	nonsteroidal antiinflammatory drugs
NTG	nitroglycerin
N/V	nausea and vomiting
O_2	oxygen
OB	obstetric
OB/GYN	obstetrician/gynecologist
OGTT	oral glucose tolerance test
OM	otitis media
OPV	oral polio vaccine
OR	operating room
ORIF	open reduction and internal fixation
OSA	obstructive sleep apnea
OT	occupational therapist (therapy)
OTC	over the counter
P	pulse
$Paco_2$	partial pressure of carbon dioxide in arterial blood
PACU	postanesthesia care unit
PAD	peripheral artery disease
Pao_2	partial pressure of oxygen in arterial blood
Pap	Papanicolaou smear
PCA	patient-controlled analgesia
PCI	percutaneous coronary intervention
PCN	penicillin
PCP	primary care provider
PCWP	pulmonary capillary wedge pressure
PD	Parkinson's disease
PE	pulmonary embolus
PEEP	positive end-expiratory pressure

PEFR	peak expiratory flow rate
PEG	percutaneous endoscopic gastrostomy tube
peri	perineal (related to perineum)
PERRL(A)	pupils equal, round, and reactive to light (accommodation)
PET	positron emission tomography
PFM	peak flow meter
PFT	pulmonary function test
pH	negative logarithm of the hydrogen ion concentration—acidity/basicity of the blood
PICC	peripherally inserted central catheter
PIDD	primary immunodeficiency disease
PIH	pregnancy-induced hypertension
PIV	peripheral IV
PKU	phenylketonuria
PM	afternoon or evening
PMH	past medical history
PO	by mouth
PO_4	phosphate
POD	postoperative day
postop	postoperatively
PPD	purified protein derivative (test for TB)
prn	as needed
PSA	prostate-specific antigen
PT	physical therapist (therapy)
PT	prothrombin time
PTH	parathyroid hormone
PTSD	posttraumatic stress disorder
PTT; aPTT	partial thromboplastin time; activated partial thromboplastin time
PVCs	premature ventricular contractions
PVR	Post-void residual
q	every (e.g., q2h)
R	right; respirations
RA	room air
RAI	radioactive iodine
RBC	red blood cell
RCA	right coronary artery
RLQ	right lower quadrant (of abdomen)
RN	registered nurse
ROM	range of motion
RPR	rapid plasma reagin (test for syphilis)
RUQ	right upper quadrant (of abdomen)
SAH	subarachnoid hemorrhage
SBAR	situation, background, assessment, recommendation
SBO	small bowel obstruction
SBP	systolic blood pressure
SCD	sequential compression device
SCI	spinal cord injury

SE	status epilepticus	TIBC	total iron binding capacity
sed rate	erythrocyte sedimentation rate	tid	3 times per day
SIADH	syndrome of inappropriate antidiuretic hormone	TLS	tumor lysis syndrome
		TPA	tissue plasminogen activator
SICU	surgical intensive care unit	TPN	total parenteral nutrition
SL	sublingual	TRUS	transrectal ultrasound
SLE	systemic lupus erythematosus	TSH	thyroid-stimulating hormone
SLP	speech language pathologist	TUMT	transurethral microwave thermotherapy
SOAP	subjective, objective, assessment, plan		
SOB	short (shortness) of breath	TUNA	transurethral needle ablation
S/P	status post	TURP	transurethral resection of the prostate
SpO$_2$	arterial oxygen saturation		
S/S	signs and symptoms	UA	urinalysis
SRMC	single room maternity care	UAP	unlicensed assistive personnel
SSRI	selective serotonin reuptake inhibitor	UDS	urinary drainage system
STAT	immediately	US	ultrasound
STEMI	ST segment elevation myocardial infarction	UTI	urinary tract infection
		VDRL	Venereal Disease Research Laboratory (test for syphilis)
STI	sexually transmitted infection		
Subcut	Subcutaneous	VP	ventriculoperitoneal
T&A	tonsillectomy and adenoidectomy	$\dot{V}/\dot{Q}$	ventilation-perfusion
TB	tuberculosis	$\dot{V}/\dot{Q}$ scan	ventilation-perfusion scan (of lungs)
T&C	type and crossmatch	VS	vital signs
Td	tetanus/diphtheria (vaccine)	VSD	ventricular septal defect
TED	thromboembolic deterrent	V$_T$	tidal volume
TENS	transcutaneous electrical nerve stimulation	VTE	venous thromboembolism
		WBC	white blood cell
TIA	transient ischemic attack	WNL	within normal limits

Illustration Credits

Case Study 5

(p. 24) From Ignatavicius DD, Workman ML: *Medical-surgical nursing*, ed. 6, St. Louis, 2010, Saunders.

Case Study 8

(p. 41) Modified from Lilley LL, Rainforth Collins S, Harrington S, et al: *Pharmacology and the Nursing Process*, ed. 6, St. Louis, 2011, Mosby.

Case Study 9

(p. 43) From Lewis SL, Dirksen SR, Heitkemper MM, et al: *Medical-Surgical Nursing: assessment and management of clinical problems*, ed. 8, St. Louis, 2011, Mosby.

Case Study 12

(p. 56) From Jarvis, C.: *Physical Examination and Health Assessment*, ed. 6, St. Louis, 2012, Saunders.

Case Study 13

(p. 62) Modified from Fuller JK: *Surgical technology: principles and practice*, ed. 5, St. Louis, 2010, Saunders.

Case Study 14

(p. 67) Modified from Huszar R: *Basic dysrhythmias: interpretation and management—revised reprint*, ed. 3, St. Louis, 2007, Mosby.

Case Study 15

(p. 75) From Gray Morris D: *Calculate with confidence*, ed. 5, St. Louis, 2010, Mosby.

Case Study 25

(p. 126) Modified from Linton AL: *Introduction to medical-surgical nursing*, ed. 4, St. Louis, 2007, Saunders.

Case Study 29

(p. 145, both figures) From Brown M, Mulholland JM: *Drug calculations: process and problems for clinical practice*, ed. 8, St. Louis, 2008, Mosby.

Case Study 30

(p. 151) From Macklin, D., Chernecky, C., & Infortuna, M.H.: *Math for Clinical Practice*, ed. 2, St. Louis, 2011, Mosby.

Case Study 31

(p. 158) From Aehlert B: *ECGs made easy*, ed. 4, St. Louis, 2011, Mosby/JEMS.

Case Study 48

(p. 234) From Gray Morris D: *Calculate with confidence*, ed. 5, St. Louis, 2010, Mosby.

Case Study 53

(p. 256) From Lewis SL, Dirksen SR, Heitkemper MM, et al: *Medical-surgical nursing: assessment and management of clinical problems*, ed. 8, St. Louis, 2011, Mosby.

Case Study 56

(p. 273) From Kee, J.L., Marshall, S.M., Turner, S., & Eberly, D.: *Clinical Calculations*, ed. 6, St. Louis, 2009, Saunders.

Case Study 57

(p. 277) From Lewis SL, Dirksen SR, Heitkemper MM, et al: *Medical-surgical nursing: assessment and management of clinical problems*, ed. 8, St. Louis, 2011, Mosby.

Case Study 71

(p. 337) From Ignatavicius DD, Workman ML: *Medical-surgical nursing*, ed. 7, St. Louis, 2013, Saunders.

Case Study 72

(p. 344) From Urden LD, Stacy KM, Lough ME: *Critical care nursing: diagnosis and management*, ed. 6, St. Louis, 2010, Mosby.

Case Study 75

(p. 356) From Lewis SL, Dirksen SR, Heitkemper MM, et al: *Medical-surgical nursing: assessment and management of clinical problems*, ed. 8, St. Louis, 2011, Mosby.

Case Study 91

(p. 424) From Potter, P.A., Perry, A.G., Stockert, P., & Hall, A.: *Basic Nursing*, ed. 7, St. Louis, 2011, Mosby.

Case Study 96

(p. 454) From Gray Morris D: *Calculate with confidence*, ed. 5, St. Louis, 2010, Mosby.

Case Study 98

(p. 462) Modified from Ignatavicius DD, Workman ML: *Medical-surgical nursing*, ed. 6, St. Louis, 2010, Saunders.

Case Study 103

(p. 494) From Aehlert B: *ECGs made easy*, ed. 4, St. Louis, 2011, Mosby/JEMS.

Case Study 104

(p. 500, both figures) From Gray Morris D: *Calculate with confidence*, ed. 5, St. Louis, 2010, Mosby.

Case Study 107

(p. 512) Modified from Ignatavicius DD, Workman ML: *Medical-surgical nursing*, ed. 7, St. Louis, 2010, Saunders.

Case Study 117

(p. 558) From Gray Morris D: *Calculate with confidence*, ed. 5, St. Louis, 2010, Mosby.

Case Study 123

(p. 594) From Gray Morris D: *Calculate with confidence*, ed. 5, St. Louis, 2010, Mosby.

Case Study 125

(p. 604) From Workman, M.L., LaCharity, L.A., & Kruchko, S.L.: *Understanding Pharmacology*, St. Louis, 2011, Saunders.

Case Study 126

(p. 610) Modified from Harkreader H, Hogan MA: *Fundamentals of nursing: caring and clinical judgment*, ed. 2, St. Louis, 2004, Saunders.

Case Study 127

(p. 611) From Lilley LL, Rainforth Collins S, Harrington S, et al: *Pharmacology and the Nursing Process*, ed. 7, St. Louis, 2011, Mosby.

Case Study 128

(p. 619) From Perry SE, Hockenberry MJ, Lowdermilk DL, et al: *Maternal child nursing care*, ed. 4, St. Louis, 2010, Mosby.

Case Study 130

(p. 628) Modified from Perry SE, Hockenberry MJ, Lowdermilk DL, et al: *Maternal child nursing care*, ed. 4, St. Louis, 2010, Mosby.

Case Study 133

(p. 641) From Perry SE, Hockenberry MJ, Lowdermilk DL, et al: *Maternal child nursing care*, ed. 4, St. Louis, 2010, Mosby.